Imaging in Musculoskeletal and Sports Medicine

Imaging in Musculoskeletal and Sports Medicine

BRIAN HALPERN, MD
Sports Medicine
The Hospital for Special Surgery
New York, New York

STANLEY A. HERRING, MD
Physiatry and Sports Medicine
Puget Sound Sports and Spine Physicians
Seattle, Washington

DAVID ALTCHEK, MD
Orthopaedic Surgery and Sports Medicine
The Hospital for Special Surgery
New York, New York

RICHARD HERZOG, MD
Department of Radiology
Hospital of the University of Pennsylvania
Philadelphia, Pennsylvania

**Blackwell
Science**

Blackwell Science
Editorial offices:

350 Main Street, Malden, Massachusetts 02148 USA
Osney Mead, Oxford OX2 0E1, England
25 John Street, London WC1N 2BL, England
23 Ainslie Place, Edinburgh EH3 6AJ, Scotland
54 University Street, Carlton, Victoria 3053, Australia

Other editorial offices:

Blackwell Wissenschafts-Verlag, GmbH Kurfürstendamm 57,
    10707 Berlin, Germany
Zehetnergasse 6, A-1140 Vienna, Austria

Distributors:
USA
    Blackwell Science, Inc.
    Commerce Place
    350 Main Street
    Malden, Massachusetts 02148
    (Telephone orders: 800-215-1000 or 617-388-8250;
        fax orders: 617-388-8270)

Canada
    Copp Clark Professional
    200 Adelaide Street, West, 3rd Floor
    Toronto, Ontario M5H 1W7
    (Telephone orders: 416-597-1616 or 1-800-815-9417; fax:
        416-597-1617)

Australia
    Blackwell Science Pty., Ltd.
    54 University Street
    Carlton, Victoria 3053
    (Telephone orders: 03-9347-0300; fax orders: 03-9349-3016)

Outside North America and Australia
    Blackwell Science, Ltd.
    c/o Marston Book Services, Ltd.
    P.O. Box 269
    Abingdon
    Oxon OX14 4YN
    England
    (Telephone orders: 44-01235-465500; fax orders:
        44-01235-465555)

Acquisitions: Jim Krosschell
Production: Textbook Writers Associates, Inc.
Manufacturing: Lisa Flanagan

Typeset by Braun-Brumfield, Inc.
Printed and bound by Braun-Brumfield, Inc.

© 1997 by Brian Halpern and Stanley Herring

Printed in the United States of America

97 98 99 00   5 4 3 2 1

Library of Congress Cataloging-in-Publication Data

Imaging in musculoskeletal and sports medicine / [edited by]
    Brian Halpern . . . [et al.].
        p.   cm.
    Includes bibliographical references and index.
    ISBN 0-86542-418-7 (sewn)
    1. Sports injuries—Imaging.   I. Halpern, Brian.
    [DNLM: 1. Athletic Injuries—diagnosis.   2. Diagnostic
        Imaging.
    QT 261 I31 1997]
    RD97.I43   1997
    617.1'027—dc21
    DNLM/DLC
    for Library of Congress   97-12111
                                                        CIP

The Blackwell Science logo is a trade mark of Blackwell Science Ltd., registered at the United Kingdom Trade Marks Registry.

To our families
The most important and enduring images of all

Contents

Contributors

RICHARD J. BORGATTI JR. MD, *Brielle Orthopedics, Brick, New Jersey; Clinical Instructor, Family Medicine, University of Medicine and Dentistry of New Jersey, Robert Wood Johnson Medical Center, New Brunswick, New Jersey*

MICHAEL A. CATALANO MD, *Director, Center for Fitness Medicine, Boulder, Colorado*

LEIGH ANN CURL MD, *Sports Medicine and Shoulder Service, The Hospital for Special Surgery, New York, New York*

JONATHAN T. DELAND MD, *Attending Physician, The Hospital for Special Surgery; Assistant Professor, Cornell University Medical College, New York, New York*

WAYNE P. FOSTER MD, *Associate, Department of Otolaryngology, Head and Neck Surgery, Geisinger Medical Center, Danville, Pennsylvania*

GREGORY GASTALDO MD, *Medical Director of Athletic Medicine, Princeton University, Princeton, New Jersey*

BRIAN HALPERN MD, *Assistant Attending Physician, The Hospital for Special Surgery; Director of Sports Medicine, University of Medicine and Dentistry of New Jersey, Robert Wood Johnson Medical School, Department of Family Medicine; Associate Team Physician, New York Mets, New York, New York*

JOHN M. HENDERSON DO, FAAFP, *Director, Primary Care Sports Medicine, Hughston Sports Medicine Center, Columbus, Georgia*

STANLEY A. HERRING MD, *Clinical Associate Professor, Department of Rehabilitation Medicine, Department of Orthopaedic Surgery, University of Washington; Team Physician, Seattle Seahawks, Seattle, Washington*

DAVID O. HOUGH MD, (deceased) *Professor of Family Practice, Director of Sports Medicine, Michigan State University, East Lansing, Michigan*

BARBARA KADELL MD, *Clinical Professor of Radiologic Sciences, UCLA School of Medicine, Los Angeles, California*

SHELDON KAPLAN MD, *Radiologist, New Jersey Diagnostic Imaging, Brick, New Jersey*

J. BRUCE KNEELAND MD, *Associate Professor of Radiology, Hospital of the University of Pennsylvania, Philadelphia, Pennsylvania*

JAMES A. KRCIK MD, *Resident, Internal Medicine and Pediatrics, Rush-Presbyterian-St. Luke's Medical Center, Chicago, Illinois*

KATHERINE LUDWIN MBBS, MRCP, FRCR, *Department of Academic Radiology, Queen's Medical Centre, Nottingham, England*

ROGER L. McCOY II MD, *Arizona Orthopaedic and Sports Medicine Specialists, Phoenix, Arizona*

DOUGLAS B. McKEAG MD, MS, *Coordinator of Sports Medicine, Michigan State University Team Physician, Michigan State University, East Lansing, Michigan*

LANCE A. MARKBREITER MD, *Orthopaedic Surgeon Specializing in Foot and Ankle Surgery, Shore Orthopaedics, Tinton Falls, New Jersey; Monmouth Medical Center, Long Branch, New Jersey; Riverview Medical Center, Red Bank, New Jersey*

JEFF MITCHINSON MD, *Department of Radiology, St. Joseph Hospital, Tawas City, Michigan*

ROBERT MONACO MD, MPH, *Director, Sports Medicine, Rutgers University; Clinical Assistant Professor, Department of Family Medicine, Robert Wood Johnson Medical School, New Brunswick, New Jersey*

RANDOLPH PEARSON MD, *Associate Professor of Family Practice, Team Physician, Michigan State University, East Lansing, Michigan; Director, MSU/St. Lawrence Family Practice Residency, Lansing, Michigan*

HOLLIS G. POTTER MD, *Assistant Attending Radiologist, The Hospital for Special Surgery/New York Hospital; Assistant Professor of Radiology, Cornell University Medical College, New York, New York*

JAMES C. PUFFER MD, *Professor and Chief, Division of Family Medicine, UCLA Center for the Health Sciences, Los Angeles, California*

E. LEE RICE DO, *President and Medical Director, San Diego Sports Medicine and Family Health Center, San Diego, California*

DONALD ROSEN MD, *Attending Radiologist, Medical Center at Princeton, Princeton, New Jersey*

ALICE SCHEFF MD, *Assistant Professor of Radiology, Hospital of the University of Pennsylvania, Philadelphia, Pennsylvania*

KEITH L. STANLEY MD, *Eastern Oklahoma Orthopedic Center, Inc./Sports Medicine Center, Affiliate Clinical Faculty Professor, Oklahoma University College of Medicine; Team Physician, Tulsa University, Tulsa, Oklahoma*

PAUL R. STRICKER MD, *Assistant Professor of Pediatrics and Orthopedics, Department of Pediatrics, Vanderbilt University Medical Center, Nashville, Tennessee*

EUGENE TRYCIECKY DO, *Associate Professor of Radiology, Michigan State University, East Lansing, Michigan*

STUART M. WEINSTEIN MD, *Puget Sound Sports and Spine Physicians; Clinical Assistant Professor, Department of Rehabilitation Medicine, University of Washington, Seattle, Washington*

THOMAS L. WICKIEWICZ MD, FACS, *Chief, Sports Medicine and Shoulder Service, Associate Attending Orthopaedic Surgeon, The Hospital for Special Surgery, New York, New York*

WILLIAM W. WOODRUFF MD, *Clinical Assistant Professor, Department of Radiology, Jefferson Medical College, Thomas Jefferson University, Philadelphia, Pennsylvania; Associate, Division of Special Imaging, Clinical Supervisor, MRI, Department of Radiology, Geisinger Medical Center, Danville, Pennsylvania*

Preface

The practice of medicine continues to evolve rapidly with change often driven by technology. This is certainly the case with imaging studies, where new and continuously upgraded tests offer the practitioner a remarkable array of choices. The increasing utilization of these helpful (and sometimes costly) diagnostic imaging studies requires a concomitant increase in the clinician's knowledge regarding the selection and interpretation of these studies.

This textbook presents to the primary care and specialist provider a basis from which to determine appropriate musculoskeletal imaging. The relevant science of the imaging techniques and the specifics of how to order each test are discussed in conjunction with the all-important area of how to interpret the images. Analysis of imaging studies is supplemented with treatment plans based on the results of the testing ordered.

The organization of the chapters in this textbook is based on anatomy. Within each chapter, an attempt has been made to provide multiple images for common clinical entities. Hopefully, this will provide a useful tool to all practitioners involved in making decisions about imaging in musculoskeletal and sports medicine.

This endeavor required significant effort to produce the text and multiple correlating images. Our appreciation is extended to our editors, authors, and busy experts, who gave their valuable time to create this unique work. Thanks also go out to Mary Benard at Blackwell Science for gently riding herd on all of us to help get this project completed. We hope you enjoy the textbook.

B. H.
S. H.

CHAPTER *1*

Epidemiology of Sports Injuries

KEITH L. STANLEY

*S*tudies in the epidemiology of human illness and disease have long been a part of medical science. The epidemiologic studies as they relate to sports injuries have been much slower in developing. Sports medicine physicians and scientists have recognized the importance of knowledge derived from epidemiologic studies. This is especially pertinent in identifying injuries, determining etiologic factors, designating appropriate imaging studies, and developing strategies for prevention and treatment.

In its simplest definition, *epidemiology* is the study of the distribution and determinants of disease (1). An expanded version by Duncan is as follows: "Epidemiology is the study of the distribution and determinants of the varying rates of diseases, injuries, or other health states in human populations" (2).

A control or comparison group must be present for a study to be epidemiologic. To make a comparison, you need to develop a rate that is expressed as

$$\text{Rate} = \frac{\text{events}}{\text{population at risk}}$$

When reviewing epidemiologic studies, one needs to determine if the study is reporting *incidence rate* versus *prevalence rate*:

$$\text{Incidence rate} = \frac{\text{number of new cases of injury over a period of time}}{\text{population at risk}}$$

$$\text{Prevalence rate} = \frac{\text{total number of cases of injury at a given time}}{\text{total population}}$$

Another set of terms to be understood is *retrospective* versus *prospective*. Most studies in sports injury epidemiology are retrospective (i.e., they look back in time). More studies are now being done prospectively (i.e., the study group is followed forward in time).

One may ask why epidemiologic data are important to sports medicine? This is best summarized by McKeag and Hough (3), as enumerated below:

1. Identify causes of injuries.
2. Provide a more accurate picture of clinical reality.
3. Determine the effectiveness of preventative measures.
4. Monitor the health of athletes, which will assist in rational medical planning.
5. Quantify the risks of various types, frequencies, and intensities of exercise activities.
6. Provide an overview of long-term injury trends in specific sports.

There have been attempts to standardize the reporting of sports injuries. The most precise way to report sports injuries is case rates per 1000 athlete-exposures. An *athlete-exposure* is defined as one athlete participation in one practice or game where there is a possibility of sustaining an athletic injury (3). See the example below.

High School Football

50 players × 4 weekly practices	= 200 athlete-exposures
35 players × 1 Friday night game	= 35 athlete-exposures
Total athlete-exposures for week	= 235

Three major reporting systems that track athletic injuries currently use the athlete-exposure as their mechanism of data collection. They are the National Athletic Injury/Illness Reporting System (NAIRS), the National Collegiate Athletic Association Injury Surveillance System (NCAA-ISS), and the Athletic Injury Monitoring System (AIMS) (3).

Efforts have been made to standardize a reporting system so that epidemiologic studies are reported accurately and have application on a broader scale. If there is not a clear definition of injury, criteria for selection of subjects, and a proper denominator (i.e., population at risk), then these studies basically are only case reports.

One major weakness that still loomes even in current studies is the definition of a *reportable injury*. In general, most definitions incorporate all of the following:

1. The injury occurs in a scheduled practice or competition.
2. The injury requires medical attention.
3. The injury results in restriction or exclusion of the athlete from the remaining practice or competition or the following one or more days (4).

With the preceding definition, there remain significant injuries that will not be reported. This may be due to the fact that the injury occurs on a weekend and is not followed or reported by the supervising personnel or that the athlete actually keeps that information from the supervising coach or athletic trainer.

The person responsible for reporting remains a major variable in the recording of sports injuries. The reporting can be different when a coach versus an athletic trainer reports the injury. A coach may under-report injuries, whereas more highly trained medical personnel may even in some cases over-report.

The impact and importance of epidemiology to sports medicine can be monumental. Understanding of sports medicine epidemiology has served as the impetus for rule changes, for developing preventive training programs, and for developing new equipment or modifying existing equipment. It has further identified health issues that are pertinent to populations other than athletes.

The following review of the current and recent past literature is intended to offer the reader insight as to injury trends. This also may aid in understanding of specific injuries in a given sport. Overall, the goal is to raise readers' awareness in reviewing epidemiologic studies as well as to help physicians develop criteria for selecting proper imaging studies.

Injuries in American football are among the most studied and reported sports injuries. Among 5- to 14-year-olds, football required more emergency room visits (453.9 visits per 100,000 participants) than any other organized sport (5).

Study of catastrophic injuries and fatalities related to high school and college football from 1982 to 1988 found that football led the list of the most reported catastrophic injuries. These numbered 187 at the high school level and 50 at the collegiate level, and 73 of these injuries were fatal. When calculated as a rate per 100,000 participants per year, the football rate of catastrophic injury was 3.3; this was exceeded, though, by ice hockey at 4.5 and gymnastics at 3.7 (7).

To gain a perspective on the incidence of injury in football, one must consider the approximate population involved and identify injury trends within the sport. Mueller and Schindler reported that approximately 1.8 million athletes play football from high school to the professional level in the United States (8). Injury rates in football have been reported to occur in anywhere from 35% to 81% of participants (35.2% NATA Research Committee Report) (9,10).

In an extensive study by Rice on data collected from 1979 through 1987, football had a 54.8% injury rate per 100 athletes per season. Expressed as an injury rate per 1000 athletic exposure, football lists at 12.2%. This is probably the best study not only for football but also for multiple sports at the high school level, accurately reporting injury rates per 1000 athletic exposures (4) (Table 1-1).

While there are many inconsistencies with football studies (definition of injury and collection of data techniques), it is clear that football generates a high injury rate. This forces a large volume of injuries on the physician, who must then be cognizant of economy and outcome when deciding on imaging and treatment options.

The importance of these data lies in the attention they direct toward possible preventive measures and also to evaluate the current medical supervision of this particular sport. As is well known, many rule changes have come about in football as a result of studies showing certain tackling techniques putting football play-

T A B L E   **1-1**

Injury Data Analysis, 1979–1987

Rank and Sport	Number of Seasons	Total Athletes	Injury Rate per 100 Athletes per Season	Injury Rate per 1000 Athletic Exposures	Significant Injury Rate per 1000 Athletic Exposures	Major Injury Rate per 1000 Athletic Exposures	Percent of Different Athletes Injured
1. Cross-country, girls	57	604	56.3	15.9	3.2	1.0	34.3
2. Wrestling	46	1,494	50.9	12.8	2.6	0.9	31.4
3. Soccer, girls	52	1,272	45.5	12.6	3.2	0.6	33.1
4. Football	61	3,695	54.8	12.2	2.9	0.7	33.6
5. Gymnastics, girls	30	526	37.5	10.2	3.0	0.9	27.2
6. Soccer, boys	64	1,807	38.2	10.0	2.0	0.2	27.2
7. Cross-country, boys	58	1,180	34.2	9.6	2.2	0.5	23.4
8. Basketball, girls	86	1,501	31.4	6.6	1.7	0.5	22.9
9. Track, girls	56	1,764	22.3	6.1	1.4	0.3	16.7
10. Volleyball, girls	62	1,410	21.5	6.0	1.1	0.3	17.1
11. Basketball, boys	102	1,584	31.3	5.8	1.4	0.3	25.4
12. Baseball	69	1,503	22.4	5.5	1.2	0.3	18.0
13. Softball, girls	66	1,293	18.7	4.9	1.2	0.3	15.3
14. Track, boys	57	2,140	16.5	4.5	1.1	0.2	13.4
15. Swimming, girls	19	520	14.2	3.9	1.0	0.3	10.8
16. Tennis, coed	48	1,552	6.8	1.9	0.4	0.1	5.6
17. Swimming, boys	31	1,017	5.0	1.3	0.5	0.2	4.7
18. Golf, coed	41	737	1.4	0.7	0.0	0.0	1.4
TOTALS	1,005	25,599					

SOURCE: Reproduced by permission from Rice SG. Epidemiology and mechanisms of sports medicine. Teitz CC, Decker BC, eds. Scientific foundations of sports medicine 1989:3–23.

ers at risk for spine injury or with particular blocking techniques resulting in unnecessary risk to the knee, as reported by Thompson et al (15). Making changes in the contact allowed in football did cause a reduction of 15% in injuries when schools were compared with their own previous records. In another study by Halpern et al, injuries to the knee and ankle accounted for 25% of all injuries and 33% of all medical costs (16). It was postulated that this had some relation to the type of shoe that was worn (i.e., high top versus soccer style or a long versus a short cleat). Such efforts to study cause and effect can lead to preventive measures that can have a major impact on injury patterns in the sport of football. Data also have shown that playing surfaces may have an impact on injury rates.

At issue is the type of medical coverage available to a given level of sport participation.

Commonly discussed at sports medicine meetings is the high level of medical coverage that occurs at the professional and collegiate levels. This diminishes at the high school, junior high school, and little league levels. Lindamen reports from the Michigan State High State Athletic Association that only 61% of the schools that responded to a survey report having a physician available for at least one team at some time during the year (18). This was a very generous study in that a school was considered to have a team physician if a physician was present for at least one practice or contest during the entire year. Lindamen further noted that while NATA reports that 60% of football injuries occur during practice (9), his survey indicated that only 1% of the high schools had physicians available during practice (18).

The value of these studies is to indicate the problem areas concerning coverage of a high-

TABLE 1-2

Site of Injuries as a Percentage of All Injuries by Study, High School Football Players, United States

Site of Injury	Hale	Olson	Culpepper	Pritchett	Moretz
Head/neck	6	9.7	7.6	11.3	5.8
Shoulder	10	9.3	13.3	—	6.6
Upper arm		1.2	1.4	—	
Elbow	3	1.6	3.4	—	2.5
Lower arm	4	0.8	2.0	—	0.4
Hand/fingers/wrists	16	12.8	14.7	—	10.0
Upper extremity	—	—	—	35.5	19.5
Chest/ribs/abdomen	—	5.4	4.1	—	—
Back	5	2.3	4.9	7.7	5.4
Pelvis/groin/hip	3	—	2.8	7.4	12.0
Upper leg	10	4.3	4.6	—	3.7
Knee	13	36.5	22.2	12.7	22.0
Lower leg	8	2.5	4.0	—	—
Ankle/foot	12	11.6	15.1	—	22.0
Lower extremity	—	—	—	20.0	—
Other	10	0.8	0.2	5.4	9.5
Total injuries	885	257	1877	1849	241
(N)	(NS)	(4500)	(NS)	(3501)	(903)

SOURCE: Reproduced by permission from Halpern B, Thompson N, Curl WW, et al. High school football injuries: identifying the risk factors. Am J Sports Med 1987;15:316–320.

risk sport such as football. Also of value is an understanding of the most likely body part injured in a given sport. Halpern et al showed in a review of five studies that the percentages of injury are highest to the knee in the sport of football (16) (Table 1-2). Thus choices of imaging for the knee become a high priority. Hand, finger, and wrist injuries also were reported at high rates, as were injuries of the ankle and shoulder.

Soccer injuries also have epidemiologic significance, since soccer is considered to be the most popular game in the world. It is estimated that 40 million people play soccer. Hoy et al in a 1-year study found that 39% of a total 1839 sports injuries seen in emergency departments were soccer related (21).

The level of play may have an impact on injury incidence and patterns. In a Danish study, division-level players had an injury incidence of 18.5 per 1000 hours, but at series level, the incidence was only 11.9 per 1000 hours. The lower extremity was involved in 84% of all injuries, ankle sprains being the most common (36%)

(22). This study also demonstrated a higher level of injury incidence in game participation at the division level, but for the lower series level, injuries were more common at practice.

In a large study of 13,130 sports injury patients over 7 years, foot and ankle injuries were the most common injuries (greater than 50%) not only in soccer but also in gymnastics, volleyball, and martial arts (23). Further, most of the injuries were seen in the 10- to 19- and 20- to 29-year-old age groups. In males, the 10- to 19-year-old age group led, and in females, the 20- to 29-year-old age group led. Throughout the 7-year study, injury rates within age groups and within gender categories remained constant (23).

Twenty-eight percent of the epiphyseal injuries in children and adolescence were reported to be from the sport of soccer. Most of these were of the distal epiphysis of the lower extremity (24).

Skill level appears to play a role in injury incidence, although reporting methodology may account for the apparent differences. Poulsen et al found that lower-skilled players had a higher incidence of injury, but when the number of games played was assessed, there was no difference in the severity or frequency of injuries (25).

Although many epidemiologic soccer studies have been published, reporting methods vary, and many do not have a clearly defined control. One can make some general conclusions about injuries in soccer, however. Most injuries are acute, overuse injuries have the longest recovery time, and most injuries are to the lower extremity.

Another sport of epidemiologic significance is running. Worldwide, the popularity of running has grown since the early 1970s (27). Many countries have seen increases of up to 100%. In the United States alone, there are an estimated 30 million runners (27).

Injury rates seem to be affected by the specificity of the group of runners concerned (27). In reviewing studies on running injuries, it is important to determine the age group being studied, whether they are competitive versus recreational runners, and whether they are male or female.

Brody reported an overall injury rate of 60% in his study of 3000 runners (28). In a review of published studies on runners, Burnet et al indicated that 25% to 40% of runners sustained at least one of the common injuries to the knee. The foot was the second most common area of injury (29).

As with studies of other sports, the definitions of what constitutes a running injury vary. Variations also exist in runners' characteristics, research design, and length of study (27).

The length of study is important when reporting injury evidence in running based on per-year occurrence. If a study does not follow the athletes over an entire 12-month period, the data may be biased.

In studies of high school athletes, careful observations are necessary. Rice found female cross-country athletes to have the highest incidence of injury. Interestingly, male cross-country athletes ranked seventh (4) (see Table 1-1).

The etiology of running injuries is multifactorial. A worn-out or improperly fitted running shoe may contribute to injury (31). Burnet et al reported that leg-length discrepancy was the major contributing factor to running injuries (29). Poor biomechanics, errors in training such as a too rapid increase in mileage, excessive hill training, and anatomic variations are also factors to be observed (27,29,31).

Other sports have been less investigated. However, Brust et al found in children's ice hockey that illegal checks and violations were associated with 66% of injuries during games, yet in only 14% of these cases were penalties accessed. Checking from behind was believed to be most significant (33).

In a study of collegiate rodeo athletes, it was found that these athletes face an 89% potential for injury per season. Most of these injuries (92%) occurred in athletes involved in rough stock and steer wrestling events, while only 8% of injuries occurred in roping and female events (34).

A small study comparing spine injuries in gymnasts and swimmers demonstrated a higher incidence in gymnasts, as well as an increase in injury incidence in the more elite gymnasts (35) (Table 1-3).

In a study that evaluated sports injuries serious enough to require hospitalization in a pediatric emergency room, 13% of admissions for trauma were sports related. This study was conducted over a 2-year period, with 142 patients hospitalized with sports injuries (36) (Table 1-4).

Davis et al also confirmed what many other studies have reported finding: a higher incidence of injury in the 13- to 19-year-old age group and greater injury occurrence in male rather than female athletes (36).

Backx et al, in their study of 1818 school children aged 8 to 17 years participating in a variety of sports, attempted to characterize high-risk persons and high-risk sports (37). This review of the epidemiologic literature of sports

T A B L E **1-3**

Spine Changes in Female Gymnasts and Swimmers

	Number	Spondy-lolysis	Abnormal Disk
Gymnasts			
Pre-elite	11	1	0
Elite	14	3	3
National/ Olympic	8	1	5
Swimmers			
AA/AAA	8	0	1
National	11	0	2

SOURCE: Adapted by permission from Goldstein JD, Berger PE, Windler GE, Jackson DW. Spine injuries in gymnasts and swimmers: an epidemiologic investigation. Am J Sports Med 1991;19:463–468.

T A B L E   1-4

Hospitalization from Sports Injuries

Fractures	77%
Abdominal injuries	7%
Multiple trauma	5%
Cerebral contusion or hemorrhages	5%
Dislocations	3%

SOURCE: Davis JM, Cuppermann N, Fleischer G. Serious sports injuries requiring hospitalization: pediatric emergency department. Am J Dis Child 1993;147: 1001–1004.

injuries has identified several issues to be discussed.

There are differences in injuries based on level of expertise and intensity of activity. Differences in injury rates comparing practices and competitions also were found. The length of practice was discovered to have an impact on injury rates as well.

Age, gender, and sports specificity affect injury rates (38). Football has high injury rates. In all running sports, the knee and ankle are injured most commonly. Hand injuries are more likely in sports where a ball is being thrown or caught or if a racket or stick is used (39). Hand injuries are also more common in hand contact sports such as martial arts or boxing. Gymnasts, cheerleaders, and swimmers may have more shoulder and spine complaints. Baseball players are likely to have higher incidences of upper extremity injuries.

Even though general trends may be identified, the sports medicine physician must realize that injury types can cross the lines of usual cause and effect.

The epidemiology of sports injuries is both an interesting and confusing study. Hopefully, sports medicine physicians in the future will continue to work cooperatively to standardize research design, data collection, definitions and terminology, and reporting systems. This is vital to clarifying the confusing data presented in epidemiologic literature.

As this text progresses through the imaging and anatomy of injuries, hopefully, an understanding of the epidemiologic literature will be helpful in decision making. The accuracy of diagnosis depends heavily on patient history and clinical evaluation by the physician, but the proper selection of imaging also remains vital. Cost-effectiveness is also a factor to be considered. This text should assist the sports medicine physician in being efficient and accurate in sports injury evaluation.

REFERENCES

1. Morton RF, Hebel JR. Study guide to epidemiology and biostatistics. Baltimore: University Park Press, 1979:1–153.

2. Duncan DF. Epidemiology: basis for disease prevention and health promotion. New York: Macmillan, 1988.

3. McKeag DB, Hough DO. Epidemiology of athletic injuries: primary care sports medicine. Dubuque, IA: Brown and Benchmark, 1993:63–73.

4. Rice SG. Epidemiology and mechanisms of sports injuries. In: Teitz CC, Decker BC, eds. Scientific foundations of sports medicine. Philadelphia: WB Saunders, 1989:3–23.

5. Wilkins KE. Epidemiology of shoulder injuries. In: Stanitski CL, DeLee JC, Drez D, eds. Pediatric and adolescent sports medicine. Philadelphia: WB Saunders, 1994:175–182.

6. Goldbert B, Rosenthal PP, Nicholas JA. Injuries in football. Phys Sports Med 1994;12:122–132.

7. Mueller FO, Cantu RC. Catastrophic injuries and fatalities in high school and college sports, fall 1982–spring 1988. Med Sci Sports Exerc 1990; 22:737–741.

8. Mueller FO, Schindler RD. Annual survey of football injury research 1931–1990. In: Proceedings of the 68th Meeting of the American Football Coaches Association, 1991:70–75.

9. NATA Research Committee report (public relations): athletic training, 1989:60–69.

10. Garick JG, Requa RK. Injuries in high school. Sports Pediatr 1978;61:465–468.

11. Canale E, Sisk TD, Freeman BL. A chronicle of injuries of an American. Am J Sports Med 1991; 9:384–389.

12. Zemper ED. Injury rates in a national sample of college football teams: a two-year prospective study. Phys Sports Med 1989;17:100–115.

13. McLain LG, Reynolds S. Sports injuries in a high school. Pediatrics 1989;84:446–450.

14. Karpakka J. American football injuries in Finland. Br J Sports Med 1993;27:135–137.

15. Thompson N, Halpern D, Curl WW, et al. High school football injuries evaluation. Am J Sports Med 1987;15:117–124.

16. Halpern B, Thompson N, Curl WW, et al. High

school football injuries: identifying the risk factors. Am J Sports Med 1987;15:316–320.

17. Powell JW, Schootman M. A multivariate risk analysis of selected playing surfaces in the National Football League: 1980–1989. Am J Sports Med 1992;20:686–692.

18. Lindamen LM. Physician care for interscholastic athletes. Am J Sports Med 1991;19:82–87.

19. Olson OC. The Spokane study: high school football injuries. Phys Sports Med 1979;7:75–82.

20. Culpepper MI, Niemann KMW. High school football injuries in Birmingham, Alabama. South Med J 1983;76:873–878.

21. Hoy K, Linblad BE, Terkelsen CJ, Helleand HE. European soccer injuries: a prospective epidemiologic and socio-economic study. Am J Sports Med 1992;20:318–322.

22. Nielsen AB, Yde J. Epidemiology in traumatology of injuries in soccer. Am J Sports Med 1989; 17:803–806.

23. Tenvergert EM, Ten Duis HF, Clasen HJ. Trends in sports injuries 1982–1988: an indepth study on four types of sports. J Sports Med Phys Fitness 1992;32:214–220.

24. Krueger-Franke M, Siebert CH, Pfoerringer W. Sports-related epiphyseal injuries of the lower extremity: an epidemiologic study. J Sports Med Phys Fitness 1992;32:106–111.

25. Poulsen TD, Freund KG, Madsen F, Sandvej K. Injuries in high skilled and low skilled soccer: a perspective study. Br J Sports Med 1991;25: 151–153.

26. Baxter-Jones A, Maffulin N, Helms P. Low injury rates in elite athletes. Arch Dis Childhood 1993; 68:130–132.

27. VanMechelen W. Running injuries: a review of the epidemiologic literature. Sports Med 1992;14: 320–335.

28. Brody DM. Running injuries. Clin Symp 1980;32: 2–36.

29. Burnet ME, Cook SD, Brinker MR, et al. A survey of running injuries in 1505 competitive and recreational runners. J Sports Med Phys Fitness 1990;30:307–315.

30. Watson MD, Dimartino PP. Incidents of injuries in high school track in field athletes and relation to performance ability. Am J Sports Med 1987; 15:251–254.

31. Cook SD, Brinker MR, Pouche DM. Running shoes: the relationship to running injuries. Sports Med 1990;10:1–8.

32. Garrik JG. Epidemiology of sports injuries in the pediatric athlete. In: Sullivan JA, Grana WA, eds. Pediatric athlete. Park Ridge, IL: American Academy of Orthopedic Surgeons, 1991:123–132.

33. Brust JD, Leonard BJ, Pheley A, Roberts WO. Children's ice hockey injuries. Am J Dis Child 1992;146:741–747.

34. Meyers MC, Elledge JR, Sterling JC, Tolsen H. Injuries in intercollegiate rodeo athletes. Am J Sports Med 1990;18:87–91.

35. Goldstein JD, Berger PE, Windler GE, Jackson DW. Spine injuries in gymnasts and swimmers: an epidemiologic investigation. Am J Sports Med 1991;19:463–468.

36. Davis JM, Cuppermann N, Fleischer G. Serious sports injuries requiring hospitalization: pediatric emergency department. Am J Dis Child 1993; 147:1001–1004.

37. Backx FJG, Beijer HJM, Bol E, et al. Injuries in high risk persons and high risk sports in a longitudinal study of 1818 school children. Am J Sports Med 1991;19:124–130.

38. Dehaven KE, Lintner DM. Athletic injuries: comparison by age, sport, and gender. Am J Sports Med 1986;14:218–224.

39. Amadio PC. Epidemiology of hand and wrist injuries in sports. Hand Clinics: Philadelphia: WB Saunders Co. 1990;6:379–381.

CHAPTER 2

Basic Principles of Medical Imaging: Applications to Sports Medicine

J. BRUCE KNEELAND

ALICE SCHEFF

To look inside the living body was for many centuries just a dream of physicians. Only with the discovery of x-rays by Roentgen in 1895 did we begin to make any real progress toward this goal.

Medical imaging includes all the different techniques for visualizing the internal anatomy of the body that have been developed over the last century. All these techniques are relatively safe and painless and, when used appropriately, can provide valuable information to assist in the clinical management of patients. The purpose of this chapter is to explain the basic principles of each of the commonly used imaging techniques so as to serve as a foundation for subsequent chapters that detail their clinical applications.

Plain Films/Fluoroscopy

Plain films or radiographs, which are also colloquially but inaccurately called "x-rays," are films that have been exposed to x-rays. X-rays are a portion of the electromagnetic spectrum (photons) with short wavelengths and high energy. The plain film is a map of the spatial distribution (i.e., the *projection*) of the attenuation (absorption or scattering) of x-rays along a line through the anatomy between the source of the x-rays and the film. Contrast on the film is determined by the differential attenuation of x-rays by different tissues. All soft tissues attenuate x-rays to about the same degree, although fat attenuates the beam less than the "water-dense" tissues such as muscle. Gas, as in the lungs or bowel loops, attenuates the x-rays considerably less than soft tissues, whereas bone attenuates the x-rays to a considerably greater degree. Metal found in orthopedic appliances attenuates the x-rays almost completely. The film is generally processed so that areas of high exposure to the x-ray beam (i.e., weak x-ray attenuation) appear dark on the film, whereas areas of low exposure (i.e., strongly attenuated x-ray beam) appear bright (Fig. 2-1).

Plain films are inexpensive and readily available. The potentially harmful side effect of x-rays is the capacity to damage the DNA of cells, with the resulting induction of mutations in the germ cells and carcinogenesis in somatic cell lines. For this reason, even though the risk from a single plain film is minute, it is important to limit the total number of plain films to that which can be reasonably expected to give clinically relevant information and to not obtain plain films out of habit. The major disadvantage to the use of plain films from the point of view of diagnostic information is that although they permit sharp delineation of the bones, they permit only a very limited evaluation of soft tissues. Thus plain films are very useful for displaying the integrity and alignment of the bones but for soft tissues can display only such abnormalities as gas, calcification, and glass or metallic foreign bodies.

The use of a contrast agent in conjunction

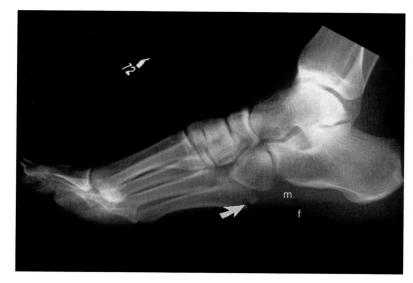

F I G U R E **2-1**

Lateral plain film of the foot and ankle. The bones are seen as the bright areas on the films. The surrounding soft tissue is barely visible on this rather dark film and appears gray, although it is possible to distinguish between the subcutaneous fat (*f*) that appears darker and the water density of muscle (*m*). The thick, linear lucency at the base of the fifth metatarsal (*arrow*) represents a subacute fracture.

with plain films is simply an extension of these same principles. A contrast agent can be any substance that is placed within the body in order to alter the attenuation of the x-rays. These contrast agents include barium sulfate, various iodine-containing compounds, and air. Iodine and barium sulfate attenuate the x-ray beam far better than soft tissues, whereas air attenuates it far less well. The major use of contrast agents in the musculoskeletal system in conjunction with plain films is the intra-articular injection of iodinated compounds (arthrography), which outline the structures within the joint that otherwise cannot be seen with x-rays. Due to the emergence of magnetic resonance imaging (MRI) (see below) as well as the moderately invasive nature of arthrography, it is only used infrequently in this era.

Fluoroscopy also uses an x-ray beam to form a map of attenuation of the tissues. It differs from the plain film in that the x-rays do not strike film but instead strike an electronic image intensifier that is much more sensitive to x-rays than film. Thus a much lower intensity x-ray beam can be used to form the image, although there is a considerable decrease in image quality. The relatively low intensity makes it feasible to generate the x-ray beam continuously. Fluoroscopy is used primarily to monitor the performance of certain types of procedures such as athroscopy or the closed reduction of fractures. It also can be used to visualize the bones during either active or passive motion.

The risk to the patient from fluoroscopy is the same as that of plain films, namely, exposure to the potentially harmful effects of x-rays. Thus

it is important to minimize the actual time the x-ray beam is on. This is also important to protect the fluoroscopist as well as the patient because, unlike plain films, there is also risk to the physician performing the study. Although the exposure from one examination is very small, the cumulative effect of performing many studies can be quite significant. It is imperative that the physician performing the studies take every precaution to minimize exposure to x-rays, including using only modern fluoroscopic equipment and wearing adequate shielding (lead apron, gloves, thyroid shield, and protective eyewear).

Computed Tomography (CT Scanning)

CT scanning uses x-rays to form cross-sectional images of the anatomic region of interest. It differs from plain films in two major ways. First, it forms a cross-sectional rather than a projection image. For this reason, it is referred to as a *tomographic* technique. Second, it forms a digital image rather than a direct image on the film from exposure of the x-ray beam.

As mentioned earlier, plain films are a projection technique in which the attenuation of the x-ray beam along a line through the anatomy is indicated qualitatively on the film by the degree of its exposure. CT scanning quantitatively measures the attenuation of the x-ray beam along lines through an anatomic region in multiple directions. From these values it is possible to calculate (*reconstruct*) a two-dimensional array of numbers that corresponds to the spatial distribution of attenuation in the anatomic cross section.

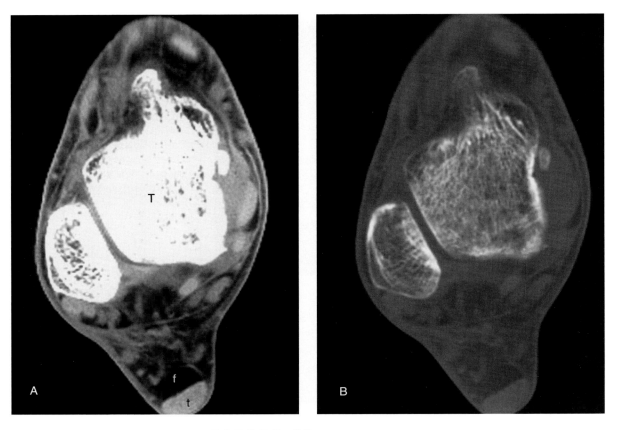

F I G U R E   **2-2**
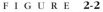

CT images of the ankle obtained through the talar dome and displayed with both narrow (A) and wide (B) window widths. The contrast between tendon (*t*) and the surrounding fat (*f*) is much more evident in the image with the narrow window width. The trabecular detail as seen in the talus (*T*) is much more evident in the image with the wide window width.

This array of CT numbers is converted to an image by assigning an intensity ranging from black through shades of gray up to white to each number (Fig. 2-2). These shades of intensity ranging from black to white are called the *gray scale*. More precisely, each shade of intensity is assigned to a specified range of CT numbers in a manner such that the intensity is roughly proportional to the magnitude of the numbers (i.e., smaller numbers are assigned intensities of black and darker gray, while higher numbers are given intensities of lighter gray and white). All CT numbers outside this range are assigned to either white or black depending on whether they are above or below the specified range. The range of numbers to which the gray scale is assigned is called the *window width,* and the center of the range is called the *level*. For images in which it is desirable to emphasize small differences in CT numbers between different tissues, a narrow window width is chosen (see Fig. 2-2A). Conversely, if it is desirable to visualize a wide range of CT numbers (e.g., bone and soft tissues) at the same time, a wide window width encompassing many CT numbers is chosen (see Fig. 2-2B). The window level is generally chosen to be near the center of the CT numbers of the structures of interest.

Each element of the two-dimensional array of CT numbers to which an intensity has been assigned in the image is called a *pixel* (picture element) or, more precisely, a *voxel* (volume element) to underscore the fact that these two-dimensional sections always have a finite thickness ranging from about 1 to 10 mm. The thickness of the plane (voxel) is always larger than the dimensions of the voxel in the plane of the section.

Because the CT number is a measure of the attenuation of x-rays and the gray scale is mapped so that the higher-attenuation pixels are displayed with brighter intensity similar to the usual display of attenuation on a plain film, the contrast properties of CT images are qualitatively similar to those of plain films, although CT is more sensitive to small contrast differences. Thus the calcified portions of bone are well visualized, while the display of soft tissues is much more limited, although considerably better than that obtained with plain films.

The orientation of the planes of section is limited by the physical geometry of the scanning gantry, and in general, images can only be acquired easily in the transverse plane (i.e., perpendicular to the long axis of the body), although in some cases it is possible to position an extremity so as to acquire images in other planes. It is also possible to *re-format* the image data into images oriented along other planes (e.g., sagittal and coronal) (Fig. 2-3). The resolution of these re-formatted images, however, is inferior to that of images acquired directly because the thickness (depth) of the cross section is much greater than the dimension of the voxel in the originally acquired plane of section.

CT scanning is often performed in conjunction with the intravenous or intra-articular injection of iodinated contrast material. Differences in attenuation and hence in "intensity" that are seen on the CT images with the intravenous injection of contrast material result from regional differences in perfusion of the tissues as well as differences in the passage of contrast material out of the capillaries into the surrounding interstitium. Regions with sufficient blood flow will demonstrate an increase in attenuation, whereas those with minimal or no blood flow will show little or no increase in attenuation. Despite the rather pronounced differences in blood flow that exist among different tissues, contrast-enhanced CT scans still demonstrate rather limited contrast within the soft tissues that is in general inferior to that of MRI (see below).

The intra-articular injection of contrast material performed in conjunction with CT scanning (a procedure called a *CT-arthrogram*) serves a purpose similar to plain-film arthrography, namely, to outline and hence make visible soft tissue structures that would otherwise not be seen. Its major advantage over that of an ordinary arthrogram is that it permits visualization of the structures in cross section. This is particularly helpful in regions of complex anatomy where overlap on projection images can lead to confusion. An additional advantage of this technique that has been noted is that the distension of the joint by contrast material may render certain structures more visible. This latter is particularly true for the insertion site of the joint capsule and labrum on the glenoid.

The risks associated with CT scanning are the same as those associated with plain films, namely, the exposure to x-rays. The dose resulting from a CT scan, however, is only slightly

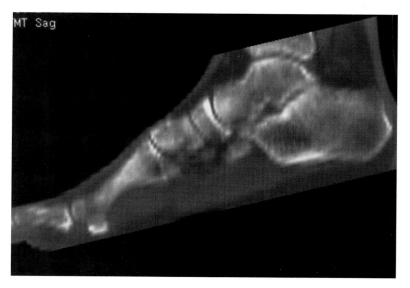

FIGURE **2-3**

Sagittal re-formatting of the axial CT sections from a study of the ankle. Note the ridges present at the margins of the bones that result from finite thickness of the original axial images that serve as the basis for this sagittal re-formatting.

more than would result from obtaining routine plain films of the region. If intravenous iodinated contrast material is used, there is a low incidence of minor reactions to the contrast material and a very small probability of a life-threatening or fatal reaction. The incidence of contrast material reactions can be reduced considerably by the use of the more expensive nonionic agents. Because of this considerably greater expense, the appropriate use of these nonionic agents is currently a matter of ongoing debate.

The incidence of serious complications following the intra-articular injection of contrast material is very low, although a transient inflammatory response of the synovium resulting in increased pain is not uncommon. The most common serious complication is that of intra-articular infection.

Nuclear Medicine (Radiotracer Imaging)

Nuclear medicine studies utilize radioactive tracers to demonstrate physiologic changes. In contrast to other imaging modalities, the radiopharmaceuticals are administered internally, and the emitted high-energy (gamma) photons are detected by specialized cameras in dynamic, planar, and tomographic modes. The appearance of a scan reflects the normal biodistribution of a radiotracer and superimposed pathophysiologic processes.

Contemporary radiotracer imaging was launched approximately 35 years ago with the development of the Anger gamma camera and recognition that technetium-99m is an ideal tracer for biomedical imaging. Although imaging applications have become increasingly sophisticated with the advent of computer technology, the original principles hold, namely, detection of gamma radiation emitted from a patient and conversion of that information into an image that maps the spatial location and intensity of the emitted protons.

Simply, the typical imaging system consists of a complex detector system (camera head), a computer console, an image printer, and a patient imaging table. When a patient is positioned for imaging, emitted gamma rays pass through the collimator and may interact with the thallium-activated sodium iodide crystal in the camera head. This interaction may result in ejection of an orbital electron (photoelectric absorption), producing a pulse of fluorescent light (scintilla-

tion event) proportional in intensity to the energy of the gamma ray. Photomultiplier tubes adjacent to the crystal detect this light and convert it into an amplified electric signal. The pulse height analyzer discriminates voltage signals emerging from the photomultiplier tubes, recording those known to correspond to the photopeak of the isotope being imaged and discarding those derived from background, scatter radiation, or interfering isotopes. The resulting image that appears on the computer screen will reflect information from the patient and the overall quality control and resolution of the imaging system. Since the image reflects statistically significant photon flux from the patient, system nonuniformity, nonlinear camera response, and improper imaging parameters will degrade the observed output. Image enhancement techniques may improve lesion contrast and complement comparative regional quantification. Specialized image acquisition including pinhole collimation can improve resolution.

The radionuclides used most frequently in nuclear medicine imaging are short-lived isotopes that emit gamma rays ranging in energy from approximately 80 to 365 keV. However, specialized detector systems employed in positron-emission tomography (PET) can accurately detect higher-energy photons (511 keV).

Technetium-99m pertechnetate (140 keV, 6-hour half-life) is the most versatile clinical isotope. Readily coupled to carriers that direct the radiotracer to specific organ systems, technetium-99m is widely available and easily imaged by the Anger camera system because it decays by isomeric transition. Other clinically useful isotopes include indium-111, thallium-201, gallium-67, xenon-133, krypton-81M, iodine-123, and iodine-131.

The risks associated with radiotracer imaging are the same as those associated with exposure to x-rays. The dose resulting from a nuclear medicine procedure ranges from less than that of a plain film to comparable to that of a CT scan. There is minimal risk of an allergic reaction. In short, the benefit-to-risk ratio is very high, the procedures are readily tolerated, and the physiologic information is unique and complementary to anatomic studies.

In the evaluation of musculoskeletal disorders, bone scans, gallium scans, and tagged leukocyte scans frequently are requested as initial screening procedures or to narrow the differential considerations. When questions pertain to the appendicular skeleton and involve recent

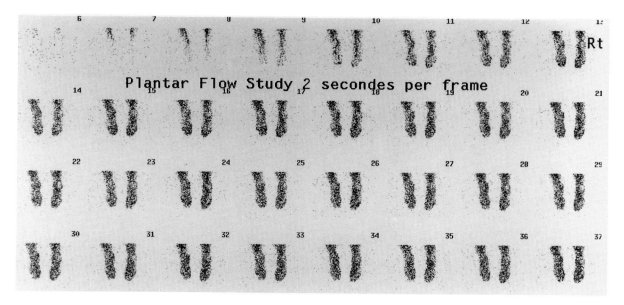

F I G U R E 2-4

Multiple planar images of both feet obtained during the flow phase of a radionuclide study. Images were obtained every 2 seconds. The feet are viewed as if looking from the sole with the toes at the bottom of each image. (Courtesy of Dr. Ron Korn of the Division of Nuclear Medicine at the Hospital of the University of Pennsylvania.)

trauma or possible associated inflammation, triple-phase bone scanning is performed. This consists of the following (Figs. 2-4 and 2-5):

1. A *flow phase* (dynamic image acquisition, centered on the painful body part, throughout tracer injection)
2. Static *blood pool* or soft tissue images, obtained immediately after tracer injection
3. Static *bone images,* obtained approximately 3 hours following tracer administration

Increased blood flow and soft tissue uptake may reflect hyperemia, a vascular lesion, or inflammation. Increased tracer uptake on the bone images, termed *hot lesions,* reflects reactive bone remodeling secondary to numerous conditions, including trauma, fracture, tumor, osteomyelitis, arthritis, biomechanical stress, Paget's disease, metabolic bone disease, fibrous dysplasia, enchondroma, and infarction. Decreased tracer uptake relative to the adjacent normal or hot bone is termed a *cold* or *photopenic lesion* and may be observed in the acute phase of ischemic necrosis or infarction, at sites of aggressive osteolytic tumors, and occasionally in early osteomyelitis and septic arthritis, especially in children.

Cross-sectional tomographic imaging can be performed throughout the axial and appendicular skeleton. Termed *single photon emission computed tomography* (SPECT), this technique provides sectional images in coronal, sagittal, and transaxial planes analogous to CT scans or MRI. Enhanced image contrast improves lesion detection and localization and frequently resolves abnormalities faintly perceived or poorly localized by the standard two-dimensional planar images.

Sonography

Sonography, also referred to as *ultrasound,* uses high-frequency pulses of sound to form cross-sectional images of the body. The frequency of the sound is typically in the range of 3 to 10 MHz, which is well outside the range of human hearing (2–20,000 Hz). Pulses of sound are generated by a transducer placed on the surface of the body and are reflected to varying degrees by the underlying tissues back to the transducer, where they are detected. An image of the reflected pulses is generated in which the intensity of the image is proportional to the strength of the reflected signal at each distance from the transducer (Fig. 2-6). There is always some degree of reflection from the internal structure of any organ, but the largest reflections are at the

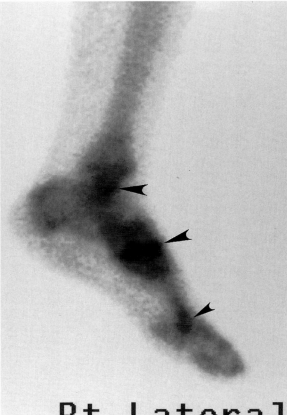

Rt Lateral

F I G U R E   2-5
Planar image of the foot and ankle in the lateral view obtained as part of the static images of a radionuclide study. The increased intensity seen at several regions of the ankle and foot (*arrowheads*) in this patient results from osteoarthritis and illustrates the nonspecific nature of this finding. (Courtesy of Dr. Ron Korn, Philadelphia.)

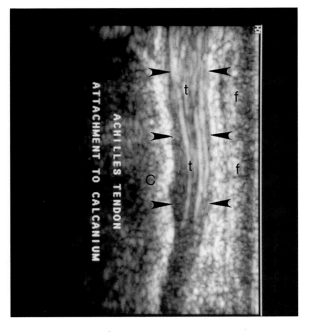

F I G U R E   2-6
High-resolution sonogram of the insertion of the Achilles tendon (*t*) on the calcaneus (*C*) imaged in the sagittal plane. The margins of the tendon are indicated by arrowheads. The subcutaneous fat (*f*) has a demonstrably different echo texture from that of the tendon. Note the bright signals at the boundaries between fat and tendon and tendon and calcaneus. The apparent reflections from deep to the surface of the calcaneus are artifactual inasmuch as there is no penetration of the ultrasound into the calcaneus. (Courtesy of Dr. Beverly Coleman, Philadelphia.)

interfaces between different types of tissue, whether at the interface between normal and abnormal tissue within an organ or at the interface between tissues of different organs. This large reflection arises because of a significant difference between the properties of the different tissues with respect to the transmission of the ultrasonic pulses. Conversely, the more uniform a tissue, the smaller is the degree of internal reflections and the greater is the transmission of the ultrasonic pulse.

As a rule, the higher the frequency of the ultrasound, the greater is the attainable resolution but the smaller is the depth of penetration of the sound from the skin surface. Ultrasound is unable to penetrate the surfaces of bones, with the result that the internal structures of bones and joints cannot be evaluated with this technique. Sonography can visualize the superficial soft tissues of the musculoskeletal system and has been used to detect the presence of degeneration or tears within the tendons, especially within the tendons of the rotator cuff.

Sonography is inexpensive, readily available, and completely safe. Its major disadvantages include both the relatively limited amount of the musculoskeletal system that can be visualized with ultrasound and the strong dependence of the accuracy of sonographic examinations on the skill of the operator. For these reasons, MRI has been used primarily for evaluation of the musculoskeletal system in the United States, although it has received considerably more utilization in Europe. With continuing financial pressures in the United States, however, the use of sonography for evaluation of the musculoskeletal system may well increase.

Magnetic Resonance Imaging

Magnetic resonance imaging (MRI) is a method of forming cross-sectional images of the body. It is the most complex and most expensive imaging technique that is in widespread clinical use. It is also a cross-sectional as well as a digital imaging technique. These carry the same implications for this technique that they carried for CT scanning. MRI takes advantage of the fact that when the nucleus of the hydrogen atom (i.e., a proton) is placed in a strong magnetic field, it can be excited with high-frequency magnetic fields (at the *resonant* frequency) and in turn emit a magnetic field of the same high frequency that can be detected. The resonant frequency is determined by a constant that is peculiar to each nucleus called the *gyromagnetic ratio* and the strength of the magnetic field at the nucleus. Although the phenomenon of resonance is induced in all the hydrogen nuclei, the emitted signal can only be detected in imaging systems from those hydrogen nuclei which are present in "free" water molecules (i.e., those which are not bound to macromolecules) and to

a lesser degree from those in the light-weight alkyl side chains of the fatty acids. Both these sources of hydrogen nuclei are referred to as *mobile protons*.

To actually form an image, an additional magnetic field called a *gradient field* must be superimposed on the static field. This alters the value of the magnetic field at each point in space so that the frequency of the magnetic field emitted by the nucleus is different at each location. This positional dependence of the frequency of the emitted field permits determination of the strength of the signal from each location in space and hence the formation of an image. This method of forming an image permits the plane of section to be taken in any direction as opposed to being largely limited to the transverse plane, as is the case with CT (Fig. 2-7).

The contrast of the MRI image is determined primarily by the concentration of the unbound water, called the *spin* or *proton density*, and the magnitude of two properties of the nuclei taken in bulk, called *T1* and *T2 relaxation times*. The relaxation times characterize the time dependence of the components of the bulk magnetization that lie parallel and perpendicular to the static field. It is not necessary to understand the precise nature of these relaxation times to understand the contrast properties of MRI. Rather,

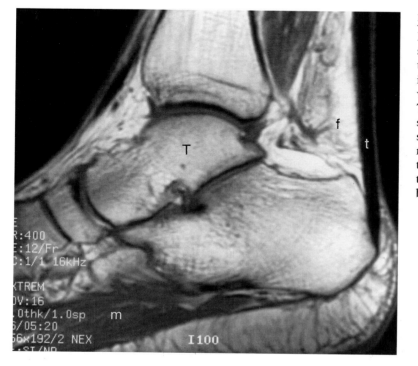

FIGURE 2-7

MRI of the ankle obtained in the sagittal plane through the insertion of the Achilles tendon. The image was obtained using a T1-weighted spin-echo sequence. The contrast among the soft tissues [fat (*f*) versus tendon (*t*) versus muscle (*m*)] is quite pronounced. Cortical bone is seen as the low signal rim surrounding the high signal marrow of each bone (*T* = talus).

it is important to understand that the presence of disease generally will increase the magnitude of relaxation times of the tissue at the site of the disease and hence create contrast between normal and abnormal tissues. This increase in relaxation times results from an alteration of the relationship between the free water molecules and the macromolecules within the tissue. The precise method by which the nuclei are excited, called a *pulse sequence,* can be adjusted so as to create differences in one of the three parameters (T1, T2, proton density), the predominant factor contributing to the image contrast. In these cases, the images are described as T1-weighted, T2-weighted, or proton density–weighted images (Figs. 2-7 and 2-8). It should always be borne in mind that although these terms denote the major factor influencing the contrast of the image, all three factors are always present to some degree in all the sequences that are used clinically.

In addition to describing a sequence as T1, T2, or proton density weighted, there are large classes of sequences that are given such names as *spin echo, fast* or *turbo spin echo, gradient echo,* and *inversion recovery.* Although the parameters of any of these sequences can be adjusted so as to make the images, T1, T2, or proton density weighted, there remain significant differences among them. In addition, there are subclasses of sequences, especially within the gradient-echo class, that have different properties as well as carry different names from one manufacturer's system to the next.

The spin-echo sequence is the mainstay of clinical MRI, particularly of the musculoskeletal system. It is a versatile sequence whose contrast properties are well understood and whose timing parameters can be altered readily to achieve the appropriate contrast. An important feature of the spin-echo sequence that is also true for most of the other sequences is that longer T1 times cause a decrease in signal intensity that is most evident on T1-weighted images, while longer T2 times result in an increase in signal intensity that is most evident on T2-weighted images. The

F I G U R E   **2-8**

MRI images of the knee obtained in the sagittal plane with proton density–weighted (A) and T2-weighted (B) spin-echo sequences. There is a linear focus of high signal within the posterior horn of the medial meniscus (*arrowhead*) that represents a tear. Compare the appearance of the normal anterior horn, which demonstrates a uniform low signal (*arrow*). The tear is much better demonstrated in the proton density–weighted image. Note also the presence of a small amount of joint fluid (*fl*) that is better depicted in the T2-weighted image.

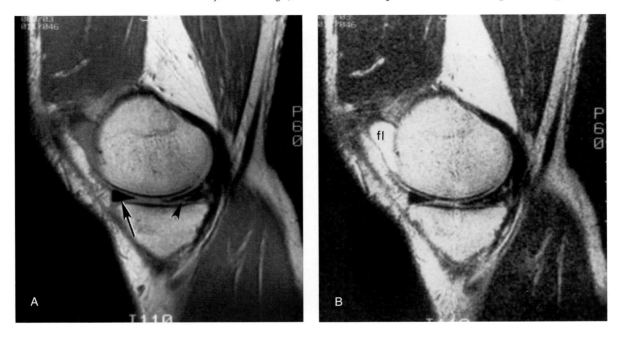

major disadvantage of this sequence is the length of time required for image acquisition (2–10 minutes), especially for T2-weighted sequences (approximately 10 minutes). In regard to image acquisition, it should be understood that all the images are being generated simultaneously during the sequence rather than sequentially, as is the case with CT scanning. For this reason, motion at any time during the sequence ruins the entire set of images.

The fast-spin-echo sequence has contrast properties that are similar to those of the spin-echo sequence but which permit much more rapid acquisition of T2-weighted images (approximately 2–3 minutes). There are some subtle differences between the spin-echo and fast-spin-echo sequences, however, that include increased signal from fat on T2-weighted images and a subtle loss of spatial detail on T1-weighted and proton density–weighted images.

Gradient-echo sequences have some properties that are similar to those of spin-echo sequences, but there are several major differences

between gradient-echo and spin-echo images. First, there can be a significant loss of signal at the boundaries between different tissues, such as the interface between cancellous bone and marrow (Fig. 2-9). This causes the marrow fat to appear darker than the subcutaneous fat. Second, gradient-echo sequences permit the rapid acquisition of sequential images either from a series of different locations or from the same location in rapid temporal sequence. This latter property is useful for studies obtained following the injection of intravenous contrast agents, as described below. Although the image quality of these techniques is inferior to that obtained with spin-echo imaging, they often yield valuable information. Finally, gradient-echo sequences permit much thinner sections through what is called a *three-dimensional* or *volumetric image acquisition*. These thinner sections are sometimes of value in the detection or characterization of disease. Thus this sequence is frequently used in the imaging of the cervical spine, where it is particularly useful for the evaluation of the

F I G U R E   **2-9**

MRI images of the knee obtained in the sagittal plane with a proton density–weighted spin-echo sequence using 3-mm-thick sections (A) and a three-dimensional gradient-echo sequence using 1.5-mm-thick sections (B). A small tear is seen on the superior surface of the posterior horn of the medial meniscus in the gradient-echo image (*arrowhead*) that is not seen in the spin-echo image. Note also the similar appearance of the marrow fat in the distal femur (*F*) and the subcutaneous fat in the spin-echo image and the relatively darker signal of the marrow fat in the distal femur compared with subcutaneous fat (*f*) in the gradient-echo image.

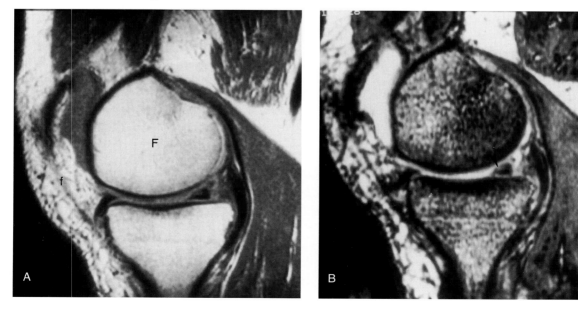

neural foramina because of their small size, although the loss of signal at the interface between the bone and the adjacent soft tissues may make the bony structures appear larger and hence the neural foramina smaller than they actually are.

The inversion-recovery sequence is almost always used to suppress the signal from fat and to maximize the contrast differences arising from differences in relaxation times. The rationale behind suppressing the signal from fat is that on T2-weighted images abnormal tissues generally display bright signal, while fat also displays bright signal. To increase the conspicuity of the abnormal tissue, it is useful to reduce the bright signal from fat, especially if it lies adjacent to the abnormal tissue. When used in this manner, the inversion-recovery sequence is called the *STIR sequence* (short TI inversion recovery). The STIR sequence is the most sensitive sequence to the presence of disease, but it is less efficient than the spin-echo sequence (i.e., a much smaller portion of anatomy can be studied in a given amount of time than with the spin-echo sequence), and its images are grainier. Other techniques also can be used to reduce the signal from fat. These generally permit more efficient imaging but exhibit less effective suppression of the signal from fat and less overall contrast than the STIR sequence.

It is valuable for clinicians to have some understanding of the MRI appearance of both normal and abnormal tissues in the musculoskeletal system as well as the basis for their appearance (see Figs. 2-7 through 2-9). The cortical and cancellous portions of the bones have no mobile protons and appear dark with all sequences. Thus these structures are only detectable because of the signal from the surrounding tissue. The tendons and ligaments, which are composed predominantly of dense fibrous tissue, have only a small number of mobile protons and likewise appear dark on all sequences. Fibrocartilage likewise has few mobile protons and appears dark on all sequences. Muscle has a medium to low signal with all sequences. Subcutaneous fat appears bright on T1-weighted sequences, moderately bright on proton density–weighted and T2-weighted sequences, and completely dark on the STIR sequence. Marrow fat has an appearance similar to subcutaneous fat on spin-echo sequences but, as noted earlier, displays considerably less signal on gradient-echo sequences. Fluid seen within the joints, whether normal or abnormal in amount, appears darker than muscle on T1-weighted images and brighter than fat on T2-weighted images.

Most of the abnormalities of the tendons, ligaments, and fibrocartilaginous structures are seen as diffuse or focal areas of increased signal within those structures on all the sequences as an alteration of the size or contour or continuity of the structure. Some abnormalities are seen better on some sequences than others. Thus, for instance, tears of the menisci generally are best seen on the proton density–weighted sequences, whereas tears of the ligaments are often best seen on the T2-weighted sequences. As noted previously, abnormalities within the marrow fat, such as fractures, osteonecrosis, infection, or tumor, generally will appear darker than the marrow fat on T1-weighted images and brighter than the fat on T2-weighted sequences. The conspicuity of the lesions on T2-weighted images can be enhanced by the use of techniques that reduce the signal from fat. Abnormalities in the muscle and other soft tissues surrounding the joint such as edema fluid or discrete cystic collections such as synovial cysts or ganglia generally appear darker than muscle on T1-weighted images and brighter than muscle on T2-weighted and STIR sequences. Hemorrhage may exhibit the same pattern or may differ depending on age and other factors and can appear both bright on T1-weighted images and/or dark on T2-weighted images depending on the age of the bleed.

Contrast agents are also used with MRI. Contrast agents in MRI are paramagnetic substances that act primarily by shortening the T1 relaxation time of the protons in the immediate vicinity of the agents. The agents by themselves do not emit an MRI signal. Shortening the T1 relaxation time has the effect of increasing the signal intensity on T1-weighted images. These agents often are used in conjunction with fat-suppression techniques (but not with the STIR sequence) to increase the conspicuity of the contrast enhancement by suppressing the bright signal from adjacent fat.

Contrast agents can be administered intravenously or injected intra-articularly. The pharmacokinetics of these agents are similar to those seen with the iodinated contrast agents used with CT scanning. Thus the differential effects on the signal intensity of different tissues reflect regional differences in perfusion of the tissues and in leakage of contrast material from the capillaries into the interstitium. In the musculoskeletal system, intravenous MRI contrast agents are used most commonly to help distinguish between recurrent disk herniation and fibrosis in the postoperative lumbar spine and occasionally to further delineate some cases of infection involving either the spine or the extremities. The intra-articular injection of contrast material serves the same function as in CT scanning, namely, to outline the margin of certain anatomic structures that are otherwise difficult to visualize and to distend the joint capsule, thus separating these structures. MR-arthrography has been applied to many different areas but finds its greatest use in evaluation of the labrum and glenohumeral ligaments in patients with instability of the shoulder.

MRI is in general quite safe. Several classes of patients, however, are at potential risk and should not undergo MRI. These include

1. Patients with cardiac pacemakers or neurostimulatory devices
2. Patients with intracranial aneurysmal clips, unless it is unequivocally known that their clips are nonmagnetic
3. Patients with radiographically visible intraorbital metallic fragments
4. Patients with certain types of prostheses (this list is rather long and cannot be given here; if the patient has any type of prosthesis, the feasibility of performing an MRI study should be discussed with the personnel of the MRI facility at the time of scheduling)

Relative contraindications to MRI include any recent surgery, pregnancy, claustrophobia, and any reason that the patient cannot remain motionless for periods of up to 10 minutes. Most orthopedic appliances (screws, plates, joint prostheses) do not pose a threat to the patient's well-being, although they may degrade the image quality significantly.

Contrast agents used in MRI are quite safe. The incidence of both minor and major reactions is exceedingly small and much less than that of the routine iodinated contrast agents used with plain films or CT scans.

The Future of Imaging

New techniques of imaging may evolve in the future, and the technology of all the imaging techniques currently available will continue to evolve and their capabilities will be enhanced. This latter is especially true for MRI. In an era of significant financial constraints, however, there will be increasing emphasis on justifying the use of any imaging technique, whether it is new, represents an enhancement of current techniques, or simply applies old techniques to a disease to which it has not been applied in the past, if it increases the cost of the patient's evaluation. Indeed, the value of even seemingly well-established clinical applications of MRI is currently being challenged by third-party payors. The value of any imaging technique can only be demonstrated by well-controlled, prospective outcome studies, and it is highly probable that such studies will be mandatory prior to the introduction of either new techniques or major enhancements to current techniques into widespread clinical practice.

CHAPTER *3*

Imaging of Head Injuries in Sports

ROGER L. MCCOY II

DOUGLAS B. MCKEAG

KATHERINE LUDWIN

JEFF MITCHINSON

JAMES A. KRCIK

The possibility of athletic head injuries, although usually infrequent, can occur in all sports such as gymnastics, skiing, rugby, ice hockey, football, and boxing. The incidence of head injury in the United States is approximately 200 injuries per 100,000 people per year (1). The projected incidence of concussions in high school football is estimated at around 2000 cases per 100,000 players (2). Data from the National Football Head and Neck Registry (3) have shown an average of about 5 to 10 deaths per year from intracranial hemorrhage from 1977 to 1987 (Fig. 3-1). From 1980 through 1984, there were 33 deaths, for a risk rate of 0.65 per 100,000 participants per year. Other data show an estimated rate of head injury to be about 250,000 per year in contact sports (3,4).

Another important statistic shows that in high school football players there is a 20% risk of minor head injury each year of play and that an athlete who has sustained one head injury may be at a fourfold greater risk for sustaining repeated head injuries during that same season (5). Besides the concerns with intracerebral hemorrhage from one of these acute injuries, the primary care sports physician also needs to be concerned with the *second-impact syndrome* (6–8). This is defined as a young athlete who has sustained a repeat concussion within a short period of time and suffers severe brain edema and a fatal outcome very shortly after the next head injury.

At present, no specific guidelines exist that dictate the exact timing of neuroradiologic studies and whether or not such studies are necessary for each minor head injury that occurs in sports. Several grading systems and treatment guidelines exist with regard to head injuries suffered during sporting activities. Because of this, the utilization of radiologic techniques tends to vary and depend on the individual, the physician, and each specific incident. Utilizing these different grading systems, we attempt in this chapter to devise a point system to aid the primary care sports medicine physician in choosing the appropriate radiologic technique when confronted with a minor head injury in athletics. Secondarily, this chapter describes several different types of head injuries and also compares different radiologic techniques while discussing their strengths and weaknesses.

Mechanisms and Biomechanical Forces of Head Injury

The cranial vault is a fixed space containing brain, spinal fluid, extracellular fluid, and blood.

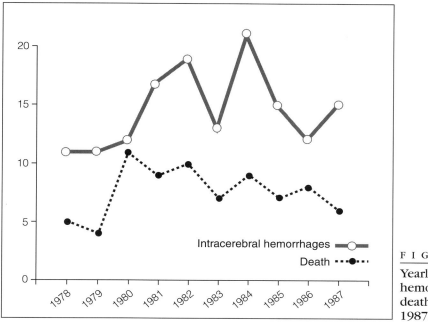

F I G U R E   **3-1**

Yearly occurrence of intracranial hemorrhage and head injury deaths from football, 1977 to 1987.

In this closed environment, the cerebrospinal fluid (CSF) provides protection and a shock-absorbing cushion to help convert external compressive stresses and forces through the skull and distribute them in a uniform fashion (4). These external forces can be either compressive, tensile, or shearing in nature. In particular, shearing forces tend to be tolerated poorly by neural tissue.

When the head of an athlete is in the resting position and is struck by a force, whether it be an opponent's football helmet or a left hook, injury to the brain occurs beneath the point of the cranial impact, resulting in a *coup injury* (9). In the case of an athlete in motion, as may occur in an equestrian's or a gymnast's fall, each striking his or her moving head with a nonmoving object (i.e., the ground), the area of injury tends to occur at the opposite side from the cranial impact, creating a *contracoup injury*. If the athlete sustains a skull fracture, whether it be linear or depressed, the forces of coup and contracoup injuries no longer apply, and one may find brain tissue injured directly below the site of the fracture (10). It is also important to realize that the head can receive accelerative forces not only from a direct contact but also when it is set in motion from impulsive loading. This may occur, for instance, when violent blows are directed to the anterior/posterior thorax while the head remains freely mobile. With an understanding of these mechanisms, combined with primate and fluid percussion animal studies over the past two decades, five parallel pathologic components can be identified: 1) focal injury, 2) diffuse axonal injury, 3) selective neuronal injury, 4) diffuse microvascular injury with loss of cerebrovascular autoregulation and brain swelling, and 5) superimposed hypoxia/ischemia (11). All these features have been reproduced in studies of acceleration without impact, and at least the first four can be documented to occur in mild head injuries in humans. It is these head injuries that the primary care sports medicine physician will be dealing with. It is rare that hypoxic and ischemic head injuries will be encountered in the sports medicine setting.

Head Injury Classification

The basic understanding of available radiologic techniques will be covered elsewhere in this book. Hence we will investigate the various head injuries that the primary care sports medicine physician may encounter. There are several different types of head injuries, including one or more of the several intracranial lesions. Intracranial lesions can be separated into hemorrhagic and nonhemorrhagic. These can be either diffuse or focal and can occur in extra-axial or intra-axial locations. Extra-axial lesions include subdural hematomas, epidural hematomas, and subarachnoid hemorrhages. Intra-axial lesions include contusions, cerebral infarctions, diffuse brain injuries, cerebral herniations, and cerebral edema (Fig. 3-2). Other related conditions are mild cerebral concussion, second-impact syndrome, and postconcussion syndrome. Although cardiovascular events account for the leading cause of athletic death, intracranial hemorrhages, especially acute subdural hematomas, account for the majority of the remaining deaths (12).

Extra-Axial Lesions

Epidural Hematoma

An epidural hematoma results from a tear of the middle meningeal artery, which runs along the temporal bone outside of the dura mater. The temporal bone is fractured in 75% to 90% of cases (13). Epidural hematomas also can arise from disruption of the meningeal emissary veins or venous sinuses. The most common locations are the temporal, frontal, and occipital regions (12).

Early recognition of this lesion is critical because the mass effect from the rapidly bleeding meningeal artery produces brain herniation that results in death of the athlete. This type of lesion, often associated with a temporal fracture, may present with a brief period of unconsciousness followed by a lucid period and then deterioration into a state of unconsciousness, coma, and death often in as little as 15 to 30 minutes. Since death is due to herniation and there is usually no significant injury to the brain itself, proper recognition and early treatment can result in normal neurologic recovery (10).

Characteristically, biconvex lentiform mass forms in the epidural space that compresses the underlying brain, creating a sharply demarcated lesion that is confined by the dura's adherence to the skull. Epidural hematomas generally are seen as hyperdense extracranial masses in this epidural location (12) (Fig. 3-3). Since delayed arterial epidural bleeds occasionally may escape detection on the initial CT scan, a second CT scan may be indicated if symptoms are delayed in onset and the first CT scan is negative.

F I G U R E   **3-2**

Types of intracranial hemorrhage and brain herniation.

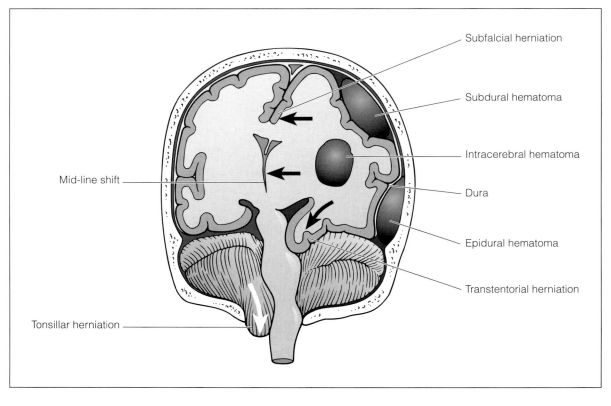

Subfalcial herniation

Subdural hematoma

Intracerebral hematoma

Mid-line shift

Dura

Epidural hematoma

Transtentorial herniation

Tonsillar herniation

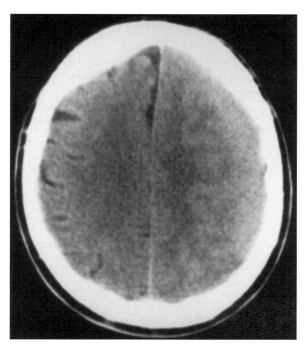

F I G U R E **3-3**

Epidural hematoma (*arrows*).

Subdural Hematoma

Most athletes with a subdural hematoma usually have sustained some form of unconsciousness, and a radiologic and neurosurgical referral is obvious. Occasionally, however, a football player or boxer may regain consciousness long enough to walk off the playing field or out of the ring only to collapse later as the hematoma evolves. Subdural hematomas usually result from damage to the superficial veins or venous sinuses within the subdural space. The blood that is released tends to spread and conform to the underlying cerebral hemispheres and occasionally is seen with additional parenchymal injury. Frequently, much of the mass effect that accompanies subdural hematomas is due to brain injury and not the hematoma itself. It is also important to remember that the possibility of concurrent intracerebral lesions or a contralateral subdural hematoma may exist with acute subdural hematomas.

On CT scans, acute subdural hematomas classically appear as a bright, hyperdense, crescent-shaped lesion located between the calvarium and the underlying cortex. If undetected, the hematoma may become isodense with the brain parenchyma on CT scans done 2 to 5

weeks later. The isodense subdural hematoma may be diagnosed from a shift of midline structures, effacement of the ipsilateral cortical sulci, or ipsilateral ventricular compression as reflections of mass effect (12) (Fig. 3-4). If bilateral isodense lesions occur, they may be hard to detect on CT scans. However, they are easy to see on magnetic resonance imaging (MRI), which may be needed for more sensitive diagnoses (Fig. 3-5). Because subdural or epidural hematomas may evolve slowly, it is usually prudent to have the athlete observed for 24 hours. If headaches or other symptoms persist, a CT scan or MRI should be ordered.

Subarachnoid Hemorrhage

Traumatic subarachnoid hemorrhage usually results from tears of small subarachnoid vessels from congenital vascular lesions such as an aneurysm or arteriovenous malformation. If a lesion is not a ruptured congenital vascular lesion but rather a normal subarachnoid vessel, the bleed is usually of less clinical significance than a subdural or epidural hematoma and in most cases has no serious clinical sequelae. On CT scan, increased density within the basal cisterns,

F I G U R E **3-4**

Isodense subdural hematoma causing left-sided cerebral edema with loss of usually distinct cortical sulci.

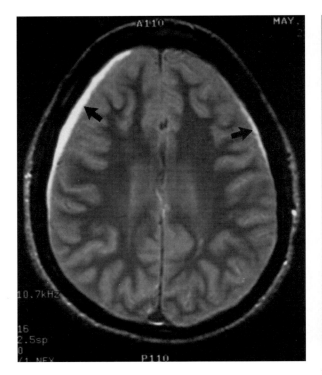

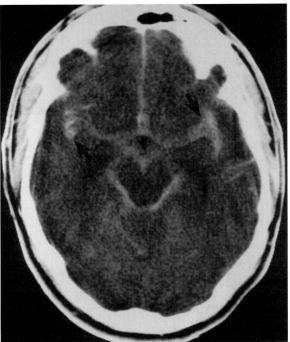

FIGURE **3-5**
Bilateral subdural hematomas on MRI (*arrows*).

FIGURE **3-6**
Diffuse subarachnoid hemorrhage (*arrows*).

interhemispheric fissures, and sulci is observed (Fig. 3-6). In addition, interventricular hemorrhages can accompany any head trauma with a subarachnoid bleed. This presents on CT scan as increased density in the ventricular system (12). As with previous head trauma, a CT scan is more expedient than an MRI and more efficient in evaluation of acute bleeds.

FIGURE **3-7**
Right frontal lobe, hyperdense, intracerebral hematoma/contusion (*arrow*).

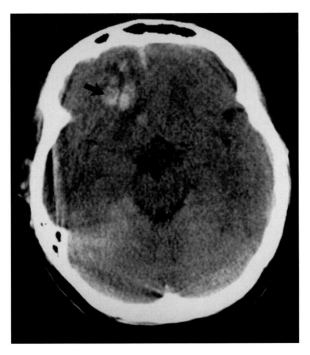

Intra-Axial Lesions

Contusion

As mentioned earlier, contusions and lacerations may develop at the point of impact or at a point opposite the impact. Common sites include the posterior portion of the frontal lobes and the anterior portion of the temporal lobes. Contusions often are found beneath depressed skull fractures as well. The CT scan of these injuries usually reveals a heterogeneous, bright (hyperdense) lesion surrounded by an irregular, marginated, hypodense component (Fig. 3-7). The dark (hypodense) zone usually represents edematous, possibly necrotic brain tissue, with the hyperdense area representing the hemorrhage itself. Frequently, small contusions may be difficult to detect on CT scan (12).

Intracerebral Hematoma

Shearing forces or rapid deceleration injuries may result in blood vessels being lacerated, producing intraparenchymal bleeding and resulting in intracerebral hematomas. The most common site of these injuries is in the frontal-temporal areas, but they also may be seen in parietal and occipital lobes. The majority of these hematomas remain superficial. Deeper intraparenchymal lesions may be difficult to detect, and the areas to be suspicious of include the corpus callosum, internal capsule, and upper brain stem. Intracerebral hematomas usually develop rapidly and appear on CT scan as homogeneous, hyperdense lesions with smooth but irregular margins. Again, hypodense, dark areas can form around the hematoma, usually caused by edema in the surrounding tissues.

Cerebral Edema

Swelling in the cerebral cortex can arise from increased brain water content (edema) or increased cerebral blood volume. The existence of edema poorly correlates with the severity of the injury but, when severe, may be associated with deterioration due to the resulting mass effect. Typically, this is seen in children and adolescents, especially when the edema is diffuse and bilateral. Acute traumatic cerebral edema is often a result of transient loss of vasomotor tone causing vasodilatation and vascular engorgement, which leads to increased blood volume and edema. Initially, there is very little to no brain tissue injury. CT findings include bilateral compression of the ventricles, obliteration of cortical sulci, and effacement of the basal cisterns (12) (Fig. 3-8).

Mild Cerebral Concussion

The Committee of Head Injury Nomenclature of the Congress of Neurological Surgeons (1966) defines *concussion* as a clinical syndrome characterized by immediate and transient post-traumatic impairment of neural functions such as alteration of consciousness and disturbance of vision or equilibrium due to brain stem involvement. This definition may not coincide with the mild concussion observed in sports-related head injuries, wherein the athlete remains conscious

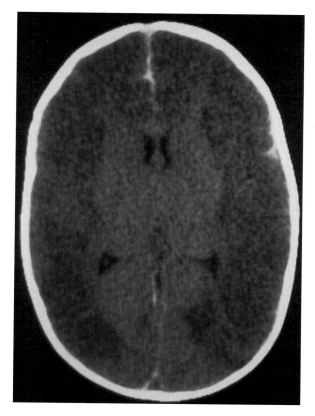

F I G U R E   3-8

Global cerebral edema.

but may show a temporary injury associated with neurologic dysfunction. Most of these injuries are minor and tend to go unnoticed or at least are not brought to the attention of medical personnel. However, since this is the most common form of brain injury seen in sports medicine, it is imperative that the primary care sports medicine physician understands the spectrum of presenting symptoms. Table 3-1 displays different grading systems that have been devised for categorizing the mild cerebral concussions that can occur in athletes. Clearly, there is no universal agreement on the definition of *concussion* or its degree of severity. Attempts have been made to define concussions on the basis of duration of unconsciousness or post-traumatic amnesia, and some have combined both in their grading systems. All, however, present criteria that progress from a mild to severe concussion by graded steps. Some include recommendations on the return to play with their grading systems. With no unanimity in grading systems, the decision to utilize radiologic techniques to

TABLE 3-1

Comparison of Classifications of Concussion

Torg	Kulund	Nelson
Grade 1 "Bell rung" Short-term confusion Unsteady gait Dazed appearance Loss of consciousness (LOC) Posttraumatic amnesia	**Mild** Stunned, dazed No confusion, dizziness No nausea, visual disturbance Feels well after 1 or 2 min Coordination	**Grade 0** Head struck or moved rapidly Not stunned or dazed initially Subsequently complains of headache and difficulty in concentrating
Grade 2 Posttraumatic amnesia Vertigo	**Moderate** LOC Mental confusion Retrograde amnesia Tinnitus, dizziness Skill recovery may be rapid	**Grade 1** Stunned or dazed initially No LOC or amnesia "Bell rung" Sensorium quickly clears (>1 min)
Grade 3 Posttraumatic amnesia Retrograde amnesia Vertigo	**Severe** Longer LOC Headache, confusion Posttraumatic amnesia Retrograde amnesia	**Grade 2** Headache, cloudy sensorium >1 min No LOC May have tinnitus, amnesia May be irritable, hyperexcitable, confused, dizzy
Grade 4 Immediate, transient LOC		
Grade 5 Paralytic coma Cardiorespiratory arrest		**Grade 3** LOC < 1 min Not comatose (arousable with noxious stimuli) Demonstrates grade 2 symptoms during recovery
Grade 6 Death		
		Grade 4 LOC > 1 min Not comatose Demonstrates grade 2 symptoms during recovery

Colorado Medical Society	
Grade 1 (mild)	Confusion without amnesia; no loss of consciousness
Grade 2 (moderate)	Confusion with amnesia; no loss of consciousness
Grade 3 (severe)	Loss of consciousness

Syndromes of Cerebral Concussion (Ommayce and Gennerelli)

I. Confusion → N1 consciousness without amnesia
II. Confusion → confusion + amnesia → N1 consciousness with posttraumatic amnesia only
III. Confusion + amnesia → N1 consciousness with posttraumatic amnesia + retrograde amnesia

Severity of Concussion (Cantu)

Grade 1 (mild)	No LOC, PTA* 30 min
Grade 2 (moderate)	LOC < 5 min or PTA > 30 min
Grade 3 (severe)	LOC ≥ 5 min or PTA ≥ 24 hr

*Posttraumatic amnesia.

define focal brain injuries also will be vague if based on these grading systems alone. Further research is ongoing to describe and better categorize the head injuries seen in athletics so that a more distinctive and more universal grading system may be developed (AMSSM Concussion Outcome Study).

Second-Impact Syndrome

There have been well-documented cases of repeated minor head injury causing brain swelling and fatal outcomes (6–8). The majority of these have occurred in apparently unrelated, minor instances of brain injury that often goes unnoticed by coaching or medical personnel. It is believed that the initial minor head injury is followed by a second injury that compounds the effects of persisting conditions from the initial injury. This may lead to autoregulatory dysfunction, cerebrovascular congestion, and subsequent serious intracranial hypertension and potentially death. Since all documented cases portray these athletes as having only minor persistent symptoms from the initial head injury (e.g., headache, poor concentration), recommendations for return to play have been conservative and require resolution of all symptoms prior to returning to full contact (13). Presently, no studies have shown findings that can help predict onset of second-impact syndrome.

Postconcussion Syndrome

Patients or athletes with concussions may report a variety of symptoms, including headaches, dizziness, memory problems, irritability, difficulty sleeping, and lack of concentration. Usually these symptoms resolve spontaneously in a short period of time. However, in some people symptoms persist, resulting in what has been labeled as the *postconcussion* or *post-traumatic syndrome*. The exact etiology of postconcussion syndrome is not known exactly, but headache and dizziness seem to be typical components of the syndrome. The headaches are usually diffuse and can be aggravated by any type of movement, anxiety, or stress. The dizziness may be accompanied by feelings of unsteadiness, which also can be exacerbated by movement or any changes in position. Nausea and vomiting do occur and can accompany these symptoms. Focal areas of neuronal loss and small lesions of the brain stem have been identified with MRI

and brain stem evoked potentials as possible causes, yet further study is needed and continues to be done in this area (14). MRI has shown a variety of abnormalities in the frontal and temporal regions with normal CT scans after normal head injuries. We must note that not all athletes with postconcussion syndrome are indicated for imaging studies. The individual patient needs to be assessed for the severity and prolongation of symptoms as to whether such studies as MRI or CT will help in management.

Radiographic Techniques

Plain skull radiography, CT scans, and MRI are utilized by physicians today in the evaluation of head trauma. Each technique has strengths and weaknesses, as detailed below. Newer techniques such as positron-emission tomographic (PET) scans, brain scan evoked potentials, and single photon emission computed tomographic (SPECT) scans may be used to study brain function and the cerebral blood flow that supports this function. However, these functional tests presently are not practical and/or are not widely available for the acutely brain-injured patient.

Skull radiography was used primarily to determine skull fractures (Fig. 3-9) and has since been replaced by CT scans, which are able to diagnose intracranial lesions requiring surgical intervention. Fractures located near the vertex of the cranium or other areas that CT scanning may not delineate sometimes can be found on plain radiographs. There is no evidence that missing these lesions is clinically significant in the absence of an associated intra- or extra-axial lesion. CT scans, therefore, have largely replaced plain films for this reason. The standard cerebral CT scan for the acute head trauma patient consists of 10 to 14 axial non-contrast-enhanced images made parallel to the skull base. Slice thickness in the adult is about 5 mm through the posterior fossa and 10 mm through the supratentorial region. "Bone windows" also can be obtained to detect fractures. A study can be completed in less than 5 minutes (12). Average cost of a head CT scan ranges from $500 to $700, which, if the scan is used to rule out catastrophic injury or to discharge a patient from the emergency department, saving an observation stay, is quite cost-effective. In certain circumstances, a CT scan may detect an unsuspected cervical spine fracture. One study demonstrated that in patients with an intracranial hemorrhage or skull fracture de-

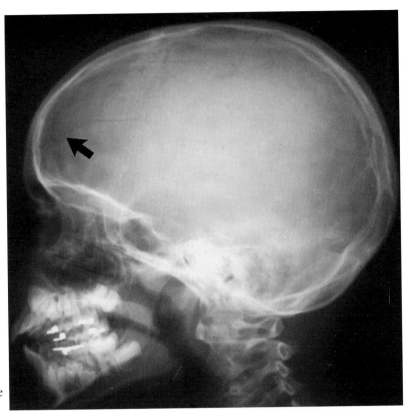

F I G U R E   **3-9**

Frontal   linear   skull   fracture (*arrow*).

tected on the initial head CT scan with extensions to the first three cervical vertebrae, 4 of 50 (8%) patients also were shown to have fractures of the C1 and C2 vertebrae that were missed on plain neck films (15). If high neck pain is present, it may be wise to extend the CT scan into these upper cervical vertebrae at the physician's discretion. MRI, on the other hand, is not being used presently for the acute head injury secondary to time and cost-effectiveness. MRI does provide superior imaging in a spectrum of intracranial pathology but does not show acute bleeding as well as CT. MRI is good to assess minor head trauma 2 to 3 days after head injury. It may aid in the assessment of sequelae and prediction of future post-injury sequelae.

Comparisons and Utilization of Radiographic Techniques

With knowledge of head injuries and the modes of radiographic techniques, we will investigate when each modality will aid the primary care sports medicine physician. Presently, the CT scan clearly has replaced plain skull radiogra-phy to assess minor to severe head injury and acute head trauma. Plain skull radiography is limited primarily to the determination of fractures. Several studies have shown that only 3% to 5% of head-injured patients are diagnosed with skull fractures utilizing plain skull radiography and that only 0.4% to 2.0% of skull fractures are clinically significant (16). Furthermore, a skull fracture by itself is unimportant compared with the possible underlying intracranial injury. For this, CT scan is clearly superior. In addition, assessing neurologic status has a greater predictive value in determining the existence of intracranial injury compared with skull radiography. One study demonstrated that the incidence of intracranial lesion development in those who are neurologically intact, despite their skull fracture, is as low as 0.5% (14). Since most athletic head injuries are minor and the majority of athletes neurologically intact, the need for further imaging studies can be determined based on any neurological changes of concern that may develop or persist.

The CT scan now plays a critical role in assessing head trauma when intracranial lesions are suspected clinically. Furthermore, the ability of a CT scan to display "bone windows" allows the physician to avoid plain radiographs. Indications are obvious when head-injured patients present with depressed or deteriorating levels of consciousness, persistent neurologic deficits, depressed skull fractures, or other signs of potentially serious intracranial injury. Most of these conditions indicate high-risk categories and require the use of CT scans, which may be followed by neurosurgical consultation. Symptoms such as headache, dizziness, or minor contusions and/or abrasions fall into a low-risk category requiring no neuroradiographic imaging.

However, it is the moderate-risk category that creates difficult decision making for the physician regarding which radiographic technique to utilize. Table 3-2 displays three risk categories (low, moderate, and high) with recommendations for the use of CT scanning in each. It is also suggested that in patients classified as having a moderate to severe head injury, based on the Glasgow Coma Scale, the CT scan should be given higher priority. Most minor head injuries fall under the rating scale of 13 to 15 on the Glasgow scale (Table 3-3), with anything below a 12 being moderate and below 8 being high.

T A B L E   **3-2**

A Strategy for Imaging Head Trauma Patients

Category*	Possible Findings	Recommendations
Low risk	No symptoms Headache Dizziness Scalp hematoma Scalp laceration Scalp contusion or abrasion Lack of moderate- or high-risk criteria	Observation alone; discharge patient with head injury information sheet (listing subdural precautions) and a companion to observe him or her
Moderate risk	History of change of consciousness at time of injury or later History of progressive headache Alcohol or drug intoxication Unreliable or inadequate history Age under 2 years, unless injury is trivial Post-traumatic seizure Vomiting Post-traumatic amnesia Multiple trauma Serious facial injury Signs of basilar fracture[a] Serious skull penetration or depressed fracture[b] Suspected child abuse	Extended close observation—watch for high-risk signs; consider CT scanning and neurosurgical consultation; skull series may (rarely) be helpful if positive, but normal films do not exclude intracranial injury
High risk	Depressed level of consciousness not clearly due to alcohol, drugs, or other cause, e.g., metabolic or seizure disorder Focal neurologic signs Decreasing level of consciousness Penetrating skull injury or palpable depressed fracture	Patient is candidate for neurosurgical consultation, emergency CT scanning, or both

*Physician assessment of the severity of injury may warrant reassignment to a higher risk group. Any single criterion from a higher risk group warrants assignment of the patient to the highest risk group applicable.

[a]Signs of basilar fracture include drainage of cerebrospinal fluid from ear or nose, hematotympanum, Battle's sign, and "raccoon eyes."

[b]Factors associated with open and depressed fractures include gunshot, missile, or shrapnel wounds; scalp injury from firm, pointed object (including animal teeth); penetrating injury of eyelid or globe; object stuck in head; assault (definite or suspected) with any object; leakage of cerebrospinal fluid; and signs of basilar fracture.

SOURCE: Reproduced with permission from Masters SJ, McClean PM, Arcarese JS, et al. Skull x-ray examinations after head trauma: recommendations by a multidisciplinary panel and validation study. N Engl J Med 1987;316:84.

T A B L E 3-3

The Glasgow Coma Scale

Response	Points
Eye opening	
Spontaneous	4
To verbal command	3
To pain	2
None	1
Best motor response	
Obeys verbal command	6
Localizes pain	5
Withdraws from pain	4
Decorticate posturing	3
Decerebrate posturing	2
No response	1
Best verbal response	
Oriented and converses	5
Disoriented and converses	4
Inappropriate words	3
Incomprehensible sounds	2
No response	1
SCORE	3–15

Since the vast majority of sports-related head injuries fall in the minor grouping on the Glasgow Coma Scale (13 to 15), the decision to utilize radiographic techniques after injury still can be confusing for the primary care physician. Research exists to support the early and frequent use of CT scans routinely as a cost-effective measure, since an injured athlete with a normal neurologic examination and a negative CT scan can be discharged safely with almost no risk of an intracranial lesion being present (17,18). A question of when a CT scan with contrast enhancement should be used is commonly asked. A CT scan with contrast enhancement, although more expensive, does help characterize isodense intracranial hemorrhage, as well as patients with acute bleeding into an old hematoma. It also can be used in evaluating injury that has occurred 7 to 21 days after the time of initial injury (17). Other studies have attempted to prospectively and retrospectively identify prognostic signs that correlate well with positive findings on CT scans. These studies have shown that most patients and athletes with minor head injury with no focal neurologic findings also have a very low risk of intracranial lesions requiring surgical attention and hence can be discharged home safely with observation without imaging (19). However, retrograde amnesia,

prolonged loss of consciousness, and the combination of amnesia, vomiting, and headache in patients 40 years of age or older are prognostic symptoms that correlate statistically with positive findings on CT scans (20–23).

It is in light of the confusion as to the prognostic value of certain radiographic techniques that CT scans and MRI are compared. At present, MRI is not recommended in the initial diagnosis of acute head trauma when attempting to rule out the need for surgical intervention. In some of the more severe head injuries, the need for a CT scan is quite obvious. One may ask the question, since most sports-related head injuries are minor, as to which radiologic technique will aid in safely returning the athlete to his or her respective sport. Comparatively, CT scan is superior in detecting subarachnoid hemorrhages and bony fractures (24); however, MRI seems to be more sensitive for contusions, brain stem injuries, and diffuse axonal injuries. One study performed on approximately 58 patients showed that patients who were discharged from the emergency department with normal neurologic examinations after routine evaluation and who had both CT and low-field MRI showed 10% more intracranial lesions on MRI than on CT scans (25). However, none of these added lesions required further treatment, and the patients did not deteriorate or need extended hospital stays.

Although the lesions discovered by MRI that were missed by CT scan did not affect the initial treatment of the patient and discharge from the hospital, studies have shown that these lesions may be related in some way to the neuropsychological deficits found in some mild head injury patients. In studies where neuropsychological testing was performed along with imaging studies, one showed a possible relationship between the localization of lesions seen on MRI and the neuropsychological assessments displaying deficits found in the patients. Assessments on the neuropsychological examinations displaying some low-functioning cognitive capabilities and some memory loss were found to persist for up to 1 to 3 months. The areas of the brain responsible for these functions are in the frontal lobe and temporal lobe areas. As these areas were followed on MRI throughout the testing periods, it was found that there was noticeable improvement on the neuropsychological examinations that coincided with resolution of the lesions in the frontal and temporal lobes seen on MRI (26). Therefore, the physician may

T A B L E   **3-4**

Head Imaging Point Scale*

	0	1	2	3
Loss of consciousness	None	<10 sec	10–45 sec	>45 sec
Retrograde amnesia	None	<5 min	>5 min	>24 hr
Anterograde amnesia	None	<5 min	>5 min	>24 hr
Vomiting	—	—	2	—
Worsening agitation	—	—	2	—
Glasgow Coma Scale	15	14	13	12 or less
Skull fracture	None	—	—	Yes
Neurologic examination	Negative	—	—	Yes

Points: 0–3: no CT scan necessary; 4–7: consider CT and/or close observation of clinical condition; >8: CT scan suggested.

*These guidelines should not preclude the team physician's clinical judgment in each individual patient but rather serve as a guide in the decision making.

be able to utilize serial neuropsychological testing and/or MRI to monitor the patient's progress toward safely returning to play. However, final clearance to return to play should rest in the hands of the team physician in his or her assessment of the patient's present physical and neurologic condition.

It may then be very helpful to have guidelines for the use of specific radiologic techniques in regard to minor head injuries in sports. Some of the studies mentioned in this chapter place a certain amount of emphasis on specific signs and symptoms and their relation to the possibility of severe head injury when witnessed either in the emergency room or in the training room. Therefore, we have created a point scale based on the review of several research articles and the emphasis placed on certain prognostic signs and their correlation with either positive or negative CT findings in the hope of aiding in the decision making by the primary care physician (Table 3-4). We hope that the suggested point system will aid in choosing the proper radiologic technique in relationship to minor head injury in sports, but all final decisions should be individualized and based on the clinical judgment of the physician in each specific head injury patient. As more research and data are compiled, recommendations for the use of imaging techniques will become more specific. Until that time, however, the standard of care will support the use of early CT scanning when any concern over the athlete's condition exists.

REFERENCES

1. Borel C, Hanley D, Diringer MN, et al. Intensive management of severe head injury. Chest 1990; 98:180–189.

2. Powell JW. National estimates of concussions in high school football. NATA High School Injury Study 1986–1988. Presented at the Mild Brain Injury Summit, Washington, DC, April 16–18, 1994.

3. Torg JS, Vegso JJ, Sennett B, Das M. The National Football Head and Neck Injury Registry: 14-year report on cervical quadriplegia, 1971 through 1984. JAMA 1985;252:3439–3443.

4. Cantu RC. Head and spine injuries in the young athlete. Clin Sports Med 1988;7:459–472.

5. Gerberich SG, Priest JD, Boen JR, et al. Concussion incidences and severity in secondary school varsity football players. Am J Public Health 1975;73:1370–1375.

6. Saunders RL, Harbaugh RE. The second impact in catastrophic contact sports head trauma. JAMA 1984;252:538–539.

7. McQuillen JB, McQuillen EN, Morrow P. Trauma, sports and malignant cerebral edema. Am J Forensic Med Pathol 1988;9:12–15.

8. Kelly JB, Nichols JS, Filley CM, et al. Concussion in sports: guidelines for the prevention of catastrophic outcome. JAMA 1991;266:2867–2869.

9. Albright JP, McAuley E, Martin RK, et al. Head and neck injuries in college football: an eight-year analysis. Am J Sports Med 1985;13:147–152.

10. Cantu RC. Cerebral concussion in sport: management and prevention. Sports Med 1992;14:64–74.

11. Gennarelli TA, Segawa H, Wald U, et al. Physiological response to angular acceleration of the head. In: Grossman, Gildenberg, eds. Head injury: basic and clinical aspects. New York: Raven Press, 1982:129–140.

12. Olshaker JS, Whye DW. Head trauma. Emerg Med Clin North Am 1993;11:165–186.

13. Wilberger JE. Minor head injuries in American football: prevention of long-term sequelae. Sports Med 1993;15:338–343.

14. Cooper PR, Ho V. Role of emergency skull x-ray films in the evaluation of the head-injured patient: a retrospective study. Neurosurgery 1983;13:136–140.

15. Edwards FJ. Head injury update: the role of imaging. Emerg Med 1994;60–67.

16. Masters SJ, McClean PM, Arcarese JS, et al. Skull x-ray examinations after head trauma: recommendations by a multidisciplinary panel and validation study. N Engl J Med 1987;316:84–91.

17. Stein SC, Ross SE. Mild head injury: a plea for routine early CT scanning. J Trauma 1992;33:11–13.

18. Shackford SR, Wals SL, Ross SE, et al. The clinical utility of computed tomographic scanning and neurologic examination in the management of patients with minor head injuries. J Trauma 1992;33:385–394.

19. Mohanty SK, Thompson W, Rakower S. Are CT scans for head injury patients always necessary? J Trauma 1991;31:801–805.

20. Mikhail MG, Levitt MA, Christopher TA, Sutton MC. Intracranial injury following minor head trauma. Am J Emerg Med 1992;10:24–26.

21. Schynooll W, Overton D, Krome R, et al. A prospective study to identify high-yield criteria associated with acute intracranial computed tomography findings in head-injured patients. Am J Emerg Med 1993;11:321–326.

22. Duus BR, Boesen T, Druse DV, Nielsen DB. Prognostic signs in the evaluation of patients with minor head injury. Br J Surg 1993;80:988–991.

23. Reinus WR, Wippold FJ, Erickson KK. Practical selection criteria for noncontrast cranial computed tomography in patients with head trauma. Ann Emerg Med 1993;22:1148–1155.

24. Sklar EM, Quencer RM, Bowen BC. Magnetic resonance application in cerebral injury. Radiol Clin North Am 1992;30:353–366.

25. Doezema D, King JN, Tandberg D, et al. Magnetic resonance imaging in minor head injury. Ann Emerg Med 1991;20:1281–1285.

26. Levin HS, Amparo E, Eisenberg HM, et al. Magnetic resonance imaging and computerized tomography in relation to the neurobehavioral sequelae of mild and moderate head injuries. J Neurosurg 1987;66:706–713.

CHAPTER 4

Facial and Soft Tissue Neck Injuries

WAYNE P. FOSTER
WILLIAM W. WOODRUFF

The incidence of sports-related injuries of the head and neck is increasing due to the growing participation in more vigorous recreational activities. Although sports injuries occur most commonly in young males, the incidence of recreational injuries has increased in both sexes and in all age groups (1). The anatomic location and severity of the injury often are related to the particular sport.

Facial trauma is easily divided into three anatomic regions (inferior, medial, and lateral), each of which is commonly associated with specific sporting activities (2). The inferior area, comprised of the mandible and lower maxilla, is commonly involved in "riding activities," such as cycling, motorcycling, and horseback-riding, as well as in trauma due to contact sports such as boxing, rugby, and martial arts (2,3). The median area includes the maxillary processes, nose, orbital floor, ethmoids, and frontal sinus. Commonly it is injured in sports where collisions occur, such as soccer, basketball, rugby, and football, and where high-velocity balls are used, as in baseball, tennis, racquetball, lacrosse, and volleyball. The lateral area, formed by the zygomatic bone and its prominent arches, may be injured in contact sports or from collisions with the ground, common in skiing accidents.

Teleologically, the face acts as a physiologic "crumple zone," absorbing traumatic forces and effectively protecting intracranial vital structures (4,5). Conversely, trauma to the neck or temporal bone is more often immediately threatening to life and vital function. Evaluation and treatment will be more urgent when airway, bleeding, and circulation are not immediately apparent.

Once the patient is stabilized and a thorough history and physical examination are performed, radiographic evaluation of specific injuries can be considered. Due to availability, ease of performance, cost, and convenience, plain films of the skull and face are used in the initial workup of the patient with suspected facial trauma. Linear tomography affords improved fracture detection over plain films. Computed tomography (CT) offers at least the same fracture detection rate with superior resolution as linear tomography while providing important information regarding soft tissue injury at a decreased radiation dose rate (6). If the decision to obtain CT scans is made early in patient management, plain films may prove unnecessary.

Magnetic resonance imaging (MRI) is not used commonly as an initial evaluation in facial and neck trauma. Numerous studies have shown that MRI and CT scans are effective in detecting hemorrhagic lesions such as intracranial hemorrhage, whereas MRI is more sensitive for evaluating more prevalent nonhemorrhagic lesions and CT is more effective at delineating bony changes (7–9). Other modalities, such as ultrasound and angiography, are reserved for specific circumstances such as suspected carotid injury.

Photodocumentation is helpful in the management of facial injuries. Multiple views of the injured face should be obtained to document the injury as soon as practically possible.

Nasal Fractures

Anatomy

The nose is a pyramidal structure with its apex projecting anteriorly and its base overlying a pear-shaped opening in the midface called the *piriform aperture*. The nasal bones form the roof of the piriform aperture, articulating with each other in the midline.

The cartilaginous portion of the nose is formed by paired upper and lower lateral cartilages and the anterior portion of the nasal septum. The nasal septum, supporting the cartilaginous framework of the lower nose, is composed of the perpendicular plate of the ethmoid bone posteriorly, the quadrangular cartilage anteriorly, and the vomer bone inferiorly. Fracture or dislocation of the septum off the maxillary crest results in significant nasal airway obstruction and deformity.

Clinical Evaluation

The magnitude, direction, and concentration of a blow will determine the extent of a fracture. When evaluating a presumed nasal fracture, nasal function and aesthetics are the two criteria that demand correction. These are best determined by history and physical examination rather than by radiographic evaluation. The patient should be questioned concerning the ability to breathe through each side of the nose. The clinician also should note if the patient perceives any change in the physical shape of the nose. Additional information regarding epistaxis, pain, anosmia, or previous nasal fracture also should be obtained. Finally, associated injuries may be indicated by loss of consciousness, change in mental status, visual changes, malocclusion, clear rhinorrhea, or local sensory deficit.

The initial examination should include evaluation of the integrity of the nasal mucosa and the presence of a septal hematoma. The early examination should be performed as soon as possible after the injury because the edema and ecchymosis that develop within 4 hours of injury will obfuscate the accuracy of the physical examination. A more thorough nasal examination must follow resolution of the edema at 4 to 7 days to more accurately assess the extent of the nasal injury. With the patient comfortable, the external nose should be visualized from the frontal views and both sides in lateral and oblique views. In the frontal view, broadening, asymmetry, or curvature of the nasal dorsum may be visualized, along with nasal tip deviation. The lateral and oblique views may show dorsal humps or depressions as well as shortening of the columella or flattening of the nasal root. A thorough intranasal examination will display injuries of the septum, upper and lower lateral cartilages, and turbinates, as well as coexisting mucosal lacerations. Upon palpating the nose, crepitus or unusual motion of the cartilages may indicate fracture or dislocation of bone and/or cartilage. As with fractures elsewhere in the body, nasal fractures will be associated with point tenderness.

Radiographic Evaluation

Nasal fractures vary from simple nondisplaced linear fractures to severely comminuted fractures with marked diathesis of the nasal bones. Plain films of the skull and facial bones for routine nasal fractures can be misleading and perhaps misinterpreted by both radiologists and clinicians. Their effectiveness has been questioned because of the high incidence of false-positive and false-negative interpretations and because of the poor predictive value with regard to management (10). A markedly diastatic fracture may be misinterpreted as normal, while a normal suture line may be confused for a linear fracture. Therefore, management of a nasal fracture is best directed by the clinical evaluation, with the radiographs playing a supplemental role in the decision-making process.

On plain films, the nasal bones are best visualized with underpenetrated lateral views. Two normal linear lucencies traveling parallel to the long axis of the nasal bones, the nasociliary and nasomaxillary grooves, should not be misinterpreted as fractures. Fractures frequently, but not always, course perpendicular to the long axis (Fig. 4-1). The nasomaxillary and midline nasal suture lines, as well as developmental abnormalities, also may be misinterpreted as fractures (10).

The value of plain film evaluation of the nose and nasal septum is limited in certain circumstances. Fractures of the nasal septum and cartilaginous framework of the nose are not detectable on plain films and require tailored clinical examination for detection and treatment planning. Since cartilage comprises a greater

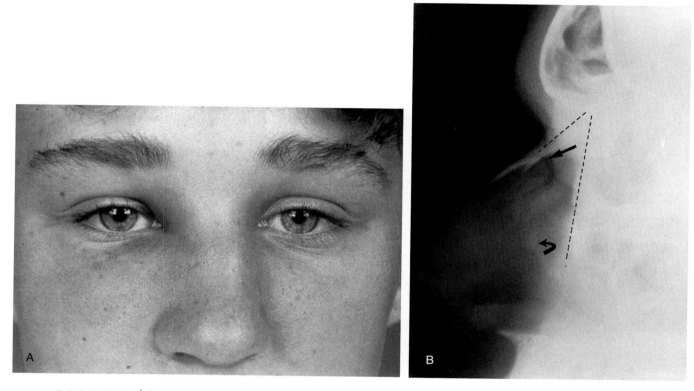

F I G U R E   **4-1**

Nasal bone fracture. (A) Gross photograph shows leftward deviation of the nasal bridge. (B) Lateral nasal bone film demonstrates a subtle lucency (*straight arrow*) perpendicular to the nasal bridge. Note the normal nasociliary grooves (*curved arrow*), depicted as lucencies that are oriented parallel to the long axis of the nasal bridge.

amount of the nose in children than in adults, plain film evaluation is even less useful in the pediatric nose.

Because treatment of nasal fractures is directed toward correcting functional and aesthetic defects, which are both poorly evaluated with radiographs, one may argue against the use of routine plain films for nasal fractures. However, when more extensive injury is suspected, further evaluation with CT scans, including axial and coronal views, should be considered.

Nasoethmoid Complex Fractures

When the force of the blow is directed downward at the nasal root, the nasoethmoid complex may be completely separated from the frontal bone and depressed inward. This results in the classic collapsed appearance of the nasal dorsum and upward-turned tip (Fig. 4-2). A widened interorbital distance (telecanthus) re-

sults from avulsion of the lacrimal bone by the medial canthal tendon. A nasoethmoid complex fracture is commonly associated with a cerebrospinal fluid (CSF) leak secondary to fracture of the cribriform plate.

When a nasoethmoid complex fracture is suspected, a high-resolution CT scan with axial and coronal planes with "bone windows" best evaluates this region and the surrounding pathology (see Fig. 4-2).

Zygoma Fractures

Anatomy

The zygoma, or malar bone, creates the lateral-most prominence of the midface. This bone provides the inferolateral orbital rim and supero-lateral roof of the maxillary sinus. A zygoma fracture, commonly known as a *tripod fracture,*

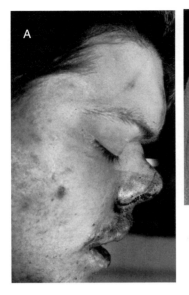

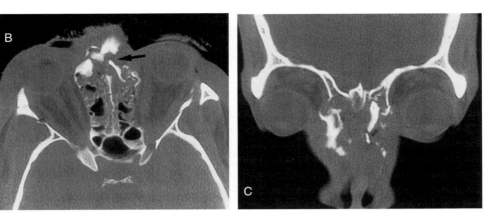

FIGURE 4-2

Nasoethmoid complex fracture. (A) Gross photograph demonstrates deepening of the nasofrontal angle with depression of the nasal dorsum and upward rotation of the nasal tip. (B) Axial CT scan shows a comminuted, depressed fracture of the nasoethmoid complex (*arrow*). Note the displaced fracture of the left lateral orbital wall. (C) Coronal view delineates the comminuted nasoethmoid complex fracture with a fracture through the cribriform plate.

is more appropriately termed a *quadripod fracture* because of its four articulations (Fig. 4-3A). Posteriorly, the zygoma articulates with the zygomatic arch of the temporal bone (zygomaticotemporal suture) laterally and the greater wing of the sphenoid (sphenozygomatic suture) medially. The zygoma articulates medially with the maxilla (zygomaticomaxillary suture line). Superiorly, the zygoma articulates with the zygomatic process of the frontal bone (zygomaticofrontal suture), completing the orbital rim.

Clinical Evaluation

The zygoma is the second most common isolated facial fracture (after the isolated nasal fracture) and the most common fracture to be associated with other facial fractures. The isolated zygoma fracture is associated most commonly with a blow from a right-handed closed fist resulting in a left zygomatic fracture.

Within several hours of the injury, edema and hematoma with ecchymosis of the lids, conjunctiva, and sclera and swelling over the face obscure the clinical picture. These signs, along with displacement of the lateral canthal tendon, depression of the globe, retraction of the lower lid, and a sunken appearance of the upper lid, are classic for a zygoma fracture. The patient may have pain on opening the mouth and lim-

ited mouth opening because the inward buckling of the zygomatic arch may impinge on the temporalis muscle. Severe inward depression of this fracture may mechanically impinge on the coronoid process of the mandible.

On physical examination with fingers passing along the orbital rim, the zygomaticofrontal and zygomaticomaxillary joints are palpated. A step-off frequently is palpable over these two joints when the zygoma is fractured. Intraorally, the lower edge of the zygomaticomaxillary joint can be palpated. Bony step-off and point tenderness are classic for the zygoma fracture, along with flattening of the malar eminence (lateral cheek prominence) (see Fig. 4-3B).

Radiographic Evaluation

Although plain films may identify all components of a tripod fracture, CT scan more accurately assesses the site of bone discontinuity as well as any rotation or diastasis. The CT scan is the best way to re-evaluate any associated bony or soft tissue injuries. A CT scan should be obtained whenever a zygoma fracture is suspected by clinical evaluation or plain film findings (see Fig. 4-3C). An early decision to obtain a CT scan may preclude the need for plain films.

The Waters posteroanterior view, also referred to as the *occipitomental view,* rotates the

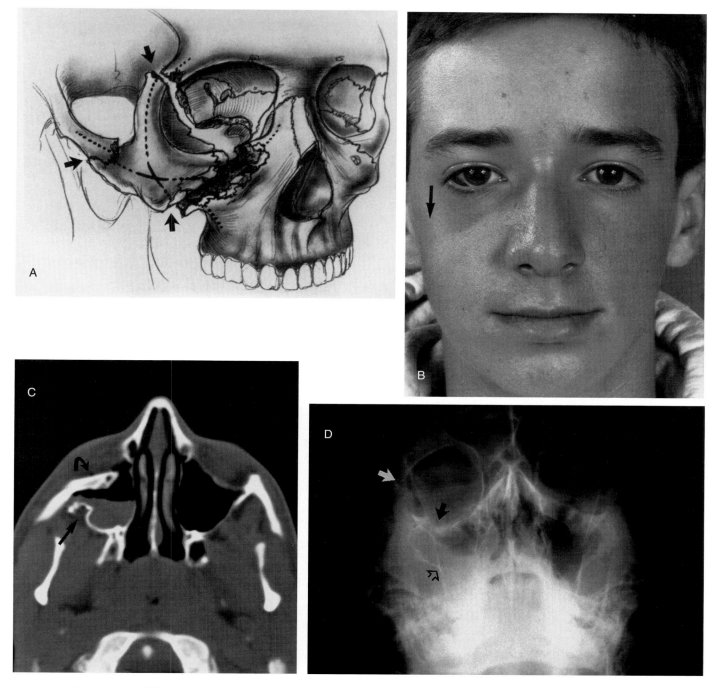

FIGURE 4-3

Tripod fracture. (A) Schematic demonstrating the components of the tripod fracture. (Reproduced with permission from Bailey BJ. Head and neck surgery–otolaryngology, vol 1. Philadelphia: JB Lippincott, 1993:976.) (B) Gross photograph shows subtle depression of the malar ridge and scleral ecchymosis. (C) Axial CT scan depicts depression and rotation of the right zygoma (*curved arrow*), a comminuted fracture of the lateral wall of the maxillary sinus (*straight arrow*), and a fluid level in the maxillary sinus. (D) Waters view shows disruption of the zygomaticofrontal suture (*white arrow*), inferior orbital rim (*solid black arrow*), and lateral maxillary sinus wall (*open black arrow*).

sphenoid ridge below the floors of the maxillary sinuses (see Fig. 4-3D). This allows visualization of the entire zygoma, orbital rims, and maxillary sinuses, including the zygomaticofrontal suture of the lateral orbital rim and the zygomatico-maxillary suture of the inferior orbital rim. A fractured zygoma is often portrayed by a diastasis or step-off at these suture sites and blood within the maxillary antrum.

When using plain films, the zygomatic arch is best evaluated using the exaggerated base view (i.e., jug handle, submentovertical, Schüller, or Pfeiffer view). The anterolateral projection also gives an excellent view of the unilateral arch free of superimposed structures.

Blowout Fractures

Anatomy

The orbital blowout fracture is a unique injury that results from force transmitted through the intact globe, transiently increasing intraorbital pressure and centrifugally displacing the weakest point of the orbit (Fig. 4-4A). The orbital floor and, less commonly, the medial orbital wall may be fractured. The thick bone of the orbital rim remains intact. The striking object is usually slightly larger than the orbital rim, such as a fist or a baseball. The orbital rim protects against objects larger than 5 cm, whereas smaller objects such as golf balls and hockey pucks are more likely to result in globe rupture (11).

The orbit is the bony cavity that encloses the globe and retrobulbar structures. It is formed by the frontal, sphenoid, zygoma, maxilla, lacrimal, and ethmoid bones. Relative to the thick bone of the orbital rim, the orbital walls are quite thin. The orbital floor measures 0.5 to 1.0 mm thick in a region located medial and slightly posterior to the midpoint of the floor (12). This is the most common location for the inferior blowout fracture. The medial wall of the orbit is composed primarily of the lamina papyracea (literally means "paper-thin plate of bone") of the ethmoid. This area is another common blowout location but less common because it is supported medially by the ethmoid labyrinth.

Several cranial nerves are of significant importance when considering orbital fractures. The optic nerve enters the orbit posteromedially through the optic foramen of the sphenoid bone. Its location is posterior to typical blowout fractures and is rarely involved, even with high-velocity trauma. The superior orbital fissure transmits the oculomotor, trochlear, abducens, and ophthalmic division of the trigeminal nerve. This area is also infrequently injured in orbital trauma. The infraorbital nerve supplies sensation to the skin of the cheek and the upper teeth and is at significant risk of injury in orbital fractures. This nerve traverses the inferior orbital canal within the floor of the orbit and is frequently injured in orbital floor trauma. The extraocular muscles and/or periorbita may become entrapped in a blowout fracture resulting in diplopia.

With an orbital blowout fracture, orbital fat frequently is forced out of the orbital confines, effectively decreasing the volume of the orbit. If this is not corrected, long-term enophthalmos results.

Clinical Evaluation

Patients with an orbital blowout fracture may present with vertical diplopia, pain, ecchymosis, visual impairment, and infraorbital hypesthesia. Although the most common cause of diplopia in an orbital fracture is orbital edema, vertical diplopia can result from either direct trauma to the inferior oblique and inferior rectus muscles by bone fragments or entrapment of these muscles when orbital contents herniate inferiorly (11,13). Diplopia is the most significant and frequent complaint of patients with orbital fractures.

Physical examination frequently reveals findings common to most orbital injuries, as well as more specific signs suggestive of blowout fractures. Subconjunctival hemorrhage, chemosis, decreased visual acuity, and a slowly reactive pupil occur in many orbital injuries. More specific signs of blowout fractures include downward displacement of the globe, vertical gaze impairment resulting in vertical diplopia, enophthalmos that may be masked by swelling in the acute state, epistaxis suggestive of lamina papyracea fracture, and infraorbital hypesthesia. A thorough ophthalmologic examination including the forced duction test is performed with early specialist consultation (11).

Any force sufficient to produce a fracture of the orbit potentially may injure the globe. The incidence of ocular complications associated with facial fractures is reported to be between 15% and 45% (14–17). This includes loss of

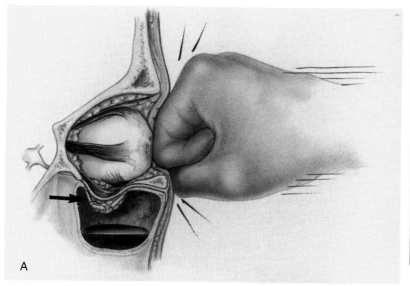

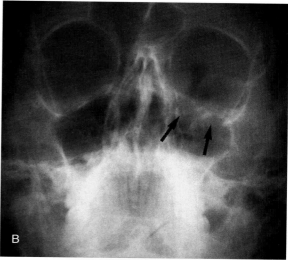

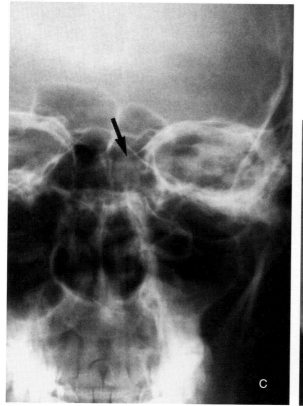

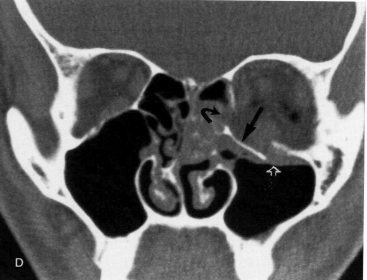

FIGURE 4-4

Orbital blowout fracture. (A) Illustration demonstrating the mechanism of action of the orbital blowout injury. (Reproduced with permission from Gean AD. Imaging of head trauma. New York: Raven Press, 1994:478.) (B) Waters view of the skull shows vague increased density (*arrows*) in the superior aspect of the left maxillary sinus, which represents the fracture deformity of the floor of the orbit and the herniated retrobulbar soft tissue. (C) Posteroanterior skull film shows asymmetric increased density (*arrow*) in the left ethmoid sinus. (D) Coronal CT scan depicts the depressed orbital floor fracture (*bold arrow*) and the herniation of soft tissue into the maxillary sinus (*open arrow*) and the ethmoid sinus (*curved arrow*).

vision due to injury to the optic nerve or its blood supply, injury to the retina, damage or dislocation of the lens, vitreous body hemorrhage, hyphema, perforation of the globe, retrobulbar hemorrhage, or damage to the iris or cornea (14–17).

Radiographic Evaluation

The initial radiographic assessment for a suspected blowout fracture may include the Waters and Caldwell views (see Fig. 4-4B). The Waters view is usually the most diagnostic plain film for the inferior blowout fracture, while the Caldwell view is most useful for the medial blowout fracture (see Fig. 4-4C). However, these studies are often nondiagnostic, with an incidence of false-negative results as high as 18% (18).

Classic radiographic signs of a blowout fracture include fragmentation of the bone of the orbital floor, depression of the bony fragments, and prolapse of orbital soft tissue into the air-filled maxillary sinus, the "teardrop sign" (13, 19). Associated findings include a fluid level in or opacification of the maxillary sinus. Orbital emphysema is seen commonly in a medial blowout fracture but not in an inferior blowout fracture (20,21). If the blowout is of the medial wall, soft tissue opacification of the adjacent ethmoid complex may be seen with a "trapdoor" appearance of the medial wall "hinged" toward the ethmoid side of the orbit (19,21,22).

Although plain films may detect blowout fractures, CT scan expectedly is more sensitive in detecting this injury and is indicated in all patients with orbital trauma to evaluate for soft tissue and associated bony injury (21). High-resolution (1–3 mm) contiguous images should be obtained in the axial and, if possible, coronal planes. An orbital floor blowout fracture can be missed easily on axial images through the orbit because the fracture is often parallel to the imaging plane. Direct coronal imaging best displays the fracture, which is perpendicular to the imaging plane (see Fig. 4-4D). The extraocular muscles, the extent of displacement of orbital contents, possible involvement of the nasolacrimal apparatus, and precise definition of the fracture margins should be assessed. A floating bony fragment within the ipsilateral maxillary sinus is a strong clue to the presence of an inferior blowout fracture on axial or coronal CT scans. The relationship of the extraocular muscles to the fracture should be assessed and is

more reliable than the attenuation values of the herniated material when diagnosing entrapment (13). Entrapment is more likely when the fracture is small and the extraocular muscles become fixed within the diastatic fragments.

MRI is useful in evaluating orbital blowout fractures, although CT remains the standard of care in evaluating orbital injury. Bony disruption is also inferable by the presence of high-intensity fat protruding into the adjacent sinus (20,21). Surface-coil MRI, with thin sections and high resolution, has been shown to be superior to CT in differentiating between herniated fat and muscle (20,21,23). T1-weighted images can characterize the nature of entrapment because the high intensity of fat contrasts with the low intensity of muscle, acute hemorrhage, and sinus fluid (24).

Medial wall blowout fractures are equally well demonstrated on CT scans in the axial or coronal planes and are much more sensitive than plain films in detecting this injury. Displacement of orbital contents and the lamina papyracea into the ethmoid sinus is demonstrated adroitly. Intraorbital emphysema may be detected (20,21).

Maxilla Fractures

Anatomy

The maxilla makes up the major portion of the midface and is responsible for most of the vertical facial growth in childhood. The maxillary bone consists of a central body and four peripheral processes: frontal, zygomatic, palatine, and alveolar. An air-filled cavity of varying size lies within the body of the maxilla. Because the thin walls of the maxillary sinus are weak, shock forces to the midface are absorbed by fracturing these walls and then distributed through the buttresses evenly to the remaining craniofacial skeleton. This cushion effect helps to protect vital structures both intracranially and extracranially.

Because the maxilla is located centrally and associated intimately with several vital soft tissue structures and nine facial bones, when fractured, numerous problems may result. The roof of the sinus is the thin bone of the orbital floor; this floor is vulnerable to blowout fractures and subsequent injury to the infraorbital nerve. Medially, the nasolacrimal system may be injured because the duct lies within the maxilla. Furthermore, the lacrimal fossa and sac are supported by the superomedial wall of the maxilla. Inferiorly, the maxilla supports the upper teeth and provides the major portion of the hard palate.

The mechanical strength of the maxilla lies in its buttresses and supporting structures. Regions of relative weakness are the foramina and the thin bone of the maxillary sinus. Laterally, the zygoma bolsters the maxilla, which in turn supports the nasal bones medially. Further support results from good dentition and firm maxillomandibular occlusion. The horizontally oriented alveolar process, usually strong and thick when good teeth are present, atrophies and weakens with poor or no dentition. The incisive and infraorbital foramina, located at the palatal midline and the zygomaticomaxillary joint, respectively, impart relative weaknesses to the maxilla.

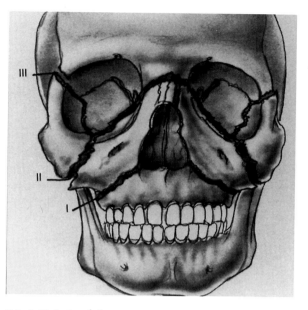

F I G U R E **4-5**

Schematic demonstrating the three Le Fort fractures. (Reproduced with permission from Bailey BJ. Head and neck surgery–otolaryngology, vol 1. Philadelphia: JB Lippincott, 1993:975.)

Clinical Evaluation

Classification

Maxillary fractures are caused by a direct midface blow or indirectly by an upward blow to the mandible. The complexity of these fractures varies from a simple bony fragment to a complex comminution with cribriform plate fracture, CSF leak, and brain injury.

In 1901, Le Fort's experiments identified and classified areas of structural weakness. In general, Le Fort fractures traverse the maxilla and the pterygoid plates to completely separate a significant maxillary segment from the craniofacial skeleton (Fig. 4-5).

The Le Fort I fracture results from a direct blow to the maxilla. The fracture extends through the maxilla and pterygoid plates. The free-floating lower maxillary fragment may be distracted a variable distance. The dentoalveolar fracture results in a loose fragment of bone with maxillary teeth attached. It is commonly caused by a concentrated blow at the level or just above the maxillary teeth. This fracture also may occur following an upward blow to the mandible transmitted through the teeth, shattering the maxilla. With either of these injuries, uncommonly there is associated maxillary division of the trigeminal nerve (V_2) or lacrimal injury.

More violent blows are necessary to result in the Le Fort II or III fractures. Pyramidal or Le

Fort II fractures lie at the superior edge of the piriform aperture and traverse the frontal process, lacrimal bone, medial floor of the orbit, infraorbital rim at the zygomaticomaxillary joint, lateral wall of the maxilla, and pterygoid plates. The ethmoid cells can be shattered and impacted if this fractured segment is driven posteriorly. V_2 and lacrimal sac injuries are not uncommon with this fracture.

A Le Fort III fracture results in complete craniofacial disjunction. This fracture extends across the floor of the orbit, zygomaticofrontal joint, and pterygoid plates. The middle third of the face is completely separated from the skull, attached only by soft tissue.

Vertical fracture of the maxilla is unusual and results from an upward midline blow to the mandible with its force transmitted through the teeth. The palate is split in the sagittal plane.

Clinical Findings

The patient suspected of midfacial fractures should be questioned, if possible, regarding preinjury occlusion, dental prostheses, previous facial trauma, and ongoing dental or orthodontic treatments. The patient with a maxillary fracture frequently will experience malocclusion. Nasal obstruction and epistaxis become apparent when the fracture involves the medial maxilla. Oral bleeding may indicate a Le Fort I or dentoalveolar fracture, whereas infraorbital hypesthesia may indicate a Le Fort II fracture.

Inspecting the fractured midface, the clinician frequently will see epistaxis; ecchymosis of the periorbita, conjunctiva, and sclera; and a subcutaneous hematoma. Intraoral inspection may reveal a laceration or ecchymosis and malocclusion with anterior open bite secondary to premature occlusion of the posterior teeth. Vertical elongation of the face may be obscured by swelling and edema in the acute phase.

Simultaneous bilateral palpation provides the most accurate examination of facial symmetry. The entire circumference of the orbital rims should be inspected for deformity and tenderness. The lateral orbital rim at the zygomaticofrontal suture is distracted and tender in a Le Fort III fracture. The inferior orbital rim may be diastatic with a Le Fort II fracture. The midface should be assessed thoroughly for mobility. By grasping the anterior maxilla at the palate and gingivobuccal sulcus with the thumb and index finger, a rocking motion will elicit any instability or crepitus in the fractured maxilla.

Radiographic Evaluation

Although the literature repeatedly refers to "pure" Le Fort fractures, rarely does a fracture follow one of the classic planes (25). More commonly, combinations of Le Fort fractures are seen.

A standard facial-sinus series consisting of Waters, Caldwell, lateral, and submentovertex views should be obtained to evaluate the midface when suspecting a fracture. The Waters view may show signs suggestive of a maxillary fracture (i.e., an air-fluid level, thickening of the sinus mucosa, infraorbital rim diathesis, orbital emphysema, frontozygomatic suture diathesis, and irregularities in the lateral maxillary sinus wall). If the patient is unable to maintain an upright position, the supine reverse Waters view can be used but generally is not as informative. The lateral view can be useful in assessing retropharyngeal soft tissue swelling or hematoma consequent to posterior maxillary displacements. The Caldwell view often demonstrates the fracture of the orbital wall and delineates the structural integrity of the premax-

illa. The submentovertex view is useful to evaluate displacement of the anterior wall of the maxilla and fractures of the zygoma, findings often associated with Le Fort III and palatal split fractures (26).

Owing to the variability of the fracture(s) and the complexity of the bony anatomy of the midface, plain film evaluation of facial fractures may be misleading, often underestimating the true extent of the injury. A CT scan is the best modality to evaluate the bony and accompanying soft tissue alterations. Coronal images may be especially useful to augment axial data in patients with complex craniofacial fractures.

Le Fort I

The floating-palate injury results in separation of the hard palate and maxillary alveolar process from the remainder of the maxilla and facial skeleton. With significant displacement, conventional radiographs can prove helpful. Because the Le Fort I fracture often results in an anterior open bite, the lateral facial view becomes helpful in delineating the posterior displacement of the hard palate. A Waters view may show the cortical disruption of the maxillary wall through or just above the alveolar process. Although an axial CT scan will reveal maxillary wall and palatal fractures, it is deficient in displaying most of the Le Fort I fracture because the horizontal orientation of the fracture is parallel to the scan plane (Fig. 4-6). The coronal CT scan is optimal because it is perpendicular to the fracture plane and clearly displays the involved vertical buttresses.

Le Fort II

Plain films may be helpful if the Le Fort II fracture is significantly displaced. Frontal films demonstrate the fracture lines along the nasion and nasal bones, as well as the inferomedial orbital rims and posterolateral maxillary walls. On lateral view, depression of the midface is seen, as well as nasion and pterygoid plate fractures. Similar findings are depicted on axial and coronal CT images.

Le Fort III

Le Fort III fracture (craniofacial disjunction) results from significantly more force than required to produce Le Fort I or II injuries. Consequently, there is a greater degree of comminution, facial

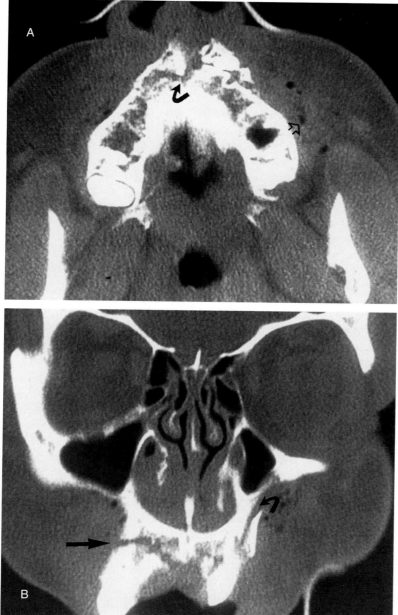

FIGURE 4-6

Le Fort I fracture. (A) Axial CT scan shows a comminuted fracture (*curved arrow*) through the anterior aspect of the maxilla. Soft tissue swelling and subcutaneous emphysema (*open arrow*). (B) Coronal CT shows the diastatic comminuted fracture through the hard palate (*straight arrow*) and maxilla (*curved arrow*).

edema, and incidence of associated intracranial injury. CT imaging is more sensitive than plain films in evaluating these extensive injuries. Classic findings on CT scans and frontal plain films include fracture lines involving the nasion, medial and lateral orbital walls, and zygoma, as well as inferior displacement of the face with vertical elongation of the orbit (20). Although coronal images greatly augment data obtained in the axial plane, the patient's clinical condition may preclude direct coronal image acquisition. If direct coronal imaging is not possible, coronal and sagittal re-creations may provide useful information. Fracture lines through the nasal arch and pterygoid plates also may be detected on lateral plain films.

Mandibular Fractures

Anatomy

The mandible forms the bony framework for the lower third of the face. Symmetric dense cortex surrounds the central trabecular bone and optimally transmits the forces of mastication. The mandible can be divided into sections, including the condyle, neck, ramus, coronoid process, angle, and body. The mandibular condyle articulates with the temporal bone superiorly at the glenoid fossa, forming the temporomandibular joint. The coronoid process is anterior to the condyle and separated from the condyle by the sigmoid notch. The temporalis muscle originates as the temporalis aponeurosis of the lateral skull and inserts on the coronoid process, where it aids in jaw closure.

The vertical portion of the mandible extends from the condyle and coronoid process to the horizontal body of the mandible. The vertical ramus and horizontal body of the mandible merge at the mandibular angle. The powerful masseter muscle, which originates from the zygomatic arch, inserts at the mandibular angle, providing strong jaw closure. The inferior alveolar nerve (V_3) and artery enter the mandible along the medial surface of the ramus as the mandibular canal. Traversing the trabecular bone of the mandible to the lateral chin region, the artery and nerve exit the mental foramen. They supply blood and sensation to the lower dentition, lip, and chin. The developing mandibles are fused at the midline, or symphysis. The area just lateral to this is called *parasymphyseal area.*

Clinical Evaluation

The mandible is the third most common facial bone to fracture. Forty percent of facial traumas include mandibular fractures. Ninety-nine percent of mandibular fractures occur in adults. A mandibular fracture in a child should raise the question of child abuse if the injury was not witnessed.

Eliciting a history depicting the events causing the injury and knowledge of the dental health of the patient are important. The preinjury relationship of the teeth, including any documented malocclusion, orthodontics, and endodontic and dental treatment, may be useful. The patient's complaints usually include inability to occlude the jaws, with pain localized to the fracture site. Areas of numbness may exist over the mentum and lower teeth because of involvement of the inferior alveolar nerve. The patient should be questioned about ability to open and close the jaws as well as any numbness or paresthesia.

Physical examination should include a thorough evaluation of the head and neck with particular attention to the mandible. Because of the rigidity and U shape of the mandible, once a fracture is detected, a second fracture or dislocation of the temporomandibular joint should be suspected. Thorough visualization and palpation both extra- and intraorally frequently will delineate the need for radiographic analysis. The most consistent finding associated with a mandibular fracture is dental malocclusion, most commonly a lateral cross-bite. Other physical findings vary with the location and severity of the fracture. An extraoral laceration, or more commonly, intraoral laceration, or ecchymosis may accompany a fracture line. Gross mobility, point tenderness, or anesthesia over the mentum further characterize the fractured mandible.

Radiographic Evaluation

When a mandibular fracture is suspected, the initial radiographic evaluation includes a mandible series and Panorex (Fig. 4-7). Although the Panorex provides the most information about the mandibular fracture, it is infrequently available in the emergency room setting and often impractical logistically. The standard mandible series, including both lateral obliques, anteroposterior, and Townes projections, likely will be the best means to evaluate the mandible radiographically in the acute setting.

Each projection in the standard mandible series demonstrates a particular area of the mandible. The lateral obliques show fractures of the body, angle, and ascending ramus. The anteroposterior view helps determine symphyseal and parasymphyseal injury and provides some information about the angle. The Townes projection is excellent to evaluate fractures and medial displacement of the condyle and moderately helpful for examining the ascending ramus, condyle, and coronoid process.

The Panorex view is obtained with the patient sitting erect with the chin on a chin rest and the x-ray source rotating around the patient's head. Most mandibular fractures and the occlusal relationship are well demonstrated. The Panorex is most helpful in evaluating the posterior third of the mandible, the region most difficult to show on a standard series. The symphysis is distorted on Panorex and may require occlusal views or an anteroposterior view to delineate symphyseal fractures.

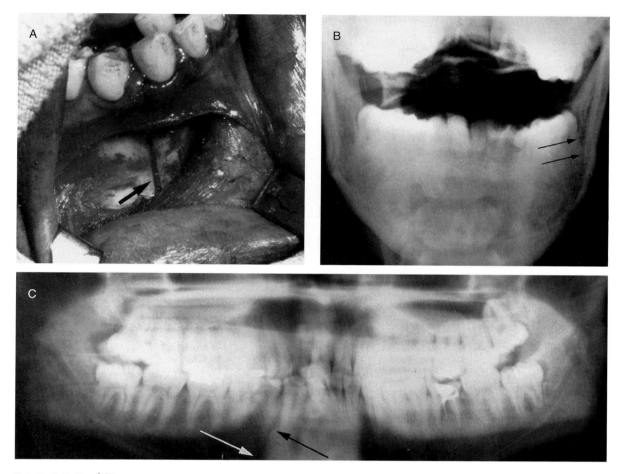

FIGURE 4-7

Body and parasymphyseal mandibular fracture. (A) Gross photograph demonstrating a parasymphyseal mandibular fracture. (B) This antero-posterior film demonstrates a fracture (*arrows*) through the posterior body of the mandible. (C) The Panorex demonstrates the parasymphy-seal fracture (*arrows*) not detected on the standard mandibular series.

Unlike most other facial fractures, CT scanning is infrequently indicated when evaluating mandibular fractures, although CT scans may augment the plain film evaluation of the condylar head and glenoid fossa. CT scan may reveal subtle fractures or deformity of the condyle, flattening or shattering of the condylar neck, or rotational derangement of the condyle referable to the glenoid fossa, all of which may not manifest on the plain film study (27) (Fig. 4-8). In the cooperative patient, images may be obtained in the axial, sagittal, or coronal plane. Re-formatted sagittal or coronal images from direct axial acquisitions may be obtained with expected loss of resolution (28).

The coronal CT scan is superior when eval-uating the position of the mandibular condyle within the glenoid fossa. Asymmetry in distance between the superior margin of the condyle and the inferior margin of the glenoid fossa indicates the presence of a dislocated condyle. Dislocation of the mandible at the temporomandibular joint (TMJ) may occur without fracture. The condyle may be extracted completely from the TMJ, most commonly displaced anteriorly. Rarely, the condyle may be impacted through the glenoid fossa and reside within the middle cranial fossa. Gas within the glenoid fossa may be the only indication of a temporal bone fracture and requires high-resolution CT scan of the temporal bone (29). MRI is the modality of choice to evaluate the TMJ meniscus.

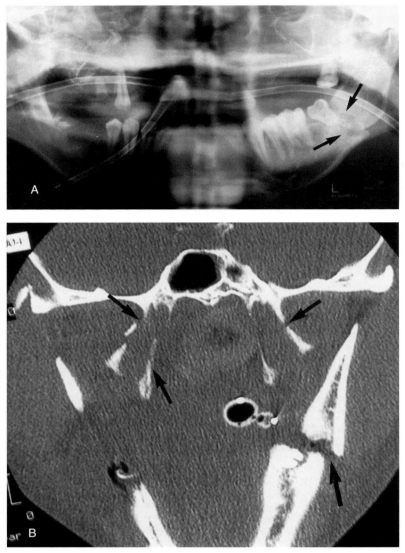

FIGURE 4-8

Posterior mandibular body fracture. (A) Panorex demonstrates a moderately diastatic fracture (*arrows*) of the posterior body of the mandible on the left. (B) Coronal CT scan confirms the findings (*large arrow*) and depicts multiple fractures (*small arrows*) of the medial and lateral pterygoid plates bilaterally.

Adjunctive films may be necessary when a mandibular fracture is diagnosed. Dental views are obtained to delineate the presence and degree of injury whenever tooth injury is suspected. When fractured teeth or fragments cannot be located, a soft tissue film of the neck and chest x-ray must be obtained to rule out a lodged or aspirated fragment.

Frontal Sinus Fractures

Anatomy

Although not present at birth, the frontal sinus typically develops to the size of a pea by 5 years of age and increases in size until growth ceases between the ages of 12 and 15 years. The final volume of the pneumatized frontal sinus averages 5 cm^3 but is highly variable, with 10% of the population developing only unilaterally and up to 4% not developing at all (30). The frontal sinus is an air-filled, mucosally lined cavity with a strong, thick anterior wall and thin posterior wall and floor. The anterior wall can withstand 800 to 2200 lb of force (approximately twice that of other facial bones) before fracturing (31). The thick anterior table acts to protect the posterior table, the anterior wall of the anterior cranial fossa. The superior sagittal sinus, dura, frontal lobe, and cribriform plate are juxtaposed to the posterior wall of the frontal sinus and can be injured secondarily when the sinus is fractured. A vertical septum commonly divides the sinus. Inferiorly, the frontal sinus drains into the middle meatus of the nasal vault via the nasofrontal recess.

Clinical Evaluation

Frontal sinus fractures may be classified into anterior wall, nasofrontal recess, and posterior wall fractures (32). Anterior wall fractures may be nondepressed, linear, or depressed, reproducing the shape of the striking object (20). The nondisplaced anterior table fracture is a rare injury and requires no surgical intervention. The most common frontal sinus fracture, the displaced anterior table fracture, requires early diagnosis and surgical reduction because it may be associated with nasofrontal or posterior table fracture.

The most common finding associated with a frontal sinus fracture is a forehead laceration over the supraorbital ridge, glabella, or lower forehead (33). Signs may include anesthesia of the supraorbital distribution, subconjunctival ecchymosis, orbital emphysema, comminution, tenderness, crepitus, or exposed bone over the glabella (34). Frequently, many findings are masked by overlying swelling; however, tenderness and crepitus usually can be elicited. Because great forces are necessary to fracture the frontal sinus, associated face and head injuries are common. The orbit, nasoethmoid complex, cranium, and maxillary sinus are the most common associated fractures. Soft tissue changes are common within the paranasal sinuses, orbit, and brain. Significant intracranial hemorrhage occurred in over 90% of patients with fractures involving the posterior wall (35).

On physical examination, the open wound should be palpated thoroughly with a sterilely gloved hand to assess the presence of a step-off deformity. The nose should be scrutinized thoroughly for a CSF leak. Any secretions from the nose should be evaluated for the bedside "halo" sign and sent to the laboratory for examination of glucose (greater than 30 mg/dL is confirmatory if the patient has a normal serum glucose level). The bedside test is performed by placing a drop of fluid on an absorbent cloth. If it contains CSF, the radial diffusion will separate into the central blood and the centrifugally migrating halo of CSF.

Radiographic Evaluation

The most useful plain film views for evaluating the frontal sinus include the Waters, Caldwell, posteroanterior, and lateral projections of the face. Radiographic evidence of frontal sinus fracture includes disruption of the sinus margins or walls, opacification of the sinus, accentuated linear densities of overlapping bone fragments, orbital emphysema, and pneumocephalus (20). Disruption of the posterior wall of the sinus may be identified on the lateral view, but assessment of this region may be difficult (25). An axial CT scan is necessary to evaluate the posterior table and thoroughly visualize the anterior table and nasofrontal duct (Fig. 4-9). Because a CT scan commonly will be obtained to rule out intracranial injury, the facial bones can be evaluated with CT, often precluding the need for plain films. A coronal CT scan will evaluate the sinus floor and nasofrontal recess. Associated orbital, ethmoid, and/or sphenoid fractures will be best visualized with combined axial and coronal CT scans.

Temporal Bone Fractures

Anatomy

The temporal bone is the most anatomically intricate structure of the body and houses numerous vital structures. The structures of most importance when evaluating a temporal bone fracture include the middle ear, cochlea, labyrinth, facial nerve, and dura mater. The inner surface of the temporal bone is covered with dura and is often torn with temporal bone fractures, resulting in CSF leakage.

Clinical Evaluation

Symptoms of temporal bone fracture may include vertigo, aural pressure, hearing loss, aural bleeding, headache, facial palsy, and unconsciousness. The otolaryngologist should be consulted as soon as the suspicion of ear or temporal bone injury is raised.

Physical examination may reveal ecchymosis behind the ear (Battle's sign) or within the ear canal or middle ear (hemotympanum). Blood within the ear canal may originate from a fracture of the external auditory canal or from a laceration on the scalp, face, or neck. The external canal should be suctioned clean so that the tympanic membrane can be visualized easily and completely. A tympanic membrane tear and hemotympanum are common but not necessarily present in fractured temporal bones.

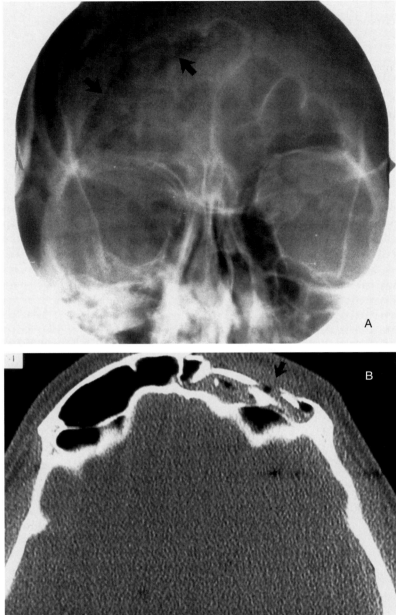

FIGURE 4-9

Frontal sinus fracture. (A) Caldwell view shows heterogeneous density within the left frontal sinus. There are alternating regions of increased and decreased density due to the overlapping and diastasis of depressed bony fragments. (B) Axial CT scan shows the depressed anterior table fractures. Importantly, the integrity of the posterior wall of the frontal sinus can be evaluated effectively with CT.

The conscious or semiconscious patient should be stimulated to ascertain movement of the face. If facial weakness is noted, every effort should be made to determine if this is a change from the initial evaluation, since facial nerve paralysis can be a surgical emergency. Nystagmus with the fast component to the unaffected side is present if the labyrinth or nerve is disrupted. Finally, CSF otorrhea or rhinorrhea indicates disruption into the cranial cavity.

Temporal bone fractures classically have been categorized as either longitudinal or transverse in orientation. Longitudinal fractures extend parallel to the long axis of the petrous ridge and classically were thought to account for 80% of temporal bone fractures. Transverse fractures are perpendicular to the long axis of the petrous temporal bone and are responsible for a majority of the remaining temporal bone fractures. Advances in imaging have led to the realization that most temporal bone fractures are complex with both longitudinal and transverse components. Longitudinal fractures usually extend through the middle ear and external auditory canal, often missing the otic capsule. Facial nerve palsy occurs in approximately 15%; this is bilateral in up to 29% (36). Transverse fractures classically extend from the jugular foramen across the internal auditory meatus, damage the cochlea, and end at the foramen lacerum or foramen spinosum. Sensorineural deafness often is associated with these fractures, whereas facial nerve paralysis occurs in approximately 50% of cases.

Radiographic Evaluation

Although the anatomy of the ear and temporal bone is exceedingly complex, the initial radiographic evaluation is straightforward. Computed tomography (CT) of the temporal bone following head trauma is indicated when there is CSF otorrhea or rhinorrhea, hearing loss, or facial nerve paralysis (37). Once a patient has stabilized from an acute injury, high-resolution CT scanning using a bone algorithm is the radiologic study of choice to evaluate potential fractures of the skull base (38) (Figs. 4-10 and 4-11). Axial and, if possible, coronal sections should be obtained. The radiologist should be informed as to the nature of the lesion so that the appropriate cuts can be made to identify fractures in all the involved areas. High-resolution CT often may demonstrate multiple fracture lines through the skull base (39). MRI scans are excellent to evaluate intracranial injuries but are not as useful for fracture identification.

Laryngeal Injuries

Anatomy

The neck contains all the elements necessary to connect and coordinate the function of the head with the rest of the body. Injury to the neck may disrupt any of these vital functions and may invoke bony, soft tissue, vascular, and central nervous systems dysfunction. Although other associated injuries may appear more impressive, correct treatment of the neck injury with preservation of the airway always should remain a first priority. Laryngeal injury from external trauma is a rare injury. External laryngeal injury accounts for 1 in 30,000 emergency room visits. Although laryngeal injury is rare, the initial management of such injuries has tremendous impact on both the immediate probability of survival of the patient and the long-term quality of life.

Generally, the structures of the upper aerodigestive tract are quite flexible and resilient, with the thyroid cartilage being relatively weak on each side of the midline (40). Its only articulation with other cartilages is with the cricoid cartilage at the cricothyroid joint (41). These structures are afforded some protection by the mandible superiorly, by the sternum inferiorly, and by the spine posteriorly. Although the spine can protect, it also can contribute to injury of the larynx, trachea, or esophagus because of its rigid nature (42).

Anatomically, several important differences exist between the upper aerodigestive tract in children and in adults. Specifically, the narrowest point of the airway in infants is at the cricoid area, whereas in adults it is at the glottic level. The cricoid in infants is located at approximately C4, and in adults it drops to the level of C7. Although the pediatric larynx is injured less often than adults, when injured, increased soft tissue damage and less frequent cartilaginous fracture are more likely because of the loose attachment of the overlying mucous membrane and increased elasticity of the cartilaginous framework. The relative cross-sectional area is decreased. This combination makes the pediatric airway especially vulnerable to compromise, particularly since medical personnel may be unimpressed with the injury's severity because of the lack of cartilaginous fracture. Also, the cartilages are more pliable in children than in adults because calcification progresses with age (42). Therefore, older patients are considered more likely to sustain comminuted laryngeal skeletal fractures. However, this theory has not been proven, since most laryngeal fractures occur in young adults, the group of patients most likely to participate in activities risking laryngeal trauma (43).

Clinical Evaluation

Although the most common and major cause of upper aerodigestive tract trauma is motor vehicle accidents, sports-related injuries to this region occur from hockey sticks, karate blows, fists, handle bars, and balls. The increased use of recreational and competition vehicles has resulted in a higher incidence of upper aerodigestive tract trauma (44). Excluding only the cervical spine, structures adjacent to the larynx are usually injured only in penetrating trauma, since they are flexible enough to avoid significant injury from blunt trauma (45).

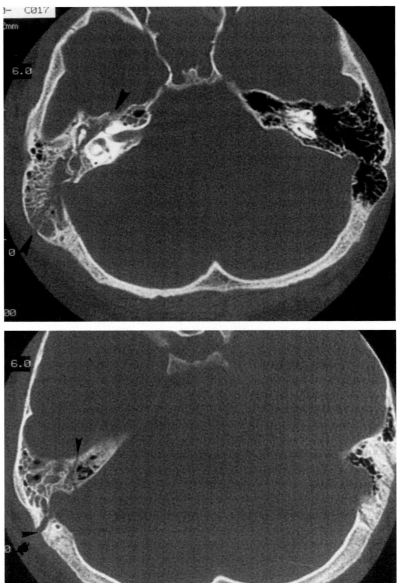

FIGURE   **4-10**

Longitudinal temporal bone fracture. Axial images demonstrate a fracture (*arrowheads*) oriented parallel to the long axis of the petrous temporal bone. Soft tissue density material fills the mastoid air cells and the middle ear cavity.

Signs and symptoms depend largely on the extent and distribution of the injury. On the patient's arrival, the first priority is to establish an airway (46). A good rule of thumb when determining the need for an immediate airway is to err on the side of caution. If time permits, early consultation with specialized personnel is warranted. Steroids may be useful if given early after the time of injury. In the controlled setting, the most conservative, reliable method of securing an airway in a patient with laryngeal injuries is local, awake tracheotomy (47). Endotracheal in-

tubation may cause further damage to the larynx, be exceedingly difficult, interfere with subsequent examination and repair of the larynx, and convert an urgent procedure to an emergent one (43). However, in certain settings, such as in the field, or in the absence of specialized personnel, endotracheal intubation may be attempted with the understanding that this procedure may precipitate the need for cricothyrotomy (48).

The pediatric patient with a laryngeal fracture is a special consideration. The child is not usually cooperative for a local awake trache-

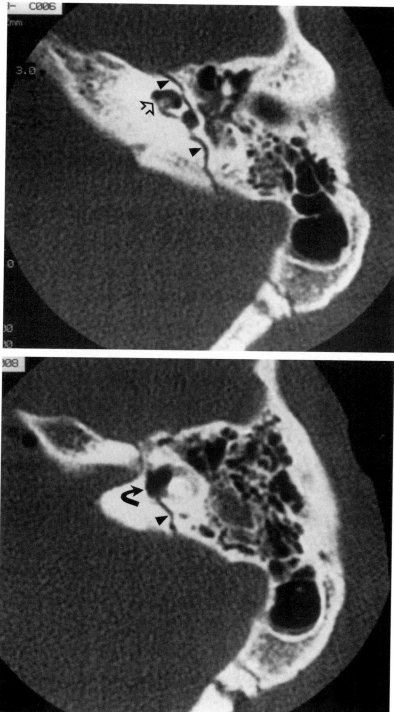

FIGURE 4-11

Transverse temporal bone fracture. Axial images show a fracture (*arrowheads*) that is perpendicular to the long axis of the petrous temporal bone. Note the gas within the cochlea (*open arrow*) and the vestibule (*curved arrow*).

otomy. Furthermore, oxygen saturation drops more rapidly than in the adult, creating a more urgent airway situation. Therefore, in the pediatric patient, rigid bronchoscopy is performed to secure the airway under direct visualization, with

tracheotomy then performed over the bronchoscope.

Once the airway is established and the patient stabilized, evaluation begins with the history taken from the patient and/or witnesses to the event. Common symptoms of laryngeal fracture include dysphagia, odynophagia, referred otalgia, hoarseness or aphonia, dyspnea, hemoptysis, stridor, and later, aspiration. Although physical examination may reveal a visible laceration, swelling, or hematoma over the anterior neck, laryngeal fractures frequently occur with minimal or no externally visible neck wounds. Palpation frequently reveals crepitus, tenderness over the thyroid or cricoid cartilage, and sometimes flattening of the thyroid prominence. Open wounds are not explored with instruments nor probed for fear of dislodging a hematoma and initiating further bleeding. The cervical spine should be palpated for bony step-offs and tenderness. Hemoptysis may reveal an injury of the upper aerodigestive system but may be difficult to evaluate because of facial bleeding.

Direct visualization of the larynx is mandatory at the first possible opportunity. Until recent years, indirect mirror examination was performed routinely and frequently did not help in the more severely traumatized patient.

Today, the widespread use of direct fiberoptic examination has allowed much improved nonoperative evaluation of the injured larynx (49). Care must be taken in the awake patient because minor trauma of the partially compromised but adequate airway can precipitate an airway obstruction and emergency. After inserting the instrument through the nose, the oro- and hypopharynx are examined. Partial motion limitation indicates structural deformity such as arytenoid dislocation, whereas complete immobility is more suggestive of recurrent laryngeal nerve injury. Failure of vocal cords to meet in the same horizontal plane may indicate a structural change in the laryngeal framework or superior laryngeal nerve injury. Any exposed cartilage is noted along with the integrity of the surrounding mucosa.

Radiographic Evaluation

Once the stable airway has been established and the patient stabilized, radiographic evaluation may be considered only if no operative urgency exists. Radiographs of the chest and neck always should be obtained. The existence of an abnormal tracheal outline, a pneumothorax, a pneumomediastinum, and cervical emphysema are important indicators of a possible breach of laryngotracheal integrity. The role of preoperative radiographic evaluation has changed dra-

matically with the widespread use of CT (47,50). Before the use of CT, plain soft tissue films, contrast laryngography, and tomogram were available to assess the soft tissues of the larynx. Frequently, these studies added little information about the integrity of the larynx not already known by examination. Plain films may identify fractures but reveal the anatomy in two dimensions and add little about the soft tissue status of the larynx. Laryngography is impossible in the acutely injured patient because of the inability to cooperate. Plain tomography lacks the soft tissue detail available on CT.

CT scan allows a noninvasive evaluation of the soft tissue and cartilaginous framework (Fig. 4-12). Its utilization in cases of severe laryngeal trauma is controversial in the literature. For the patient with a complex laryngeal injury obviously needing surgical intervention, CT may add little to the diagnostic assessment, since the patient will undergo open reduction (47). Authors with this belief state that CT should be reserved for those initially nonsurgical patients in whom laryngeal injury is suspected but not confirmed by history and physical examination. Other authors believe that CT is of particular value in the more severe cases (51,52). CT scan may identify the minimally displaced injury that if left unrepaired would lead to long-term phonatory disturbances because of disruption of the laryngeal valving mechanisms (53). When massive edema or hematoma is present, direct laryngoscopy may not be useful in determining the laryngeal framework. In this case, CT is particularly useful. If the CT scan shows no evidence of laryngeal fracture, the patient may be treated with tracheotomy and observation without exploratory surgery (47).

Cervical Arterial Injury

Anatomy

Blunt trauma to the carotid and vertebral arteries is rare but has been associated with mortality rates of 20% to 40% and permanent neurologic impairment from vascular dissection or occlusion in 40% to 80% of patients (54–56). Although carotid injury is caused most commonly by motor vehicle trauma, sport injuries from falls, hyperextension or rotational neck trauma, blunt intraoral trauma, blows from a solid object or collision with another individual, and clothes-

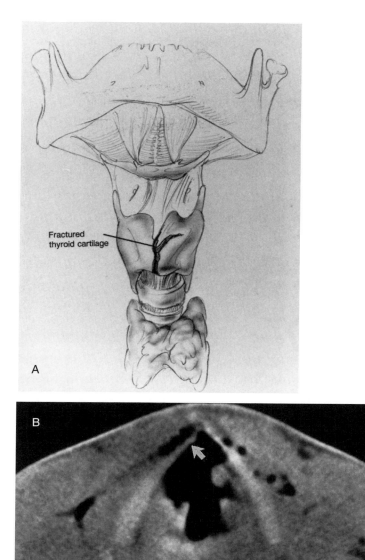

Fractured
thyroid cartilage

A

B

FIGURE   4-12

Laryngeal cartilage fracture. (A) Schematic of laryngeal cartilage fracture. (Reproduced with permission from Bailey BJ. Head and neck surgery–otolaryngology, vol 1. Philadelphia: JB Lippincott, 1993:941.) **(B) Axial CT scan shows medial displacement of the right thyroid cartilage (*arrow*) and emphysema in the surrounding fascial planes.**

line injury have been reported mechanisms (57). Vertebral artery injury has been reported following severe blunt and penetrating neck trauma or minor trauma such as rapid head turning, coughing, tennis, and yoga (58–61).

The carotid and vertebral arteries traverse the neck to provide the main blood flow to the brain. The left common carotid artery is a direct branch off the aorta, whereas the right common

carotid artery arises from the brachiocephalic trunk. Each carotid then courses upward deep to the sternocleidomastoid muscle and bifurcates into the internal and external carotid arteries at the level of the hyoid (approximately the level of C3 and C4 vertebrae). While the external carotid gives off numerous extracranial branches, the internal carotid ascends more medially, posterior to the mandible, to the skull

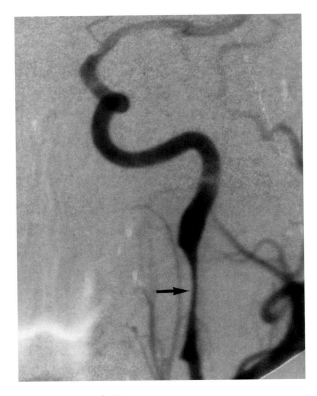

FIGURE **4-13**

Traumatic carotid dissection. Anteroposterior left common carotid arteriogram shows a focal, smoothly marginated stenosis (*arrow*) of the extracranial internal carotid artery.

base without branching. It then enters the carotid canal in the petrous portion of the temporal bone, travels above the foramen lacerum, and then traverses the cavernous sinus. The internal carotid artery terminates in the anterior and middle cerebral arteries (62).

The vertebral artery arises from the subclavian artery, passes through the neck, and enters the foramen of the transverse process of the sixth cervical vertebrae. It ascends through the transverse foramen of the first six cervical vertebrae before exiting the transverse foramen of the first cervical vertebrae. The artery then penetrates the atlanto-occipital membrane and the spinal dura, passes through the foramen magnum, and unites with the contralateral vertebral artery to form the basilar artery (58,62).

Clinical Evaluation

Arterial dissections, arterial occlusions from thrombosis, pseudoaneurysms, and carotid cav-

ernous fistulas are distinctly different entities with disparate natural histories and management strategies (63). Delays in recognition of blunt neck vascular injuries are frequent because of concomitant head injury, severe associated extracranial injuries with shock, and failure to consider the diagnosis. A high index of clinical suspicion based on careful reconstruction of injury mechanisms and physical examination should prompt screening modalities in high-risk patients because the clinical presentation of blunt cervical vascular injury is highly variable. Whenever this injury is suspected, a thorough neurologic examination with attention to cranial nerves and possible neck bruits should be performed. The clinician should look for a Horner's syndrome (miosis, anhydrosis, and ptosis) as well as for cerebellar changes. The patient may present with no significant findings, since neurologic changes may develop minutes to days after the traumatic event. Frank carotid arterial disruption, however, was uniformly fatal in one study (63).

Physical findings associated with carotid artery injuries include expanding hematoma, audible bruit, pulsatile neck mass, palpable thrill, Horner's syndrome, or any neurologic symptom not explained by another injury. The absence of any hard signs in many of these patients makes the diagnosis of such injuries particularly challenging (63).

Patients with vertebral artery dissection or occlusion usually present with pain localized in the occipital or craniocervical area ipsilateral to the damaged vessel (58). Other abnormalities may include a lateral medullary or Wallenberg's syndrome. These symptoms include nystagmus, ataxia, ipsilateral limb dysmetria, decreased pin perception to the ipsilateral face, decreased or loss of pin sensation in the contralateral limbs, and an ipsilateral Horner's syndrome (58).

Radiographic Evaluation

CT scan of the brain without contrast material should be obtained at the first sign of neurologic injury to evaluate for cerebral infarction, edema, or intracranial hemorrhage. CT can be predictive of outcome. In one study, when cerebral infarct was located on the side of an arterial injury, the mortality rate was 47% versus no deaths in 15 patients with normal CT scans (63).

To diagnose vertebral or carotid injury, conventional angiography is the most accurate means (Fig. 4-13). The entire aortic arch, brachiocephalic vessels, and extra- and intracranial course of each carotid and vertebral artery must be evaluated. These comprehensive views are essential to clearly demonstrate proximal and distal injuries, intracranial thromboembolic material, the anatomy of the collateral circulation, and bilateral injuries (58,63).

Duplex ultrasound is an underutilized means to accurately screen carotid injury. This modality can be used as a screening device in patients unable to undergo conventional angiography. False-negative results can be obtained using this modality if the injury occurs with arterial dissections of the internal carotid artery at the base of the skull because this portion of the internal carotid artery is poorly imaged by ultrasound techniques (63). However, abnormal velocity or flow within the proximal vessel can provide indirect evidence of a more distal injury (64). The most significant limitation of duplex ultrasound is an inability to visualize the distal extracranial and intracranial internal carotid artery (62).

MRI may be used to diagnose vascular injury. Magnetic resonance angiography (MRA) can effectively screen patients with suspected vascular injury in the neck and may be the first line to evaluate these vessels. Time-of-flight or phase-contrast techniques can evaluate any change in vessel caliber. Fat-saturated spin-echo techniques accurately show clot (methemoglobin) in the dissected false channels.

REFERENCES

1. Frenguelli A, Ruscito P, Bicciolo G, et al. Head and neck trauma in sporting activities: review of 208 cases. J Craniomaxillofac Surg 1991;19:178–181.

2. Peynegre R, Strunski V. Les traumatismes du tiers moyen de la face. Encycl Med Chir (Paris) Otorhino-Laryngol 1988;2:20480A.

3. Nakamura T, Gross C. Facial fracture analyses of five years of experience. Arch Otolaryngol 1973; 97:288–290.

4. Rolland A. La mandibule, point d'impact electif en traumatologie du sport. Med Sport 1982;56: 46–48.

5. Lindqvist C, Sorsa S, Hyrkas T, Santavirta S. Maxillofacial fractures sustained in bicycle accidents. Int J Oral Maxillofac Surg 1986;15:12–18.

6. Kreipke DL, Moss JJ, Franco JM, et al. Computed tomography and thin-section tomography in facial trauma. AJR 1984;142:1041–1045.

7. Gentry LR, Godersky JC, Thompson B. MR imaging of head trauma: review of the distribution and radiopathologic features of traumatic lesions. AJR 1988;150:663–672.

8. Hesselink JR, Dowd CF, Healy ME, et al. MR imaging of brain contusions: a comparative study with CT. AJR 1988;150:1133–1142.

9. Zimmerman RA, Bilaniuk LY, Hackney DB. Head injury: early results of comparing CT and high-field MR. AJR 1986;147:1215–1222.

10. DeLacey GJ, et al. The radiology of nasal injuries: problems of interpretation and clinical relevance. Br J Radiol 1977;50:412.

11. Maniglia AJ, Stepnick DW. Orbital fractures. In: English GM, ed. Otolaryngology, vol 4. Philadelphia: JB Lippincott, 1994.

12. Hammerschlag SB, Hughes S, O'Reilly GV, et al. Blowout fractures of the orbit: a comparison of computed tomography and conventional radiography with anatomical correlation. Radiology 1982;143:487–492.

13. Gean AD. Imaging of head trauma. New York: Raven Press, 1994.

14. Letsun RD. Ocular injury. Otolaryngol Clin North Am 1976;9:465.

15. Milauskas AT, Fueger GF. Serious ocular complications associated with blow-out fractures of the orbit. Am J Ophthalmol 1966;62:670.

16. Smith B, Wiggs EO. Differential diagnosis of orbital injury. Arch Ophthalmol 1973;89:484.

17. Miller GR, Tenzel RR. Ocular complications of the midface fractures. Plast Reconstr Surg 1967; 33:37.

18. Hammerschlag SB, Hughes S, O'Reilly GV, et al. Another look at blow-out fractures of the orbit. AJNR 1982;3:331–335.

19. O'Hare TH. Blow-out fractures: a review. J Emerg Med 1991;9:253–263.

20. DelBalso AM, Hall RE, Margarone JE. Radiographic evaluation of maxillofacial trauma. In: DelBalso AM, ed. Maxillofacial imaging. Philadelphia: WB Saunders, 1990:35–128.

21. Laine FJ, Conway WF, Laskin DM. Radiology of maxillofacial trauma: review article. Curr Probl Diagn Radiol 1993;22:145–188.

22. Dolan K, Jacoby C, Smoker W. The radiology of facial fractures. Radiographics 1984;4:577–663.

23. Schultz RC. Facial injuries, 3d ed. Chicago: Year Book Medical Publishers, 1988:45–72.

24. Gentry L. Facial trauma and associated brain damage. Radiol Clin North Am 1989;27:435–446.

25. Pathria MN, Blaser SI. Diagnostic imaging of craniofacial fractures. Radiol Clin North Am 1989; 27:839–853.

26. Kassel EE, Gross JS. Imaging of midfacial fractures. Neuroimaging Clin North Am 1991;1: 259–283.

27. Raustia A, Pyhtinen, Oikarinen K, Altonen M. Conventional radiographic and computed tomographic findings in cases of fracture of the mandibular condylar process. J Oral Maxillofac Surg 1990;48:1258–1262.

28. Sinn DP, Karas ND. Radiographic evaluation of facial injuries. In: Fonseca RJ, Walker RV, eds. Oral and maxillofacial trauma. Philadelphia: WB Saunders, 1991:301–322.

29. Betz B, Wiener M. Air in the temporomandibular joint fossa: CT sign of temporal bone fracture. Radiology 1991;180:463–466.

30. Owens OT, Mathog RH. Frontal sinus fractures. In: Foster CA, Sherman JE, eds. Surgery of facial bone fractures. New York: Churchill-Livingstone, 1987:13.

31. Nahum AM. The biomechanics of maxillofacial trauma. Clin Plast Surg 1975;2:59.

32. Newman MH, Travis LW. Frontal sinus fractures. Laryngoscope 1973;83:1281–1292.

33. Harris L, Marano GD, McCorkle D. Nasofrontal duct: CT in frontal sinus trauma. Radiology 1987; 165:195–198.

34. Rohrich R, Hollier L. Management of frontal sinus fractures. Clin Plast Surg 1992;19:219–232.

35. Olson E, Wright D, Hoffman H, et al. Frontal sinus fractures: evaluation of CT scans in 132 patients. AJNR 1992;13:897–902.

36. Griffin J, Altenau M, Schaefer SD. Bilateral longitudinal temporal bone fractures: a retrospective review of seventeen cases. Laryngoscope 1979; 89:1432–1435.

37. Shambaugh GE. Surgery of the ear. Philadelphia: WB Saunders, 1991.

38. Liebetrau R, Draf W, Kahle G. Temporal bone fractures: high resolution CT. J Otolaryngol 1993; 22:249–252.

39. Kinney S. Trauma to the middle ear and temporal bone. 2873–2884.

40. Cerat J, Charlin B, Brazeau-Lamontagne L, Mongeau C. Assessment of the cricoarytenoid joint: high-resolution CT scan study with histo-anatomical correlation. J Otolaryngol 1988;17:65–67.

41. Cerat J, Charlin B, Brazeau-Lamontagne L, et al. Assessment of the cricoarytenoid joint: high-resolution CT scan study with histo-anatomical correlation. J Otolaryngol 1988;17:65–67.

42. Larson DL, Cohn AM. Management of acute laryngeal injury: a critical review. J Trauma 1976; 16:858–862.

43. Schaefer SD. The treatment of acute external laryngeal injuries, "state of the art." Arch Otolaryngol Surg 1991;117:35–39.

44. O'Keefe LJ, Maw AR. The dangers of minor blunt laryngeal trauma. J Laryngol Otol 1992;106: 372–373.

45. Myers EM, Iko BO. The management of acute laryngeal trauma. J Trauma 1987;27:448–452.

46. Krekorian EA. Laryngopharyngeal injuries. Laryngoscope 1975;85:2069–2085.

47. Schaefer SD, Brown OE. Selective application of CT in the management of laryngeal trauma. Laryngoscope 1983;93:1473–1475.

48. Gussack GS, Jurkovich GJ. Treatment dilemmas in laryngotracheal trauma. J Trauma 1988;28: 1439–1444.

49. Schaefer SD, Close LG. Acute management of laryngeal trauma. Ann Otol Rhinol Laryngol 1989;98:98–104.

50. Stack BC Jr, Ridley MB. Arytenoid subluxation from blunt laryngeal trauma. Am J Otolaryngol 1994;15:68–73.

51. Fuhrman GM, Stieg FH, Buerk CA. Blunt laryngeal trauma: classification and management protocol. J. Trauma 1990;30:87–92.

52. Gussack GS, Jurkovich GJ, Luterman A. Laryngotracheal trauma: a protocol approach to a rare injury. Laryngoscope 1986;96:660–665.

53. Stanley RB, Cooper DS, Florman SH. Phonatory effects of thyroid cartilage fractures. Ann Otol Rhinol Laryngol 1987;96:493–496.

54. Krajewski L, Hertzer N. Blunt carotid artery trauma: report of two cases and review of the literature. Ann Surg 1980;191:341.

55. Fakhry S, Jaques P, Proctor H. Cervical vessel injury after blunt trauma. J Vasc Surg 1988;8:501.

56. Martin R, Eldrup-Jorgensen J, Clark D, et al. Blunt trauma to the carotid arteries. J Vasc Surg 1991; 14:789.

57. Perry M, Snyder W, Thal E. Carotid artery injuries caused by blunt trauma. Ann Surg 1980;192:74.

58. DeBehnke D, Brady W. Vertebral artery dissection due to minor neck trauma. J Emerg Med 1994;12:27–31.

59. Hilton-Jones D, Warlow C. Non-penetrating trauma and cerebral infarction in the young. Lancet 1985;1:1435–1438.

60. Herr R, Call G, Banks D. Vertebral artery dissection from neck flexion during paroxysmal coughing. Ann Emerg Med 1992;21:88–91.

61. Pryse-Phillips W. Infarction of the medulla and cervical cord after fitness exercises. Stroke 1989; 20:292–294.

62. Davis J, Zimmerman R. Injury of the carotid and vertebral arteries. Neuroradiology 1983;25:55–69.

63. Cogbill T, Moore E, Meissner M, et al. The spectrum of blunt injury to the carotid artery: a multicenter perspective. J Trauma 1994;37:473–479.

64. Hennerici M, Steinke W, Rautenberg W. High-resistance Doppler flow pattern in extracranial carotid dissection. Arch Neurol 1989;46:670.

CHAPTER 5

Principles and Practice of Imaging of Athletic Injuries to the Cervical, Thoracic, and Lumbar Spine

STUART M. WEINSTEIN

STANLEY A. HERRING

*A*thletic competition exposes the spine to both acute, dynamic overload and chronic, repetitive forces. The mechanism of these injuries can be flexion, extension, compression, rotation, or a combination of these. There is a differential propensity to certain spine injuries depending on the sport and position played within that sport. Some conditions such as spondylolysis and spondylolisthesis are found much more commonly in certain athletes (i.e., gymnasts); however, the nature of most spinal injuries is not unique to sports. Sports injuries result from the same types of problems that can occur either with other forceful traumatic events (e.g., automotive "whiplash" injury) or even without an obvious precipitant. Also, athletes are equally susceptible to "nonmechanical" etiologies of spinal pain (e.g., infection, tumor), and these always must be considered in the differential diagnosis, especially if symptoms are out of proportion to the mechanism of injury (if any) or the symptoms and signs persist despite appropriate rehabilitation measures.

This chapter will be divided into axial pain, myelopathic syndromes, and radiculopathic syndromes. Each clinical syndrome will be divided into pathomechanics and pathophysiology, clinical presentation, imaging—including when to order, what to order, typical findings, and clinical correlation—and treatment options specific to the imaging results. As with many medical, orthopedic, and neurologic conditions, no simple protocol exists that will allow the health care practitioner to confidently obtain the "right" diagnostic study at all times. In fact, usually there is not just one recognized test to confirm the clinical assessment; this is especially true when imaging spinal disorders. However, every attempt will be made to compare and contrast the various studies, with emphasis on relative diagnostic specificity and sensitivity.

Axial Pain Syndromes

Nonmechanical

Infection, Diskitis

Pathomechanics/Pathophysiology Diskitis is more common in children, possibly due to the relatively greater blood supply to the disk as compared with adults, but often an infectious etiology of diskitis in children is not discovered (1). In contrast to osteomyelitis, which is an infectious process affecting the vertebrae, usually from an extraosseous focus, diskitis is an inflammatory condition of the intervertebral disk for which the exact etiology is undetermined in the majority of cases. Trauma and avascular necrosis, both potentially causing disruption of the vertebral endplate, have been theorized to result in diskitis. Typically, the lumbar or lower thoracic disks are involved. In adults, diskitis usually results from an extension of osteomyelitis from an adjacent vertebral body; however, it also can result from an invasive procedure such as disk surgery or disk space injection. The incidence of infectious diskitis following diskography has been reported to be from 0.5% to 4.0% (2).

Clinical Presentation The presentation of diskitis may be acute and fulminant or chronic and indolent, with symptoms lasting for up to years before diagnosis. Infectious diskitis with an acute, severe presentation is most suggestive of a bacterial origin. Pain may be present at rest or precipitated by movement. A common finding in children is a refusal to stand or walk. Low back pain, an antalgic gait, and irritability are key symptoms and signs for the presence of diskitis in children. In adults or children, often there is no fever, and blood cultures are normal, except in acute bacterial disk space infection. In childhood diskitis, the erythrocyte sedimentation rate (ESR) is almost always elevated, but a normal ESR in an adult does not rule out diskitis (1).

Imaging Early diagnosis of diskitis is essential, and imaging studies typically are performed immediately on suspicion. In the acute stage, plain x-rays may be entirely normal. Later, however, typical findings include disk space narrowing and endplate sclerosis, followed by endplate erosions on both sides of the disk. In the chronic stage, vertebral body ankylosis may occur. In the past, technetium bone scan imaging was the "gold standard" test to demonstrate disk space inflammation and/or vertebral body infection, but magnetic resonance imaging (MRI) is now considered the test of choice for the evaluation of diskitis as well as osteomyelitis due to its extreme sensitivity for inflammation. Typical findings include low signal from the involved disk space and adjacent vertebrae on T1-weighted sequences and increased signal on T2-weighted sequences (Fig. 5-1A and B). Additionally, MRI allows for assessment of vertebral endplate discontinuity, paravertebral phlegmon, and the presence of spinal canal compromise due to abscess or retropulsed bone fragments. In the clinical setting of acute diskitis, the classic T2 MRI findings may not be present, and "inflammation sensitive" inversion recovery sequences may be useful (see Fig. 5-1C). Differentiating between infectious and noninfectious diskitis may be accomplished with indium-labeled leukocytes. Although the specificity of this test is quite high, the sensitivity is relatively low, possibly due to the relative avascularity of the adult intervertebral disk.

Treatment In children, the course of diskitis is usually self-limited, responding to rest and anti-inflammatory medications. The use of antibiotics in children is controversial. Diskitis resulting from infection is usually treated with antibiotics; however, the initiation of antibiotic therapy without knowing the specific organism involved is not ideal. Thus imaging may be valuable in isolating a biopsy site if the blood workup is nondiagnostic and tissue culture becomes necessary. If no organism is isolated and the clinical course is stable, then treatment with analgesics, rest, and bracing is reasonable. An extended course of broad-spectrum antibiotics may be instituted without knowing the specific organism if this "conservative" approach fails to provide benefit. Diskectomy and fusion also may be considered in the absence of a specific etiology if the patient is debilitated by pain and/or there is evidence for neurologic compromise due to abscess or retropulsed fragments within the spinal canal.

Tumor, Osteoid Osteoma

Pathomechanics/Pathophysiology This bone lesion occurs most commonly in the long bones of the lower extremity but also in the axial skeleton—slightly more frequently in the lumbar spine and equally in the thoracic and cervical spine. Although considered a benign tumor, other etiologies suggest that it results from a chronic infection or a post-traumatic reparative process. The lesion is usually small, by definition less than 2 cm (a lesion greater than 2 cm is usually considered an osteoblastoma), and histologically is sclerotic bone surrounding a nidus of osteoid, vascular tissue, and trabecular bone.

Clinical Presentation This bone lesion is found most commonly in males between the ages of 10 and 30 years, although this is variable. The pathognomonic symptoms include nocturnal exacerbation of pain, which is relieved by the use of nonsteroidal anti-inflammatory agents, classically aspirin. The favored mechanism of analgesia is postulated to be reduction in osteoma prostaglandin production (3). However, some osteoid osteomas are painless, especially early in their development (4), and with others, analgesia is not afforded by aspirin. Initially, the pain associated with osteoid osteomas may be vague and intermittent, but as the lesion matures, the pain becomes more intense and well localized. Radiating symptoms are unusual unless the lesion has irritated a nerve root. Examination find-

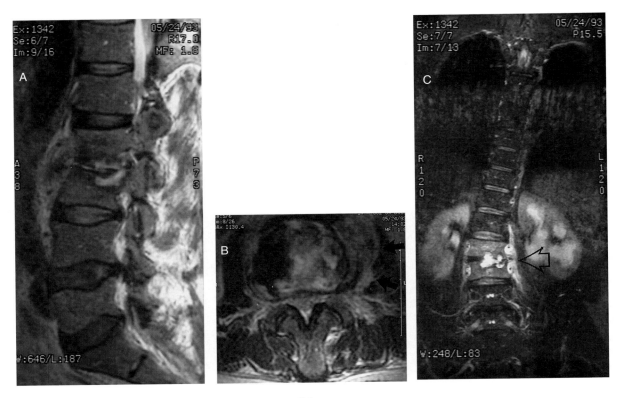

FIGURE **5-1**

MRI of L2–L3 intervertebral diskitis. Sagittal (A) and axial (B) T2-weighted images demonstrating high signal intensity from within the intervertebral disk, endplate destruction, epidural extension of infected disk material, and paravertebral abscess (*closed arrows*). (C) Coronal inversion recovery image demonstrating very high signal intensity within the intervertebral disk and adjacent vertebral bodies and abscess formation within the left psoas muscle (*open arrow*).

ings supportive of an osteoid osteoma are local tenderness, muscle spasm, and secondary scoliosis. New-onset scoliosis in a young patient should raise suspicion about this condition (5).

Imaging Plain radiographs always should be obtained when investigating for an osteoid osteoma. If visualized, the classic findings include a lucent nidus approximately 1.0 to 1.5 cm in diameter (occasionally with a central calcification) surrounded by a zone of very dense sclerotic bone. In the early stages of this tumor, x-rays may be normal, or the lesion may not be well visualized. The test of choice would then be bone scan imaging, which should reveal very intense uptake of technetium at the site of the lesion (Fig. 5-2A). Osteoid osteomas almost always occur in the posterior elements, including the pedicle, less frequently in the zygapophysial joints, and least commonly in the vertebral

body. Following plain radiographs or bone scan, limited computed tomography (CT) with thin slices (i.e., 1.0–1.5 mm) and a bone algorithm should be performed to specifically identify the nidus (see Fig. 5-2B), which confirms the diagnosis and rules out more serious neoplasms. Osteoid osteomas also can be visualized on MRI, with findings of low signal on T1-weighted sequences and increased signal on T2-weighted sequences. Although CT is usually indicated before MRI, the MRI may add useful information concerning the appearance of the spinal cord or conus in patients in whom the tumor encroaches on the epidural space.

Treatment The definitive treatment is surgical removal of the nidus and sclerotic bone. For this reason, precise localization through imaging studies is critical. Malignant transformation is rare, but recurrence of the tumor is pos-

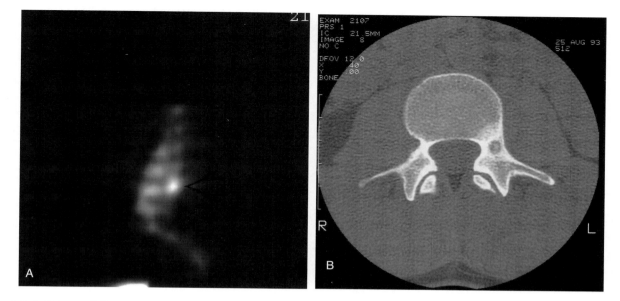

FIGURE 5-2

Osteoid osteoma. (A) SPECT bone scan imaging (sagittal) demonstrating intense abnormality at the L3 level. (B) CT imaging (bone algorithm, 1.5-mm slices) demonstrating a lesion of the left L3 pedicle with a lucent nidus containing a central calcific fleck.

sible, especially following subtotal surgical resection.

Mechanical

Fracture, Anterior Column (Vertebral Body)

Pathomechanics/Pathophysiology Fractures isolated to the vertebral body are typically compression injuries and result from an axial load with or without a flexion component. These can be subgrouped into impaction injuries, resulting in vertebral wedge compression or chip fractures; split fractures, in which the anterior half of the vertebral body is split by the intervertebral disk in either a sagittal or a coronal direction; and burst fractures with varying degrees of comminution and displacement, which have the greatest likelihood to cause spinal canal encroachment and neurologic damage. With this mechanism of injury, the posterior elements and posterior soft tissues are usually spared. Aside from the burst fracture, this single-column injury is an inherently stable fracture (6,7).

Clinical Presentation These injuries are relatively uncommon in sports but occur most frequently in the lower thoracic or upper lumbar spine and can result from a fall onto the buttocks or rigid lower extremities. There is acute, sharp pain localized to site of injury, often with associated muscle spasm. Neurologic symptoms and signs are absent unless a burst fracture has occurred with resulting compression of the distal spinal cord or cauda equina.

Imaging Plain radiographs are always required if a significant axial load injury has occurred. Both lateral and anteroposterior (AP) x-rays are necessary (Fig. 5-3A and B). If vertebral body height is maintained, then no significant compressive bony injury occurred. Loss of vertebral height, however mild, should suggest that the force of injury was great enough to potentially result in a burst fracture, and this demands further assessment with either CT utilizing stacked images and thin cuts (i.e., 1.0 to 1.5 mm) with sagittal re-formations or MRI. Additional plain film evidence for a burst component includes obvious displacement of the superoposterior portion of the vertebral body in the lateral plane (see Fig. 5-3C) and/or splaying of the pedicles in the AP plane. This finding implies that either plastic deformation or fracture of the posterior elements or pedicles must occur; thus a burst fracture is not necessarily limited to the anterior column. Computed tomography is faster to obtain, which is appealing for the acutely painful patient, and will

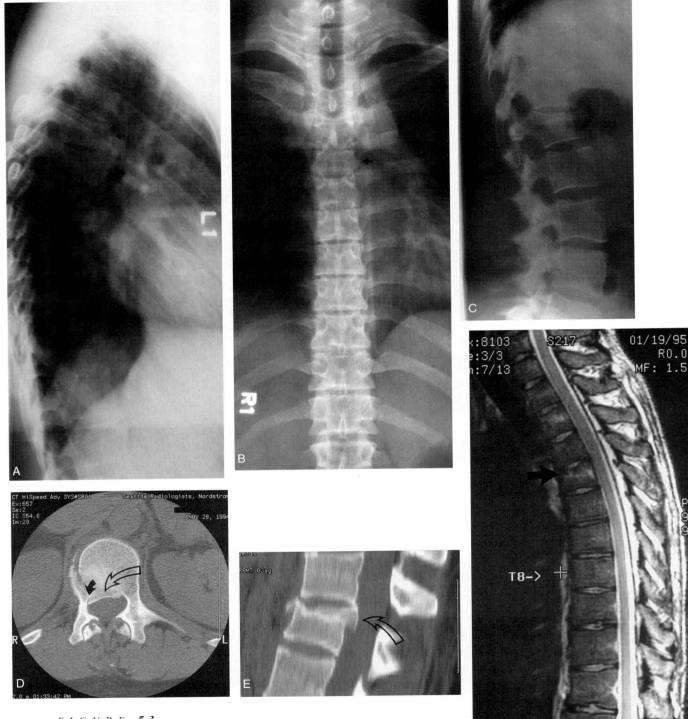

FIGURE 5-3

Anterior column fractures. T5 vertebral compression fracture, lateral (A) and plain film AP (B) views demonstrating mild anterior wedging (*closed arrow*). (C) L1 vertebral burst fracture, plain film lateral view demonstrating posterior displacement of the superoposterior portion of the vertebral body (*open arrow*). L1 vertebral burst fracture, CT axial (D) and sagittal (E) re-formations demonstrating a posterior displaced fragment of bone (*open arrows*) and a fracture extending into and impacting the base of the right pedicle (*closed arrow*). (F) T5 vertebral compression fracture, MRI, T2-weighted sagittal sequence demonstrating increased signal from within the vertebral body (*closed arrow*) without a burst component.

more clearly evaluate for both retropulsed bone into the spinal canal and the posterior elements for unsuspected bony injury than MRI (see Fig. 5-3D and E). MRI is useful in that it can identify 1) an acute fracture (increased signal on T2-weighted sequences; see Fig. 5-3F), 2) microfractures or bone contusion that might otherwise have been unrecognized if the plain x-ray was normal, 3) any retropulsed disk (and bone) fragments within the spinal canal, 4) any damage to the spinal cord or thecal sac (as determined by signal change), and 5) perivertebral soft tissue swelling. Bone scan imaging may assist in dating a plain x-ray finding of a vertebral body compression; however, bone scans can remain positive even 6 months or longer following an injury. Although MRI findings of an acute compression fracture usually resolve within 3 to 6 weeks, abnormal signal intensity in the cancellous bone associated with an acute compression fracture also may persist for several months, particularly with inversion recovery or fat-suppressed T2-weighted images.

Treatment The critical question with this mechanism of injury is whether or not a burst component is present. MRI or CT scanning is essential in this regard and will determine the appropriate course of treatment. If present, surgical stabilization or extended bracing (i.e., for up to 12 weeks) with a custom-molded body jacket in slight hyperextension is mandatory. Serial plain x-rays, once per week for 2 to 3 weeks following the acute injury, are necessary to evaluate for progressive collapse of the vertebral body or kyphosis at that spinal segment. Surgical decompression is unusual in the absence of significant or progressive neurologic deficit, and surgical stabilization is also not usually required unless progressive spinal deformity is developing.

Fracture, Posterior Column (Zygapophysial Joint, Pars Interarticularis)

Pathomechanics/Pathophysiology Posterior element injuries are found more commonly in the athletic population than in the general population because the movements of extension and extension combined with rotation are intrinsic to many sports. These posterior column injuries typically result from chronic repetitive overload as opposed to an acute traumatic event, although a single episode may bring the condition to clinical awareness.

While pure extension injury can cause spinous process impingement with resulting periostitis, rarely does spinous process fracture result. Cervical spinous process fracture at the C7 level, the so-called clay-shoveler's fracture, can occur following forceful lifting because extreme muscular contraction avulses this posterior structure. This is an inherently stable fracture and is not seen commonly in sports.

Forceful spinal extension often is associated with some degree of segmental rotation (8). Biomechanically, the lumbar zygapophysial joint and pars interarticularis can be loaded with repetitive extension and rotation. Zygapophysial joint fracture, pars stress reaction, and spondylolysis occur most commonly at the L5 level, where maximum shear across the L5–S1 spinal segment occurs. Pars injuries can develop acutely; however, the same mechanical stresses that can cause an acute fracture also can aggravate a previously asymptomatic isthmic spondylolysis. Spondylolisthesis due to pars defects can only develop when these are bilateral, usually develops at the onset of the lysis, remains stable if less than grade III (i.e., 75% listhesis), and do not typically progress past the end of adolescence. Late development or progression of this type of a spondylolisthesis is usually associated with progressive degeneration of the intervertebral disk at that segment.

Clinical Presentation Low back pain is the chief symptom and may or may not be acute. The pain is usually unilateral, unless bilateral zygapophysial joints or pars interarticulares are involved. Referred pain patterns in a sclerotomal distribution can occur. The degree of radicular involvement depends on the presence of a spondylolisthesis, with nerve root symptoms proportional to the grade of slippage. Physical examination findings for zygapophysial-mediated pain are variable; however, pain theoretically is exacerbated by extension and rotation maneuvers. The typical findings with an acute pars defect are ipsilateral pain provoked with standing on a single lower extremity and extending the spine and severe hamstring tightness. Both conditions may have associated localized muscular spasm.

Imaging Plain radiographs are always obtained if a posterior column injury is suspected, especially in the young athlete. In addition to "routine" AP and lateral x-rays, bilateral oblique x-rays are essential to evaluate both the zygapophysial joints and the pars interarticularis. Yet plain radiographs have limited specificity and sensitivity such that an acute pars or joint injury may not be visualized adequately, and even more diagnostically challenging is attempting to determine if a pars interarticularis defect on plain x-ray is indeed the source of the patient's pain complaints.

Confirmation of a symptomatic pars defect can be made by single photon emission computed tomographic (SPECT) bone scan imaging (9,10) (Fig. 5-4A–C). There is at least a twofold increase in sensitivity when utilizing SPECT versus planar imaging, and the tomographic scan allows more precise identification of a posterior location. SPECT also allows visualization of other posterior element fractures, including the zygapophysial joint; however, it is sometimes difficult to distinguish between a pars injury and a zygapophysial joint injury with SPECT. A negative (normal) SPECT bone scan almost always rules out an acute posterior element fracture; however, bone scans can remain positive for many months following an injury, so these tests are not useful for assessing the degree of "healing," even in the presence of clinical recovery.

F I G U R E   **5-4**

Spondylolysis. (A) Planar bone scan imaging (coronal), normal study. SPECT bone scan imaging (coronal, posterior) (B) and axial (C), same patient, now demonstrating an abnormality of the L5 pars interarticularis (*open arrows*). (D) CT imaging (bone algorithm, 1-mm slices) demonstrating a right L5 pars fracture without separation (*closed arrows*).

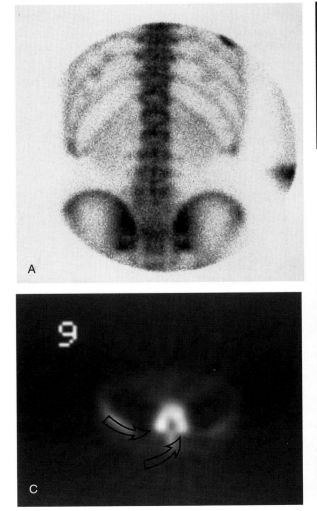

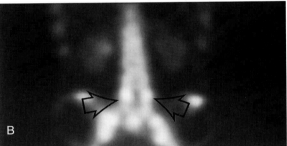

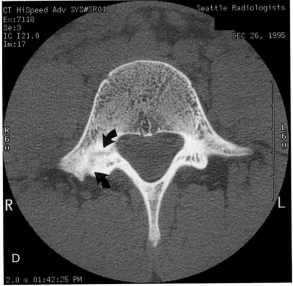

Further, the onset of a spondylolisthesis may be associated with abnormalities on SPECT anteriorly at the diskovertebral joint (11). It is debatable whether this finding is a precursor to the listhesis (i.e., internal disk derangement with the development of instability) or is secondary to the slippage. In either case, if the pars interarticularis fracture is not acute, the SPECT bone scan is not abnormal posteriorly. Limited, thin-slice (1 mm) CT utilizing a bone algorithm can be very useful in differentiating between a pars defect and a zygapophysial joint abnormality, as well as in determining the age and completeness of the pars defect, particularly if plain x-rays are equivocal. CT is especially effective in identifying a pars stress reaction (sclerotic pars without an obvious bony defect) or a defect without bony separation (see Fig. 5-4D). If the patient is less than 10 years old, standing lateral flexion and extension radiographs every 6 months through the adolescent growth spurt are indicated to monitor for the development or progression of a spondylolisthesis.

Treatment The classic treatment for an acute pars fracture as described by Steiner and Micheli has been immobilization with a Boston overlap brace in neutral degrees of lordosis 23 hours per day for a period of 6 months (12,13). However, utilizing follow-up oblique plain x-rays, true bony healing may be realized in only 18% to 32% of patients. With relative rest, pain relief is usually achieved in a much shorter period of time, from 6 to 12 weeks, without extensive rigid bracing. The most important determinant of true bony healing may be the stage of the pars abnormality at the time of presentation (14). Morita et al have demonstrated with sequential CT imaging that with limited activity and nonrigid bracing, bony union can be achieved in a large majority of patients if the pars abnormality is in the "early" stage (i.e., radiolucency without complete defect) and that even in the "progressive" stage (i.e., hairline defect or fragmentation) bony healing occurs in a large percentage if the lesion is unilateral (14). Bilateral abnormalities healed less well in both groups, but the early-stage lesions still responded better.

Frequently, healing is determined through clinical assessment alone, in order to avoid the radiation exposure. Follow-up CT scanning may be appropriate, especially if the initial study reveals an early lesion. An athlete may be kept out of competition longer if true bony healing is the goal. The degree of spondylolisthesis as determined by plain x-ray also plays a role in return to participation decision making. Greater than grade II slips (more than 50%) typically would preclude the athlete from returning to high-risk sports (e.g., gymnastics, wrestling, dance, football, pole vaulting, diving). The degree of slip and associated radicular signs and symptoms also would determine the need for surgical intervention.

Arthropathy (Zygapophysial, Uncovertebral, Costovertebral Joints)

Pathomechanics/Pathophysiology The zygapophysial, uncovertebral (present only in the cervical spine), and costovertebral joints all have pain-generating potential. The zygapophysial and costovertebral joints are innervated by the medial branch of the posterior primary rami of at least two adjacent spinal nerves. Immunohistochemical studies in animals have demonstrated the presence of both nociceptors and proprioceptors in the zygapophysial joint capsule (15–17). The uncovertebral joints are probably innervated by branches from the sinuvertebral nerve that also supply the posterior portion of the intervertebral disk. The presence and geometry of all these structures determine available segmental range of motion. In the cervical spine, the oblique orientation of the zygapophysial joints dictates that there is always coupled motion between axial rotation and lateral bending. With mechanical overload, exaggeration of coupled motion can lead to capsular strain injury, intra-articular osteochondral impaction injury, or unilateral zygapophysial dislocation, implying disruption of the joint capsule and ligamentous support structures. The uncovertebral joints, which "mature" postnatally, are present from C3 to C7, protect the intervertebral disk posterolaterally, and assist in guiding flexion and extension. The most common abnormality of these structures is degenerative arthropathy, leading to pain and/or restricted motion.

The zygapophysial joints of the thoracic spine are also oriented obliquely. The upper joints protect primarily against anterior translation, and the lower joints protect against axial rotation. Although the coupling patterns are less pronounced in the thoracic segments, joint injuries similar to those of the cervical spine can occur, except that frank joint dislocation in sports is rare. Unique to the thoracic spine is the presence of the articulating ribs. The costovertebral joint is comprised of two articulations—the head of the rib with the vertebral body at the same level and one above and the costotransverse joint, which is the articulation of the rib to the transverse process at the same level. The costovertebral and costotransverse joints and their associated ligaments serve to stiffen and strengthen the thoracic spine; however, rib and/or segmental spinal injury can alter the mechanics of these joints, resulting in pain and stiffness. True costovertebral joint dislocation is uncommon, but with capsular and/or ligamentous laxity, joint hypermobility and "subluxation" are possible.

The mechanism of injury to the lumbar zygapophysial joint is similar to that resulting in posterior element fractures (see above). Acute capsular strain injuries can result from a flexion overload injury, but repetitive extension and rotation overload can break down the articular cartilage and subchondral bone. In humans substance P receptors (a neuropeptide that mediates pain) have been identified in the subchondral bone of the zygapophysial joint (18). Although the term *facet syndrome* as it applies to the lumbar spine has been challenged (19), the finding of substance P receptors would tend to support the concept that the lumbar zygapophysial joint is a potential pain generator.

Clinical Presentation There are no physical examination findings that are pathognomonic for posterior element pain and dysfunction (20). By history, pain provocation usually occurs with movement, particularly into the posterior and posterolateral quadrants, and this often can be reproduced during the examination. Referred pain patterns are common and follow a sclerotomal distribution that has been well described (21–24). Uncovertebral joint pain also can be reproduced with motion into the lateral, posterolateral, and posterior directions. Although cervical rotation is known to occur primarily at the C1–C2 segment, restriction in rotation frequently results from uncovertebral arthropathy, which developmentally is not present rostral to C3. Costovertebral joint pathology may manifest as localized pain with trunk rotation and deep inspiration. With all the posterior column abnormalities, palpatory examination should reveal specific segmental level tenderness and possibly abnormal motion with segmental mobilization techniques (25). Radicular symptoms and signs do not occur unless, for example, joint hypertrophy causes mechanical impingement of the exiting nerve root. This would be more typical of uncovertebral arthropathy due to the close

proximity of the uncovertebral joint and the neuroforamen.

Imaging The diagnostic imaging approach for these suspected joint abnormalities is similar to that discussed for assessing fractures (see above). SPECT bone scan imaging may identify abnormal radionuclide uptake: in the cervical spine, anteriorly for uncovertebral (Fig. 5-5A and B) and posterolaterally for zygapophysial arthropathy (Fig. 5-6A and B); in the thoracic spine, posterolaterally for zygapophysial (Fig. 5-7) and costovertebral arthropathy; and in the lumbar spine, posterolaterally for zygapophysial arthropathy (Fig. 5-8A and B). A normal SPECT bone scan does not entirely rule out joint-mediated pain, but a positive scan does assist in clinical correlation. A positive scan is usually followed by a CT scan (thin cut, bone algorithm) to better define the location and severity of the abnormality (see Figs. 5-5C, 5-6C, and 5-8C). The CT scan probably should include at least one level above and below the suspected abnormal level because SPECT bone scan imaging does not allow precise spatial resolution, especially if the lesion is very abnormal with a "ballooning" effect. Although MRI can identify joint abnormalities, the definition is not nearly as clear as with CT, and SPECT and CT should be the tests of choice for this condition.

Treatment The ability of these imaging studies to identify a clinically relevant lesion also has significant implications for treatment. The use of selective injections, whether posterior element procedures (i.e., intra-articular zygapophysial joint injection, medial branch blocks, or costovertebral injection) or epidural injections for uncovertebral joint pain, depends on an accurate anatomic diagnosis for level as well as accessibility into the joint structure. Further, the injection technique should be performed under imaging control, with either fluoroscopic or CT guidance, because this minimizes technical uncertainties, provides an additional diagnostic tool (if local anesthetic is a component of the injectate), and maximizes the therapeutic potential (if corticosteroid is used).

Diskogenic (Internal Disk Disruption/ Endplate Herniation, Annular Tear Syndrome, Central Disk Herniation)

Pathomechanics/Pathophysiology It is now well accepted that at least the outer third of the intervertebral disk is innervated (26,27). The

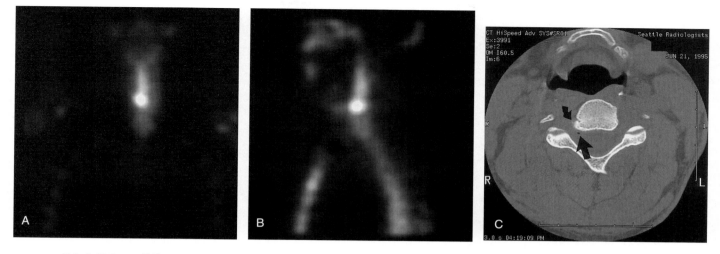

F I G U R E   **5-5**

Cervical-uncovertebral joint arthropathy. SPECT imaging (coronal, anterior) (A) and sagittal (B), demonstrating focal abnormality at the right C5–C6 level anteriorly. (C) CT imaging (bone algorithm, 1-mm slices) demonstrating right C5–C6 uncovertebral joint spurring (*curved arrow*) and small nitrogen gas bubble indicating a degenerative synovial joint (*straight arrow*).

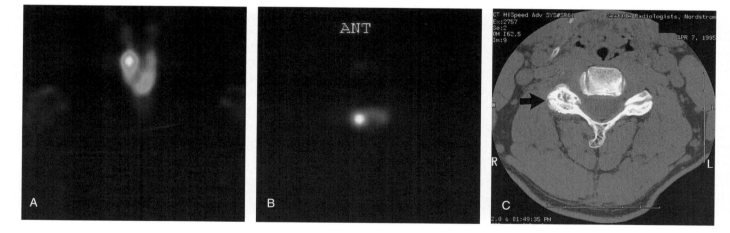

F I G U R E   **5-6**

Cervical-zygapophysial joint arthropathy. SPECT imaging (coronal, posterior) (A) and axial (B), demonstrating focal abnormality at the right C3–C4 level posterolaterally. (C) CT imaging (bone algorithm, 1-mm slices) demonstrating severe right C3–C4 zygapophysial joint arthropathy (*closed arrow*) with obliteration of the joint space, subchondral sclerosis and cyst formation, and hypertrophic changes.

sinuvertebral nerve, which contains both somatic (recurrent branch of the ventral rami) and autonomic (gray rami communicans) branches, innervates the posterior annulus fibrosus and posterior longitudinal ligament. The lateral and anterior aspects of the annulus are supplied by gray rami communicans. Both encapsulated and free nerve endings have been demonstrated in the outer annulus and posterior longitudinal ligament, suggesting both proprioceptive and nociceptive functions, respectively, the latter possibly mediated in part through substance P

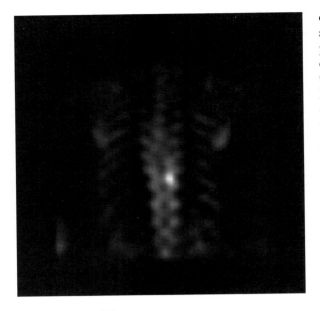

FIGURE **5-7**

Thoracic-zygapophysial joint arthropathy. SPECT imaging (coronal, posterior) demonstrating a focal abnormality at approximately the right T8–T9 level posterolaterally.

receptors (28). The vertebral endplate is not innervated, and its structure is more similar to the intervertebral disk than to the subchondral bone of the vertebral body.

There exists a continuum of intervertebral

disk pathology that may present with axial pain syndromes in the absence of radicular or myelopathic symptoms or signs, including internal disk disruption, annular tear, and central disk herniation. Degenerative disk changes are universal in humans. Although a "painless" degenerative disk can become "painful" following acute or repetitive trauma such as occurs in many sports, the pathophysiology of painful disk degeneration may still reflect changes in the annulus. In general, the lumbar disk may be more susceptible to all these conditions because of the higher loads that are borne by the lumbar spine. However, painful disk syndromes can exist throughout the spinal axis.

Internal disk disruption probably occurs secondary to an endplate injury. For example, axial load injuries such as falling onto the buttocks place the lumbar vertebral endplate at risk for fracture, allowing herniation of the nucleus pulposus into the vertebral body, the so-called acute Schmorl's node. This exposes the nuclear material to the systemic blood supply (in the highly vascularized vertebral body) and may initiate an autoimmune process ultimately leading to nuclear degradation (29). Although the endplate is not innervated, an acute inflammatory response within the vertebral body may be painful. Further, as nuclear degradation progresses, the peripheral annular fibers may deteriorate.

In general, the lumbar intervertebral disk does not tolerate rotational load well, particularly

FIGURE **5-8**

Lumbar-zygapophysial joint arthropathy. SPECT imaging (coronal, posterior) (A) and axial (B), demonstrating a focal abnormality at the left L3–L4 level posterolaterally. (C) CT (bone algorithm, 1-mm slices) demonstrating moderately severe left L3–L4 degenerative changes with joint space narrowing and periarticular hypertrophy.

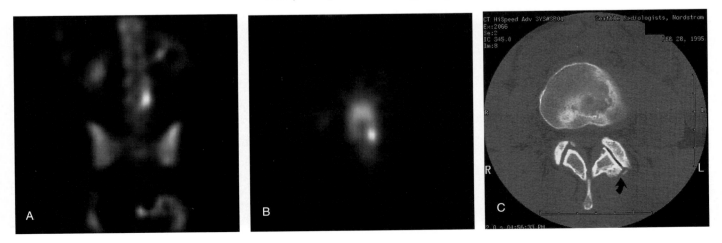

if combined with flexion postures. With greater than 3 degrees of lumbar segmental rotation, the posterior and posterolateral annulus is subject to microtrauma (30). Painful annular tear syndromes can occur in the absence of morphologic disk bulging or protrusion (31). Although the posterior longitudinal ligament is thickest posteriorly, theoretically providing greater support to the intervertebral disk, central disk bulges, protrusions, and frank herniations frequently occur. The central location typically spares the exiting nerve roots, and unless the herniation is very large or the spinal canal is relatively small, neurologic symptoms and signs are unusual.

Painful cervical disk abnormalities also occur, probably from the same common denominator of an annular tear or deterioration. In general, the cervical spine is subject to less absolute load; however, in collision sports, there is clearly a higher risk of acute overload to the cervical intervertebral disk resulting in neurologic injury (see the sections on Myelopathic and Radiculopathic Syndromes, later). The cervical spine is geometrically designed to tolerate greater physiologic range of motion than the rest of the spinal axis, especially rotation, due to the relatively greater height-diameter ratio of the cervical disk as compared with the rest of the spinal axis, the anteriorly located nucleus pulposus, the presence of the supporting uncovertebral joints (see above), and the well-developed posterior longitudinal ligament, which reduces the risk of central disk ruptures, thereby protecting the spinal cord.

Less is presently known about the thoracic intervertebral disk pathomechanics than about the rest of the spinal axis. The presence of the rib cage essentially stiffens and strengthens the thoracic spine. However, painful endplate herniations can occur from the same axial overload mechanism as occurs in the lumbar spine. The thoracic spine is subject to different biomechanical stresses than the lumbar spine, which may explain the fewer number of traumatic thoracic disk herniations. The thoracic disk is better supported posteriorly by a more robust posterior longitudinal ligament, so the subset of central disk abnormalities is also less commonly seen as compared with those of the lumbar spine.

Clinical Presentation By definition, athletes with these painful disk conditions present with localized spinal pain ranging in severity from mild to severe. The mechanism of injury is usually a fall onto the buttocks or a flexion and/or rotation injury. Although not pathognomonic, an annular tear may be suspected if a popping or tearing sensation is felt or heard. Similar to posterior element injuries, sclerotomal pain referral patterns do occur frequently (e.g., cervical disk abnormalities presenting with interscapular pain and shoulder girdle pain and lumbar disk abnormalities presenting with hip girdle pain). Physical examination findings may be misleading. In the lumbar spine, for example, depending on the acuteness of the injury, repetitive forward bending may be necessary to "load" the disk enough to provoke symptoms from an internally disrupted disk or annular tear. Symptoms stemming from a central disk protrusion or herniation and sometimes an annular tear may be worsened by trunk extension and relieved by forward bending. This seems especially true in the young athlete. Trunkal shifts are less common due to the central nature of these abnormalities. Manual examination may reveal a segmental level of focal tenderness as well as more generalized myofascial tenderness and spasm. Dural tension testing and neurologic examination are normal, although there may be significant hamstring tightness.

Imaging Modern imaging technology has indicated that subclinical intervertebral disk morphologic changes occur frequently (32–35). This implies that injuries resulting in clinical symptoms usually do not occur to a previously "normal" disk. Additionally, this fact presents a great challenge to the sports physician to determine the relevance of any abnormality visualized on imaging studies. As a result, clinical correlation between the mechanism of injury, clinical symptoms and signs, and the imaging tests is critical.

MRI is clearly the test of first choice when evaluating any of the aforementioned disk abnormalities. This imaging modality is the only noninvasive method to assess the internal architecture of the intervertebral disk. CT scanning, with or without contrast enhancement, fails to visualize the "inside" of the disk. Internal disk disruption has been most studied in the lumbar spine, and the typical MRI findings may include decreased signal intensity from the nucleus pulposus on T2-weighted sequences (36) (Fig. 5-9A), disruption of the vertebral endplate with an endplate herniation (Fig. 5-10A and B) (if acute, there is an increased T2-weighted signal intensity pattern surrounding the herniation, indicating edema), and the presence of high-signal-intensity zones in the posterior or pos-

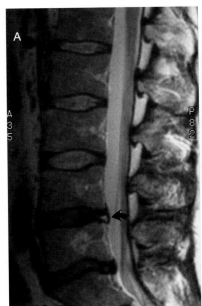

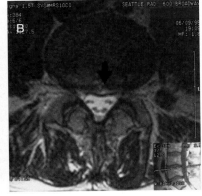

FIGURE 5-9

MRI of the high-signal-intensity zone (HSIZ) from the L4–L5 intervertebral disk. On sagittal (A) and axial (B) T2-weighted images, increased signal is seen in the posterior annulus (*closed arrows*).

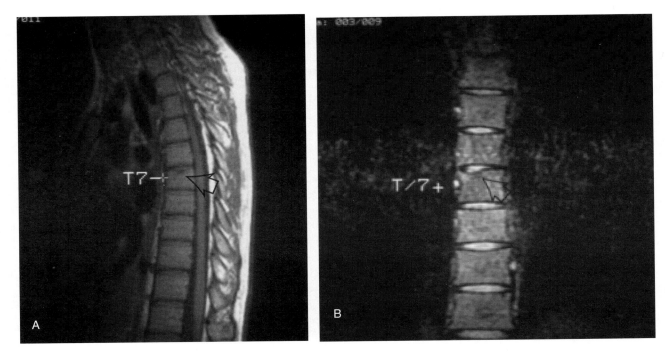

FIGURE 5-10

MRI of a thoracic endplate herniation, T7 vertebral body. On sagittal T1-weighted (A) and coronal inversion recovery (B) images, a focal right-sided T6–T7 disk protrusion is seen into the superior endplate of T7.

terolateral annulus suggesting radial annular tears on both sagittal and axial T2-weighted images (37) (see Fig. 5-9A and B).

This high-signal-intensity zone may be very sensitive and specific in regard to predicting a clinically painful disk; however, provocative diskography-CT theoretically should identify all painful annular tears (38–40). This test, however, is both controversial and not benign, with an incidence of postprocedure diskitis of up to

4%. The controversy relates to the validity of the procedure in that there exists the potential for significant examiner bias and, more important, the surgical ramifications of a "positive" result (see below). Although SPECT bone scan imaging also will identify an acute endplate herniation, it will not assess the intervertebral disk per se, so a specific diagnosis of internal disk disruption cannot be made by bone scan alone. Nevertheless, a positive SPECT scan may support an equivocal MRI in the appropriate clinical setting.

MRI is also an ideal test for evaluating a central disk protrusion or herniation (Figs. 5-11 and 5-12). The benefits of MRI versus CT are that the former is not an ionizing radiation test, it visualizes all of the lumbar disks, it provides a much clearer distinction between the posterior disk margin and the thecal sac, it allows better visualization of the spinal cord and conus, and it provides a clearer differentiation between the thecal sac and the epidural venous plexus. CT imaging of the cervical intervertebral disk is particularly difficult to interpret. Contrast-enhanced CT and diskography-CT (Fig. 5-13) usually will identify a central disk abnormality anywhere in the spinal axis, but it is an invasive procedure.

Treatment Although low back pain is considered a self-limited process, these painful disk conditions may in fact last many months to years. In general, disk-related spinal pain without radicular involvement is probably a more difficult clinical entity to treat definitively than even severe radiculopathy. In many instances, treatment for any of these conditions can progress without any diagnostic imaging if the health care provider is confident in his or her diagnosis or at least that the patient's condition is not worsening. The reasons for obtaining any of the above-mentioned studies would be lack of progress with treatment and need for alternative treatment approaches. This could include rigid bracing (in the lumbar spine), selective spinal injection (i.e., epidural steroid injection), and/or surgical consultation. A fluoroscopically guided epidural steroid injection performed at the level of pathology has the greatest chance of effectiveness; therefore, MRI would be appropriate to plan this intervention. Provocative diskography is often done only if a "positive" result would lead to a surgical recommendation, which would necessarily imply a fusion procedure (41). The pain provoked by diskography may be concordant or nonconcordant with the patient's usual pain pattern. Theoretically, leaving a nonconcordantly painful disk out of the fusion construct may lead to a failed surgery syndrome. Further, since multilevel fusions are less desirable than single-level procedures, provocative diskography may in fact

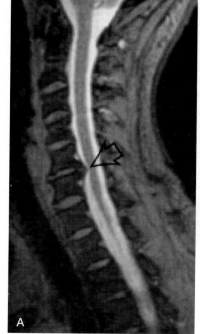

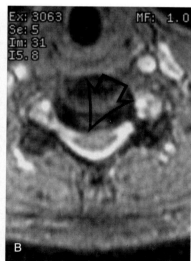

FIGURE **5-11**

MRI of a C5–C6 central disk herniation. On sagittal (A) and axial (B) T2-weighted images, a focal small central disk herniation (with associated endplate ridges) is seen that partially effaces the subarachnoid space anterior to the spinal cord (*open arrows*).

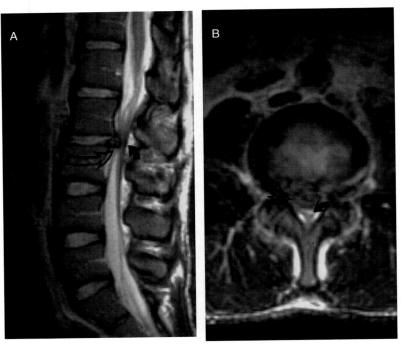

FIGURE 5-12

MRI of a L2–L3 central disk herniation. On sagittal (A) and axial (B) T2-weighted images, a very large central disk herniation (*open arrows*) is seen that markedly compresses the thecal sac (*closed arrows*).

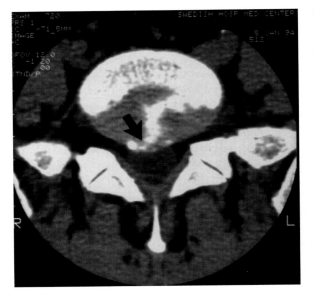

FIGURE 5-13

Postdiskogram CT, central disk herniation at the L5–S1 level. Contrast dye leakage is demonstrated centrally and right paracentrally (*closed arrow*).

be more useful in determining who is not a surgical fusion candidate. Diskectomy procedures in this diagnostic group typically do not provide a successful resolution of pain.

Myelopathic Syndromes

Transient Quadriplegia and Cervical Spinal Stenosis

Pathomechanics/Pathophysiology

Certain activities or positions in sports are at increased risk for producing a cervical spine injury, including tackling in football, takedown in wrestling, checking into the boards in hockey, soccer goalie, head-first slide in baseball, dismount in gymnastics, landing in pole vaulting, and diving. Intentional "spearing" (using the head as a weapon) has been outlawed from all levels of football, thus reducing the incidence of catastrophic spinal cord injury.

The most common spinal injury resulting in cervical spinal cord damage is fracture-dislocation. This injury results from an axial load mechanism in which the cervical spine is slightly flexed forward at the time of impact of the top of the head with the opponent's body or the ground. The resulting straightening of the cervical lordosis causes the spine to act as a segmented column, eliminating the effectiveness of the cervical musculature in absorbing the force of the impact (42). The cervical vertebrae are sandwiched between deceleration forces from the head striking a solid object and acceleration forces from the momentum of the body, which continues forward. At maximum compressive deformation, angular deformation and buckling occur. Typically, the anterior column is compressed and the posterior column is distracted, leading to an unstable fracture-dislocation.

Other mechanisms of spinal cord injury include hyperflexion, in which the posterior aspect of the intervertebral disk is subjected to excessive distraction forces with rupture of the annulus and subsequent disk herniation into the spinal canal; hyperextension, in which the posterior elements may fracture due to excessive compressive force with impingement within the spinal canal by a fragment of bone; and hyperextension without fracture but in the presence of congenital or acquired central spinal stenosis. Acquired spinal stenosis may occur from ligamentum flavum hypertrophy, a central disk protrusion, or bony osteophytes (i.e., posterior bony bar).

Additionally, physiologic cervical spinal extension results in ligamentum flavum buckling with the potential for indentation of the cervical spinal cord, narrowing of the AP diameter of the central spinal canal by up to 2 mm, and potential for compression of the spinal cord between the vertebral body and the most proximate portion of the spinolaminar line to the inferior vertebrae—the so-called pincers effect (43).

The spinal cord and its surrounding neural tissues are relatively resilient to tensile load. Within normal cervical flexion and extension range of motion, the spinal cord is not subjected to increased force because of folding and unfolding of redundant neural tissue (accounting for 75% of the range of motion) or reversible elastic deformation of neural tissue (accounting for 25% of the range of motion) (44). The spinal cord is certainly at risk with compression, as described above. Various degrees of myelopathy can result, ranging from a neurapraxic lesion such as transient quadriparesis, to spinal cord contusion, and finally, to more permanent neurologic dysfunction such as a central cord syndrome or complete quadriplegia.

Clinical Presentation

In the acute setting (e.g., on the field), it is critical to differentiate spinal cord injury from other peripheral nerve injuries such as a "burner" or "stinger" (see the section on Radiculopathic Syndromes, later). The hallmark of spinal cord injury is the involvement of two or more limbs. Various presentations may occur from complete motor and sensory loss below the injured spinal segmental level to incomplete motor and sensory symptoms only. The term *transient quadriparesis/quadriplegia* globally refers to the entire range of transient myelopathy, but its time course is strictly defined as less than 23 hours, by which time all motor and/or sensory dysfunction has cleared. However, neck pain and rigidity usually continue beyond the cessation of neurologic symptoms, especially if significant ligamentous and/or bony injury has taken place.

The incomplete sensory symptoms are often dysesthetic or paresthetic in nature. Preferential motor and/or sensory impairment of the upper as compared with the lower extremities reflects the topographic orientation of these respective axons within the cervical spinal cord. The upper extremity fibers are located most medially and are most susceptible to spinal cord edema (or hemorrhage), resulting in the typical central cord syndrome. This syndrome sometimes will manifest only with burning hands (45) and must not be confused with a "burner," which always will present unilaterally.

Imaging

With any athlete presenting with spinal cord symptoms or signs due to forceful contact or collision, a fracture-dislocation must be ruled out. Once the athlete presents to the emergency room, presumably transported with full cervical spine precautions, a lateral cervical spine x-ray is obtained; helmets are *not* removed prior to the initial x-ray (46). If no obvious instability is identified, the helmet is carefully removed, and a full series of static cervical x-rays is obtained, including AP, lateral, open mouth, and oblique views; however, static x-rays alone are inadequate to evaluate for occult instability, and depending on the athlete's neurologic status, lateral flexion-extension x-rays are performed. If neurologic signs and symptoms persist, then dynamic radiographic assessment is postponed, but it must be completed once the athlete's neurologic status has stabilized. At this point, advanced imaging techniques such as MRI and/or contrast-enhanced CT should be done to assess for spinal canal compromise by disk and/or bone, especially in the presence of myelopathy.

The presence or absence of spinal stenosis has a direct bearing on prognosis and return-to-play decisions. However, the definition and appropriate imaging of spinal stenosis are controversial. The bony dimensions of the cervical spinal canal can be determined by direct assessment from a lateral cervical spine x-ray with known magnification or from CT. Absolute canal diameter of less than 12 mm from C3 to C7 is considered abnormal and indicative of spinal stenosis, whereas measurements greater than 15 mm are normal. The *Torg ratio* has been described to indirectly assess for spinal stenosis on plain cervical spine x-rays when the magnification is unknown (47) (Fig. 5-14). The numerator of the ratio is the diameter of the spinal canal from the posterior margin of the vertebral body to the nearest point on the corresponding spinolaminar line, and the denominator is the width of vertebral body. According to Torg et al, a ratio of less than 0.8 is considered positive for the presence of spinal stenosis.

There are two significant limitations to use of the Torg ratio in determining the presence or absence of spinal stenosis. First, in general, athletes tend to have larger vertebral bodies than the average person, so the Torg ratio is skewed toward the diagnosis of spinal stenosis (i.e., ratio < 0.8). Although the Torg ratio is very sensitive (i.e., true bony spinal stenosis usually yields a Torg ratio of less than 0.8), it is not very specific (i.e., it has a high number of false-positive results), with a positive predictive value for true spinal stenosis of only 13% in professional football players (48). This is due in part to the

fact that Torg's controls were not athletes and did not have greater than average-sized vertebral bodies. Second, the ratio does not reflect the variable anatomic relationship of the neural tissue contents of the spinal canal (i.e., spinal cord and cerebrospinal fluid) to the bony canal. Even with a bony canal that measures 12 mm or less, the spinal cord may be small enough that it is neither deformed or compressed nor is the cerebrospinal fluid (CSF) cushion around the cord compromised. This could only be assessed by MRI or contrast-enhanced CT and would essentially rule out "functional" spinal stenosis (49) (Fig. 5-15).

Therefore, a more practical definition of spinal stenosis may be based on the functional reserve of the spinal canal, which is an assessment of the amount of CSF around the spinal cord and the shape of the spinal cord, which can only be measured by MRI or contrast-positive CT imaging (50,51). Although screening cervical spine x-rays are not presently recommended (52), x-rays that have been done previously revealing a magnification-corrected canal height of 12 mm or less or an abnormal Torg ratio should not be ignored and require further investigation for functional spinal stenosis (Cantu RC, personal communication, 1995).

FIGURE **5-14**

Torg ratio, an indirect assessment of cervical spinal stenosis. The ratio of the spinal canal to the vertebral body is the distance from the midpoint of the posterior aspect of the vertebral body to the nearest point on the corresponding spinolaminar line (*a*) divided by the anteroposterior width of the vertebral body (*b*). (Reprinted by permission of the publisher from Torg JS, et al. Neurapraxia of the cervical spinal cord with transient quadriplegia. J Bone Joint Surg 1986;68A:1354–1370.)

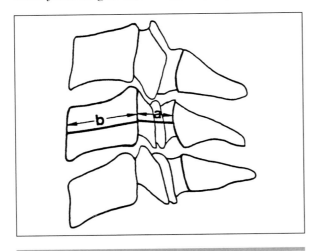

Treatment

In this discussion, the term *treatment* will be directed toward return-to-play considerations following spinal cord injury. There is no question that any degree of permanent myelopathy is an absolute contraindication to return to play, whether caused by a fracture-dislocation, spinal stenosis, or an unclear mechanism of injury. However, when reviewing return-to-play criteria following an episode of transient quadriplegia, there appears to be two divergent opinions. Torg has stated that a single episode of transient quadriplegia, in the absence of instability or spinal cord compression, does not forbode a future occurrence of permanent spinal cord injury, although it may lead to another episode of transient quadriplegia (52,53). Further, Torg has concluded that the presence of spinal stenosis, as determined by the ratio method, does not predispose an athlete to permanent myelopathy, even with a previous history of transient quadriplegia, and that tackling technique may be the most important determinant of future spinal cord injury (54). As shown previously, however, the Torg ratio, when applied to the professional

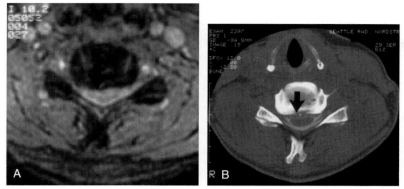

F I G U R E **5-15**

Functional spinal stenosis at the C5–C6 level. MRI (A) (axial T2-weighted, volume acquisition) and contrast-enhanced CT scan (B) demonstrating spinal canal narrowing in the AP plane to 8 to 9 mm, loss of CSF around the spinal cord, and deformation of the right half of the spinal cord due to posterior vertebral body osteophytes (*closed arrows*).

football population, significantly overestimates the presence of spinal stenosis, so Torg's conclusions that spinal stenosis does not predispose to future permanent spinal cord injury may not be valid.

Cantu agrees with Torg in that there is no evidence to suggest that one episode of transient quadriplegia in the absence of functional spinal stenosis will lead to permanent spinal cord injury and that there may be an increased risk of another episode of transient quadriparesis or quadriplegia; however, he has contrarily concluded that an athlete with a history of one episode transient quadriplegia is at risk for future permanent spinal cord injury, with or without fracture-dislocation, if an appropriate workup reveals functional spinal stenosis (49,50). In fact, both Torg and Cantu seem to agree that spinal stenosis, as judged by spinal cord deformation or compression, in a player who has sustained transient spinal myelopathy is an absolute contraindication to return to contact or collision sports. Further, there is consensus that not all athletes with Torg ratios of less than 0.8 should be restricted from contact or collision sports. Undoubtedly, many individual factors, including socioeconomic ones, contribute to the decision-making process regarding return to play. In every situation, athletes should be fully informed of their relative risk of further catastrophic injury based on their history, physical examination, and state-of-the-art imaging studies.

Radiculopathic Syndromes

Pathomechanics/Pathophysiology

The pathomechanics of sports-related radiculopathy are different in the cervical and lumbar spine. Thoracic radiculopathy is unusual in the athletic and general population and will not be discussed in this chapter. For the purposes of definition, *radiculopathy* will be used to describe radicular pain in a dermatomal distribution and/or neurologic symptoms (i.e., numbness or paresthesias) or signs (i.e., weakness in a myotomal distribution). Both of these require the presence of an anatomic defect that corresponds to the clinical presentation. The term *radiculitis* reflects radicular pain and/or radicular symptoms or signs in the absence of an obvious corresponding anatomic abnormality.

Cervical

In the cervical spine, the primary mechanism resulting in cervical radiculopathy is dynamic neuroforaminal encroachment (55). Movement of the neck into an extended and rotated posture, either from chronic repetitive activity or from an acute overload, can result in compressive neuropathy of the cervical nerve root–spinal nerve complex. The former is encountered in sports such as tennis (i.e., overhead shot and serve), and the latter is commonly encountered in collision sports such as football (i.e., tackling). The injury known as a *stinger* probably reflects cervical radiculopathy, especially in the more experienced athlete (55,56). Although the stinger has been purported to be a brachial plexus injury (57), a review of neuroanatomic features of the cervical nerve root–spinal nerve complex suggests that even in less experienced athletes (i.e., athletes with less neck strength), in whom the mechanism of the stinger is contralateral flexion, it is the C5 through C7 nerve root–spinal nerve complex that is more susceptible than the brachial plexus to tensile overload (58). Underlying degenerative changes such as uncovertebral or zygapophysial joint arthropathy narrows the intervertebral foramen and may predispose the athlete to radicular injury with movement of the neck into the posterolateral quadrants. As a rule, significant degenerative changes are restricted to the senior athlete. Cervical disk herniations are a less common cause of cervical radiculopathy in the athlete, but they certainly need to be considered, especially if significant motor dysfunction is present. The pathophysiology of weakness may include radicular compression as well as ischemia. Primary nerve root tumors also must be considered in the differential diagnosis of radiculopathy, and although there is no "mechanism" of injury, the onset of symptoms may be coincident with a spinal injury.

Lumbar

Lumbar radiculopathy is much more commonly due to disk herniation [i.e., a focal extension of disk beyond the vertebral endplate, including a disk protrusion (contained by the outer annulus fibrosus with intact posterior longitudinal ligament), a disk extrusion (noncontained), or a sequestered free fragment (no longer in contact with the parent disk)] or in some cases a disk bulge (i.e., a nonfocal or circumferential, symmetric extension of disk beyond the margin of the vertebral endplates) superimposed on a congenitally small spinal canal. A healthy lumbar disk is tolerant of compressive load but much less tolerant of shear. In particular, the annulus fibrosus can tear with excessive rotational shear. The lumbar motion segment is protected against excessive rotation by the geometry of the zygapophysial joints, except in forward flexion. The combined motion of flexion and rotation occurs commonly in sports, placing the disk at risk. Disk herniations usually occur following an acute event; however, chronic subclinical annular disruption typically leads to this final presentation. Most often lumbar disks herniate posterolaterally, where the posterior longitudinal ligament is thinnest. Central disk herniations do occur, but radiculopathy secondary to this is not common unless the spinal canal is small. Lateral (i.e., foraminal or extraforaminal) disk herniations are least common. Significant degenerative lumbar changes, more common in the senior athlete, also can result in compressive lumbar radiculopathy due to lateral recess or foraminal stenosis. Lumbar radiculitis is noncompressive nerve root dysfunction explained by the now well-accepted biochemical mediators (i.e., enzymes and neuropeptides) of pain and inflammation that exist in the nucleus pulposus and dorsal root ganglion (59,60). However, "pseudoradicular" patterns may occur secondary to myofascial pain syndromes and trigger points in the posterior hip girdle musculature. As with the cervical spine, nerve root tumors also should be considered.

Clinical Presentation

By definition, cervical radiculopathy presents with unilateral upper extremity involvement, and lumbar radiculopathy typically presents with only one lower extremity affected; however, central disk herniations and central lumbar spinal stenoses may present with bilateral lower extremity symptoms and/or signs. As stated in the section, Myelopathic Syndromes, bilateral upper extremity symptoms following a forceful cervical spine injury suggest spinal cord compromise. Similarly, bilateral lower extremity symptoms should lead one to consider more serious abnormalities, including a very large central disk herniation, severe spinal stenosis, or other space-occupying lesions such as a tumor.

In the cervical spine, a stinger most commonly affects the fifth, sixth, or seventh nerve root. Multilevel involvement is very rare. Occasionally, pain is the only presenting complaint, and without a dermatomal or myotomal distribution of symptoms, an exact segmental level of injury is difficult to determine. The duration of symptoms varies from seconds to hours, and persistent neurologic signs, almost always weakness, may remain for weeks or longer depending on the severity of nerve root injury (58).

The most commonly affected lumbar nerve roots are L5 and S1, which is reflective of the frequent involvement of the L4–L5 and L5–S1 intervertebral disks or lateral recess stenosis, respectively. Radicular pain from disk herniations usually is made worse by flexion-oriented activities; however, nerve root impingement in the lateral recess (usually by a disk extrusion or sequestered fragment) may present with symptoms aggravated by extension positions and postures. Foraminal stenosis or a lateral disk herniation at the L5–S1 level will impinge the L5 nerve root–spinal nerve complex and the L4 nerve root at the L4–L5 level. Both stenosis and lateral disk herniations present with similar symptoms, namely, pain worsened by lumbar extension postures. As with cervical radiculopathy, a wide variety and severity of symptoms and signs may occur, from lower extremity pain only to myotomal weakness only. The presence of bladder and/or bowel control dysfunction, suggestive of a cauda equina syndrome, is highly unusual but indicates an emergency situation.

Imaging

Early imaging of radiculopathy is not necessary if the following conditions are met: The athlete is young and otherwise healthy; the mechanism of injury is consistent with a radicular injury; the clinical presentation suggests single-level involvement; the neurologic status is not worsening; and the pain is not incapacitating. Nevertheless, the athlete is often managed more aggressively than the average person, especially at the elite level, such that imaging evaluation is often obtained soon after injury. The results of such testing may assist with diagnosis, treatment, prognosis, and return-to-play decisions. Imaging studies usually are obtained if the clinical picture is unclear or not improving.

The test of choice when evaluating for a disk herniation as the cause of radiculopathy is the MRI (Figs. 5-16 and 5-17). This includes central, posterolateral, and lateral disk herniations. Depending on the quality of the MRI, which includes the strength of the magnet as well as the software package, the MRI also may assist with the assessment of uncovertebral and foraminal stenoses as etiologies of cervical or lumbar

radiculopathies. The MRI also will assess for annular tears, as evidenced by a high-signal-intensity zone on T2-weighted image (see the section on Axial Pain Syndromes, Diskogenic), which may help to explain lumbar radiculitis. However, it is not possible to determine whether an annular tear is acute or chronic, since a chronic tear containing granulation tissue also demonstrates high T2-weighted signal intensity. An annular disruption potentially allows intradiskal neuroirritative substances to cause an inflammatory process about the nerve root in the absence of a compressive lesion. MRI is also the ideal imaging tool to evaluate for more unusual causes of radiculopathy, including spinal nerve tumors such as a neurofibroma (Fig. 5-18). Occasionally, a far lateral lumbar disk herniation may not be well visualized by MRI, and a lumbar diskogram with postdiskogram CT is required to demonstrate this (61). If lumbar spinal stenosis is clinically suspected, particularly in the senior athlete, a lumbar myelogram with postmyelogram CT scan may be the test of choice because bony detail will be better defined than with MRI (Fig. 5-19). Myelography and nonenhanced CT alone are ineffective in properly evaluating for spinal stenosis.

For the diagnosis of cervical and lumbar radiculopathy, the sensitivity and specificity of plain radiographs are widely accepted as low. One observational study of collegiate football players, however, reported a threefold greater

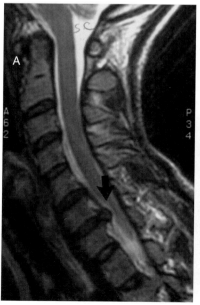
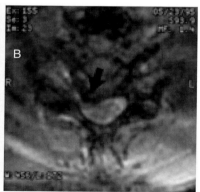

FIGURE **5-16**

MRI of a cervical disk herniation at the C6–C7 level. On sagittal (A) and axial (B) T2-weighted images, a large focal right-sided disk herniation is seen impeding the exiting C7 nerve root and deforming the lateral aspect of the spinal cord (*closed arrows*).

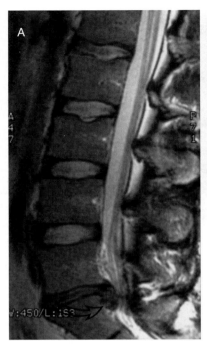

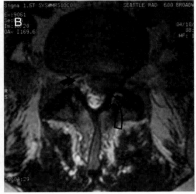

F I G U R E   **5-17**

MRI of a lumbar disk herniation at the L5–S1 level. On sagittal (A) and axial (B) T2-weighted images, a large focal left-sided herniation (*open arrows*) with a probable free fragment is seen effacing the exiting S1 nerve root. The right S1 nerve root is unimpeded (*closed arrow*).

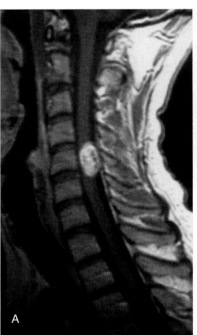

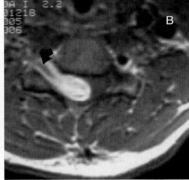

F I G U R E   **5-18**

MRI of a C6 neurofibroma. Gadolinium-enhanced sagittal (A) and axial (B) images demonstrating a large enhancing lesion in the C5–C6 neuroforamen encompassing the exiting right C6 nerve root, seen as a dark linear structure within the enhancing lesion on axial view (*closed arrow*).

likelihood of sustaining a stinger if a preparticipation lateral cervical x-ray demonstrated a Torg ratio of less than 0.8 (see section on Myelopathic Syndromes) (62). The conclusion of this study was that spinal stenosis (as determined by the Torg ratio) predisposes an athlete to sustain a stinger. Although it is intriguing to consider that a relatively simple test (i.e., lateral cervical radiograph) might allow intervention to prevent this potentially serious injury, the pathomechanical/pathoanatomic correlate is unclear. The Torg ratio, as previously discussed, was designed to assess central spinal stenosis, not foraminal stenosis. Further, the absolute values of cervical

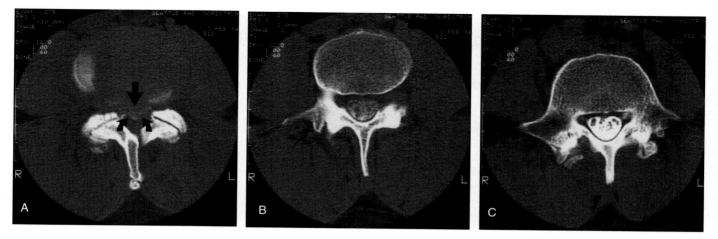

F I G U R E   5-19

Lumbar spinal stenosis, L4–L5 level. Postmyelogram CT images (bone algorithm, 3-mm slices) highlight the marked spinal stenosis at L4–L5 (due primarily to zygapophysial joint and ligamentum flavum hypertrophy) with a trace of contrast material within the thecal sac (A, *closed arrows*) and a normal amount of contrast material within the sac above (B) and below (C) the L5 level.

central diameters were not significantly different in the stinger versus control groups.

Treatment

Treatment may or may not be influenced by the results of the imaging studies. As stated earlier, disk abnormalities, including disk bulges and herniations, are found commonly in asymptomatic people, so clinical correlation is extremely important. It is worth noting, however, that Jensen et al found a very limited number of disk extrusions or free fragments by MRI in an asymptomatic population (35). Certainly, if surgery is being contemplated, a clear anatomic diagnosis is absolutely critical. However, surgery for neurologically stable or improving radiculopathy is not indicated except for pain control and possibly earlier return to play. Overall, the natural history of disk herniations is favorable, and neurologic impairment, even profound weakness, can and often does improve spontaneously. Imaging studies may allow appropriate placement of injectable corticosteroids such as epidural injections if this is being considered as a possible treatment option.

REFERENCES

1. Fibrosus D, Gdalia A, Galil A, et al. Diskitis in children. Contemp Orthop 1992;25:493–497.

2. Osti OL, Fraser RD, Vernon-Roberts B. Diskitis after diskography: the role of prophylactic antibiotics. J Bone Joint Surg 1990;72B:271–274.

3. Sherman MS, McFarland G Jr. Mechanism of pain in osteoid osteoma. South Med J 1965;58:163–166.

4. Lawrie TR, Aterman K, Sinclair AM. Painless osteoid osteoma: a report of two cases. J Bone Joint Surg 1970;52A:1357–1363.

5. Freiberger RH. Osteoid osteoma of the spine: a cause of backache and scoliosis in children and young adults. Radiology 1960;75:232–235.

6. Gertzbein SD. Spine update: classification of thoracic and lumbar fractures. Spine 1994;19:626–628.

7. White AA, Panjabi MM. Clinical biomechanics of the spine. 2nd ed. Philadelphia: JB Lippincott, 1990:215–216.

8. Bogduk N, Twomey LT. Clinical anatomy of the lumbar spine. 2nd ed. Melbourne: Churchill-Livingstone, 1991:164.

9. Collier BD, Johnson RP, Carrera GF, et al. Painful spondylolysis or spondylolisthesis studied by radiography and single photon emission computed tomography. Radiology 1985;154:207–211.

10. Bodner RJ, Heyman S, Drummond DS, Gregg JR. The use of single photon emission computed tomography (SPECT) in the diagnosis of low-back

pain in young patients. Spine 1988;13:1155–1160.

11. Lusins JO, Elting JJ, Cicoria AD, Goldsmith SJ. SPECT evaluation of lumbar spondylolysis and spondylolisthesis. Spine 1994;19:608–612.

12. Steiner ME, Micheli LJ. Treatment of spondylolysis and spondylolisthesis with the modified boston brace. Spine 1985;10:937–943.

13. Micheli LJ. Back injuries in gymnastics. Clin Sports Med 1985;4:85–93.

14. Morita T, Ikata T, Katoh S, Miyake R. Lumbar spondylolysis in children and adolescents. J Bone Joint Surg 1995;77B:620–625.

15. Yamashita T, Cavanaugh JM, El-Bohy AA, et al. Mechanosensitive afferent units in lumbar facet joint. J Bone Joint Surg 1990;72A:865–870.

16. Giles LG, Harvey AR. Immunohistochemical demonstration of nociceptors in the capsule and synovial folds of human zygapophyseal joints. Br J Rheumatol 1987;26:362–364.

17. Ashton IK, Ashton BA, Gibson SJ, et al. Morphological basis for back pain: the demonstration of nerve fibers and neuropeptides in the lumbar facet joint capsule but not in the ligamentum flavum. J Orthop Res 1992;10:72–78.

18. Beaman DN, Graziano GP, Glover RA, et al. Substance P innervation of lumbar spine facet joints. Spine 1993;18:1044–1049.

19. Carette S, Marcoux S, Truchon R, et al. A controlled trial of corticosteroid injections into the facet joints for chronic low back pain. N Engl J Med 1991;325:1002–1007.

20. Schwarzer AC, Aprill CN, Derby R, et al. Clinical features of patients with pain stemming from the lumbar zygapophysial joint: is the lumbar facet syndrome a clinical entity? Spine 1994;19:1132–1137.

21. Dwyer A, Aprill C, Bogduk N. Cervical zygapophysial joint pain patterns: I. A study in normal volunteers. Spine 1990;15:453–457.

22. Aprill C, Dwyer A, Bogduk N. Cervical zygapophysial joint pain patterns: II. A clinical correlation. Spine 1990;15:458–461.

23. Dreyfuss P, Tibiletti C, Dreyer S. Thoracic zygapophysial joint pain patterns: a study in normal volunteers. Spine 1994;19:807–811.

24. McCall IW, Park WM, O'Brien JP. Induced pain referral from posterior lumbar elements in normal subjects. Spine 1979;4:441–446.

25. Maitland GD. Vertebral manipulation. 5th ed. London: Butterworth, 1986:171–281.

26. Bogduk N, Windsor M, Inglis A. The innervation of the cervical intervertebral disk. Spine 1988;13:2–8.

27. Bogduk N, Twomey LT. Clinical anatomy of the lumbar spine. 2nd ed. Melbourne: Churchill-Livingstone, 1991:116–120.

28. Korkala O, Gronblad M, Liesi P, Karaharju E. Immunohistochemical demonstration of nociceptors in the ligamentous structures of the lumbar spine. Spine 1985;10:156–157.

29. Gertzbein SD. Degenerative disk disease of the lumbar spine: immunological implications. Clin Orthop 1971;129:68–71.

30. Farfan HF, Cossette JW, Robertson GH, et al. The effects of torsion on the lumbar intervertebral joints: the role of torsion in the production of disc degeneration. J Bone Joint Surg 1970;72A:468–497.

31. Moneta GB, Videman T, Kaivanto K, et al. Reported pain during lumbar discography as a function of anular ruptures and disc degeneration: a reanalysis of 833 discograms. Spine 1994;19:1968–1974.

32. Boden SD, Davis DO, Dina TS, et al. Abnormal magnetic resonance scans of the lumbar spine in asymptomatic subjects: a prospective investigation. J Bone Joint Surg 1990;72A:403–408.

33. Boden SD, McCowin PR, Davis DO, et al. Abnormal magnetic resonance scans of the cervical spine in asymptomatic subjects. J Bone Joint Surg 1990;72A:1178–1184.

34. Wiesel SW, Tsourmas N, Feffer HL, et al. A study of computer-assisted tomography: I. The incidence of positive CAT scans in an asymptomatic group of patients. Spine 1984;9:549–551.

35. Jensen MC, Brant-Zawadzki MN, Obuchowski N, et al. Magnetic resonance imaging of the lumbar spine in people without back pain. N Engl J Med 1994;331:69–73.

36. Panagiotacopulos ND, Pope MH, Krag MH, Block R. Water content in human intervertebral disks: I. Measurements by magnetic resonance imaging. Spine 1987;12:912–917.

37. Aprill C, Bogduk N. High-intensity zone: a diagnostic sign of painful lumbar disk on magnetic resonance imaging. Br J Radiol 1992;65:361–369.

38. Horton WC, Daftari TK. Which disk as visualized by magnetic resonance imaging is actually a

source of pain? A correlation between magnetic resonance imaging and discography. Spine 1992; 17:S164–S171.

39. Parfenchuck TA, Janssen ME. A correlation of cervical magnetic resonance imaging and diskography/computed tomographic diskograms. Spine 1994;19:2819–2825.

40. Schellhas KP, Pollei SR, Dorwart RH. Thoracic diskography: a safe and reliable technique. Spine 1994;19:2103–2109.

41. Colhoun E, McCall IW, Williams L, Pullicino VNC. Provocation diskography as a guide to planning operations of the spine. J Bone Joint Surg 1988; 70B:267–271.

42. Torg JS, Vegso JJ, O'Neill MJ, Sennett B. The epidemiologic, pathogenic, biomechanical, and cinematographic analysis of football-induced cervical spine trauma. Am J Sports Med 1990;18: 50–57.

43. Penning L. Some aspects of plain radiography of the cervical spine in chronic myelopathy. Neurology 1962;12:513–519.

44. Breig A. Biomechanics of the central nervous system: some basic normal and pathological phenomena. Stockholm: Almquist and Wiskell, 1960.

45. Maroon JC. "Burning hands" in football spinal cord injuries. JAMA 1977;238:2049–2051.

46. Prinsen RKE, Syrotuik DG, Reid DC. Position of the cervical vertebrae during helmet removal and cervical collar application in football and hockey. Clin J Sport Med 1995;5:155–161.

47. Torg JS, Pavlov H, Genuario SE, et al. Neurapraxia of the cervical spinal cord with transient quadriplegia. J Bone Joint Surg 1986;68A: 1354–1370.

48. Herzog RJ, Wiens JJ, Dillingham MF, Sontag MJ. Normal cervical spine morphometry and cervical spinal stenosis in asymptomatic professional football players: plain film radiography, multiplanar computed tomography, and magnetic resonance imaging. Spine 1991;16:S178–S186.

49. Cantu RC. Commentary. Functional cervical spinal stenosis: a contraindication to participation in contact sports. Med Sci Sports Exerc 1993;25:316–317.

50. Cantu RC. Sports medicine aspects of cervical spinal stenosis. In: Holloszy JD, ed. Exercise and sports sciences reviews. vol. 23. Baltimore: Williams & Wilkins, 1995:399–409.

51. Cantu RC. Cervical spinal stenosis: challenging an established detection method. Phys Sports Med 1993;21:57–63.

52. Torg JS, Currier B, Douglas R, et al. Symposium: spinal cord resuscitation. Contemp Orthop 1995; 30:495–509.

53. Torg JS, Glasgow SG. Criteria for return to contact activities following cervical spine injury. Clin J Sports Med 1991;1:12–26.

54. Torg JS, Sennet B, Pavlov H, et al. Spear tackler's spine: an entity precluding participation in tackle football and collision activities that expose the cervical spine to axial energy inputs. Am J Sports Med 1993;21:640–649.

55. Levitz CL, Reilly PJ, Torg JS. The pathomechanics of chronic, recurrent cervical nerve root neurapraxia: the chronic burner syndrome. Am J Sports Med 1997;25:73–76.

56. Watkins RG. Nerve injuries in football players. Clin Sports Med 1986;5:215–246.

57. Clancy WG. Brachial plexus and upper extremity peripheral nerve injuries. In: Torg JS, ed. Athletic injuries to the head, neck and face. Philadelphia: Lea and Febiger, 1982:215–220.

58. Herring SA, Weinstein SM. Electrodiagnosis in sports medicine. Phys Med Rehabil 1989;3:809–822.

59. Weinstein JN. Neurogenic and nonneurogenic pain and inflammatory mediators. Orthop Clin North Am 1991;22:235–246.

60. Saal JS, Franson RC, Dobrow R, et al. High levels of inflammatory phospholipase A2 activity in lumbar disk herniations. Spine 1990;15:674–678.

61. Jackson RP, Glah JJ. Foraminal and extraforaminal lumbar disk herniation: diagnosis and treatment. Spine 1987;12:577–585.

62. Meyer SA, Schultz KR, Callaghan JJ, et al. Cervical spinal stenosis and stinger in collegiate football players. Am J Sports Med 1994;22:158–166.

CHAPTER *6*

Imaging Chest Injuries in Sports

GREGORY GASTALDO
DONALD ROSEN

*S*ignificant injuries to the chest and thorax are relatively rare in nonmotor sports. The majority of athletic injuries to the chest and thorax are minor contusions of the muscular and skeletal outer layer. These injuries require little, if any, attention. Most injuries result from blunt trauma caused by contact with another player or from sport missiles such as baseballs, softballs, or lacrosse balls. Penetrating injuries, such as impalement with a javelin, are rare but often well publicized.

Although they occur uncommonly, certain athletic injuries to the chest are life-threatening. It is important for the sports medicine physician to be able to differentiate the life-threatening injury from the less severe injury. This chapter describes the indications for and the interpretation of diagnostic imaging in these injuries to help the practitioner recognize the sometimes subtle signs of serious injury.

Other injuries to the chest are due to repetitive physical stress and are seen almost exclusively in athletes or laborers. The sports medicine physician must be able to recognize the often vague presentation of these injuries and understand how to utilize different imaging techniques to make the right diagnosis.

Injuries to the Ribs and Sternum

Rib Fractures

Rib fractures are one of the most common athletic injuries to the chest seen by physicians. Of greatest concern to the physician are the com-plications associated with fractures of the ribs, such as pneumothorax or hemothorax, rather than the fracture itself.

Rib fractures can be broken into two broad groups, those caused by blunt external trauma and those caused by the action of muscles. The group caused by muscles can be further divided into those caused by the force of repetitive muscular contractions (stress fractures) and those caused by sudden violent muscle contraction (fracture of the first rib and avulsion fractures of the free-floating ribs).

Clinical Presentation

When blunt external trauma results in an acute rib fracture, the athlete can recall one episode of forceful trauma followed by sudden sharp pain at the site of fracture. Pain referred to the site of the fracture with anteroposterior (AP) and/or lateral compression of the thorax can help differentiate a fracture from a contusion. Crepitus and/or a step-off may be palpated at the site of fracture. The clinician should look for signs and symptoms of a complicated rib fracture such as tension pneumothorax or renal, splenic, or hepatic injury.

Violent muscular contraction has been implicated in acute fractures of the first rib. This injury has been reported in baseball, tennis, basketball, and "jive dancing" (1,2). The fracture is caused by the cephalad pull of the anterior scalene muscle against the stabilizing caudal pull of the serratus anterior and other muscles. These patients often describe feeling a "snap" in the shoulder or base of the neck and acute onset of pain.

Muscle pull also has been implicated in avulsion fractures of the free-floating ribs. These fractures are caused by violent contraction of the external obliques. Although this injury is very rare, it has been reported in baseball pitchers and batters (3,4). There is sudden onset of pain and exquisite tenderness over the distal end of the free rib, often associated with swelling and ecchymosis. This injury can be differentiated by x-ray from two other clinical entities, strain of the origin of the external obliques, which occurs commonly, and the rib-tip syndrome, which occurs less commonly.

The rib-tip syndrome or slipping-rib syndrome causes pain at the costal margin and is attributable to increased mobility of the tip of the eighth, ninth, or tenth rib (5). While not a skeletal fracture, it can be confused with a rib fracture. It almost always follows a traumatic event and is associated with pain induced by exercise, pressure, or deep inspiration. The costal cartilages of the eighth, ninth, and tenth ribs do not articulate with the sternum directly, as do the upper seven ribs. Instead, they articulate with the costal cartilage of the rib above. The costal cartilages are very thin at the site where they join the cartilage above, the tenth sometimes being only 3 to 6 mm in diameter. They are connected only by weak fibrous tissue, which, when torn, allows the costal cartilage of the rib below to sublux posteriorly, often causing a clicking sound. This injury cannot be imaged reliably. Therefore, the diagnosis is made on physical examination and supported by the relief of pain with injection of anesthetic. Injection of corticosteroids may be curative, but often resection of 3 to 4 cm of the anterior costal cartilage is necessary for cure.

Stress fractures resulting from repetitive overuse present quite differently. The athlete will experience an insidious onset of a poorly localized pain. Stress fractures of the first rib cause pain in the scapular area, shoulder, behind the clavicle, and at the base of the neck (1) (Fig. 6-1). Stress fractures of the first rib have been reported in weightlifting, baseball, volleyball, judo, tennis, and golf (1,2,6,7).

Stress fractures of the middle ribs have been reported in rowers, golfers, and tennis players, but in our experience, they are seen most commonly in rowers. They usually occur posterolaterally in the rib. This is the biomechanical site of greatest bending, caused largely by the serratus

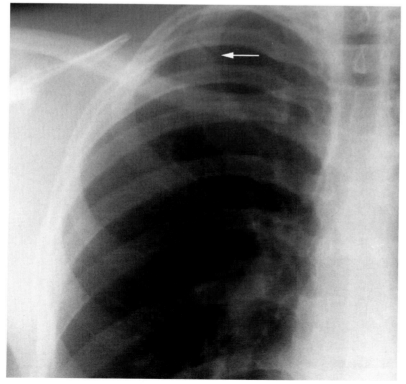

F I G U R E   **6-1**

A 31-year-old pitching coach with a 3- to 4-day history of right posterior shoulder pain. The arrow points to a minimally displaced right anterolateral first rib fracture.

anterior. The pain is often felt along the spinal border of the scapula, which can easily lead to a misdiagnosis of a rhomboid or trapezius strain (6).

Indications for Imaging

In evaluating a possible acute traumatic rib fracture, an absolute indication for a full rib series is any suspected complication such as pneumothorax, airway compromise, trauma to the great vessels, flail chest, pulmonary contusion, or renal, splenic, or hepatic injury. Acute traumatic fractures of the first three ribs carry a higher risk of trauma to the great vessels, just as fractures of ribs 10 through 12 carry a greater risk of injury to the liver, spleen, and kidneys. Suspicion of fractures in the upper or lower three ribs should be investigated with a complete rib series.

The fourth through ninth ribs are the most commonly fractured ribs and are associated with the fewest complications. In a patient with tenderness in the fourth through ninth ribs without signs or symptoms to suggest a complication, the imaging decisions are greatly affected by the risk of the athlete sustaining further trauma. The AAP Classification of Sports is helpful in this matter (Table 6-1). If the athlete wishes to return to a sport classified at or below the strenuous

class, the decision can be approached as it would in a nonathlete. The American College of Emergency Physician Cost Containment Recommendations provide reasonable indications for obtaining a full rib x-ray series in patients with possible rib fractures who are at low risk of further trauma (Table 6-2). In the absence of these indications, the presence or absence of a rib fracture does not seem to influence therapy (8). Thompson et al, in their article about the use of the rib series, stated, "Only complications influence treatment, and these are best seen on upright chest films. Because the treatment of a suspected isolated rib fracture based on either clinical or radiological findings is the same (i.e., analgesia), the additional cost of obtaining radiological confirmation of the rib fracture is not justified" (9). The upright posteroanterior (PA) and lateral chest x-rays can identify almost all complications of rib fractures and may sometimes be diagnostic of the fracture itself. However, they should not be relied on the rule out rib fractures. The single PA chest x-ray obtained on the day of the injury is the most cost-effective examination to detect the presence of significant complications of chest trauma (9).

The athlete with a suspected acute rib fracture (1–12) who participates in a sport classified as either limited contact or contact/collision

T A B L E   **6-1**

Classification of Sports

Contact		**Noncontact**		
Contact/Collision	Limited Contact/Impact	Strenuous	Moderately Strenuous	Nonstrenuous
Boxing	Baseball	Aerobic dance	Badminton	Archery
Field hockey	Basketball	Crew	Curling	Golf
Football	Bicycling	Fencing	Table tennis	Riflery
Ice hockey	Diving	Field (discus, javelin, shotput)		
Lacrosse	Field (high jump, pole vault)	Running/track		
Martial arts	Gymnastics	Swimming		
Rodeo	Horseback riding	Tennis		
Soccer	Skating (ice, roller)	Weightlifting		
Wrestling	Skiing (cross-country, downhill, water)			
	Softball			
	Squash/handball			
	Volleyball			

SOURCE: Reproduced with permission from Pediatrics 1988;81:737.

T A B L E 6-2

Indications for Rib X-ray Series from the American College of Emergency Physicians Cost Containment, Recommendations

Fractures suspected, ribs 1 to 2

Fractures suspected, ribs 9 to 12

Multiple rib fractures

Elderly patients

Pre-existing pulmonary disease

Suspected pathologic fractures

Adapted by permission from Rosen P, ed. Emergency medicine: concepts and clinical practice. 3rd ed. St. Louis: Mosby–Year Book, 1993:426.

must be approached differently. Athletes in these sports with rib fractures are at significant risk of developing complications if exposed to further trauma; thus there is a greater need to know if they have a fracture. The upright PA chest x-ray should not be relied on to rule out a rib fracture. A full rib series including coned-down views of the traumatized area should be obtained if the athlete suffered trauma judged great enough to cause a fracture and has a level of point tenderness compatible with a fracture. Although referred pain with anteroposterior (AP) compression of the chest, ecchymosis, and crepitus is slightly more specific for rib fracture than contusion (Table 6-3), it has been pointed out that the clinical impression and physical findings of rib fracture are nonspecific and unreliable (9).

A full rib series with attention to the lower ribs can differentiate avulsion fractures of the floating ribs from a strain of the origin of the external oblique or from the rib-tip syndrome (Fig. 6-2). While all three of these entities usually will heal with relative rest, an injection with lidocaine and cortisone may help alleviate symptoms (4).

With either stress fracture or acute muscular fracture of the first rib, imaging is necessary to make a definitive diagnosis in an athlete presenting with a confusing pain pattern. Proper imaging with attention to the first rib may obviate the need for other potentially expensive and invasive testing.

Stress fractures of the middle ribs can be managed without diagnostic imaging if the athlete is willing to discontinue or modify his or her training until symptoms resolve (6). However, in the competitive environment of high-level sports, athletes and coaches often find a definitive diagnosis of stress fracture helpful in planning the season for both the athlete and the team. Furthermore, confirming the suspicion of a rib stress fracture if the presentation is confusing can avoid further unnecessary evaluation.

Imaging Methods

As mentioned earlier, some clinical situations require only a PA chest x-ray. It may be relied on to rule out most complications of rib fractures that would indicate managing the patient differently. Because it can afford an adequate view of the posterior sections of the ribs that lie above the diaphragm, it can be used to diagnose fractures in these areas (Fig. 6-3).

T A B L E 6-3

Clinical Signs Correlated with Rib Fractures

Finding	No Positive Sign	Not Associated with Rib Fracture	Associated with Rib Fracture (%)
Point tenderness	86	58	28 (33)
Pain referred to site of chest compression	31	18	13 (42)
Ecchymosis	17	10	7 (41)
Splinting	40	26	14 (35)
Shortness of breath	13	9	4 (30)
Crepitus	5	3	2 (40)
Percussion	5	4	1 (20)
Abnormal breath sounds	13	9	4 (31)

Reproduced by permission from DeLuca SA, Rhea JT, O'Malley TO. Radiographic evaluation of rib fractures. AJR 1982;138:91–92.

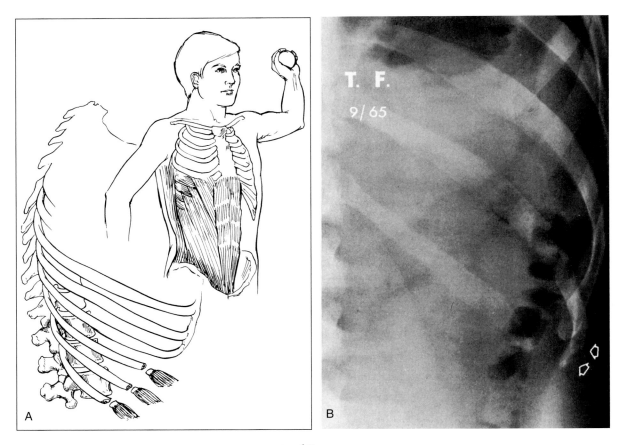

FIGURE **6-2**

(A) Drawing of avulsion of floating rib. (B) X-ray with rib detail of non-pitching side: fracture of floating ribs (*arrowheads*). (Reproduced by permission from Tullos HS, et al. Unusual lesions of the pitching arm. Clin Orthop 1972;88:169–182.)

Although fractures are seen more commonly in the posterior and middle thirds of the ribs, fractures may lie anywhere along the course of the ribs. The single PA chest x-ray is inadequate for visualization of the lateral and anterior portions of the ribs, as well as the upper and lower ribs themselves. Therefore, a proper rib series always should include more than a single projection (Fig. 6-4).

The well-accepted radiologic rib series should include 1) AP or PA views of the chest, 2) oblique views of the chest wall, 3) a separate AP view of the lower chest and upper abdomen that is well penetrated for visualization of the ribs below the diaphragm, and 4) a coned-down view of the clinically suspected location of rib injury. The AP view of the chest is taken with a large cassette, which often will include the whole bony thorax. However, in a large patient in whom the cassette cannot cover the whole thorax, the cassette should be positioned cephalad or caudad depending on the location of pain and tenderness. Because rib fractures are associated with injuries to the major organs of the chest, evaluation of the ribs should never be performed without careful inspection of the lungs and mediastinum.

Displaced rib fractures are identified most readily on the radiographs. The offset of the displaced rib is easily appreciated against the lucency of the lungs or the surrounding air (see Fig. 6-4). Sometimes displaced fractures are less obvious when there is incomplete displacement or overlap. Nondisplaced fractures are more difficult to visualize and usually are represented by lucent bands of decreased density within the ribs (Fig. 6-5). Sometimes nondisplaced fractures are seen only retrospectively secondary to

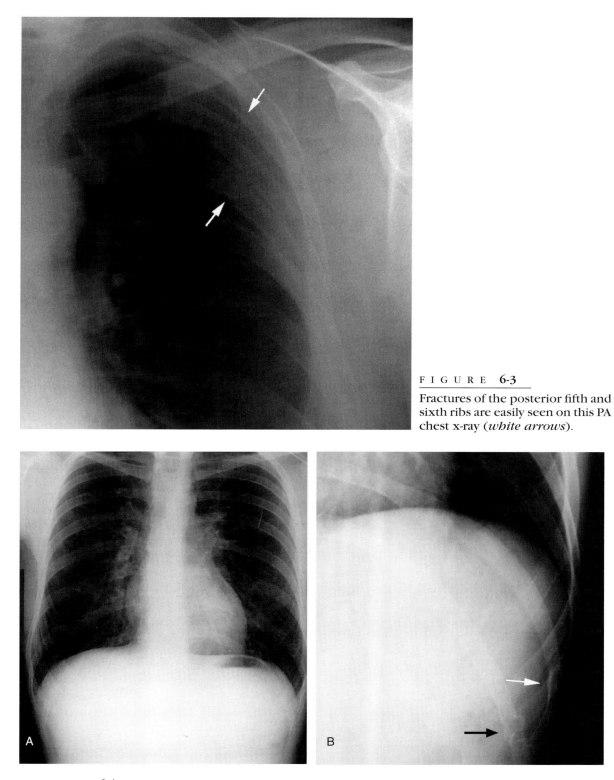

FIGURE **6-3**

Fractures of the posterior fifth and sixth ribs are easily seen on this PA chest x-ray (*white arrows*).

FIGURE **6-4**

Fracture of the tenth rib visualized more easily on a well-penetrated upper abdominal film. (A) PA chest film taken during inspiration. (B) Penetrated AP film of the lower chest and upper abdomen taken of the same patient. There are fractures of the lateral portions of the tenth and eleventh ribs (*arrows*).

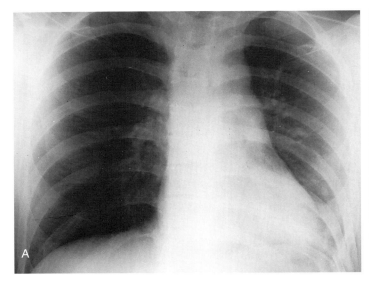

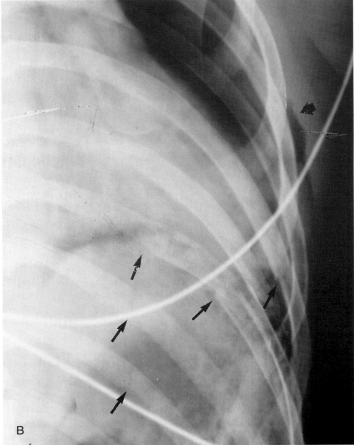

FIGURE **6-5**

Multiple left-sided rib fractures seen in a 22-year-old man injured after being thrown from a bull. (A) PA x-ray of the chest showing a left-sided pleural effusion. There is also haziness of the left lower ribs, indicating probable rib fractures. Note the difficulty in identifying the number and orientation of these fractures. (B) Oblique image of the left lower chest clearly showing linear fractures from the left seventh through twelfth ribs (*black arrows*). Also present is subcutaneous emphysema adjacent to the lateral chest wall (*black arrowhead*).

healing and callus formation (Fig. 6-6). The only sign of a nondisplaced fracture may be the surrounding soft tissue edema or hematoma. In this case, coned-down views of a suspected rib fracture may be necessary for diagnosis.

If there is a high degree of suspicion for a rib fracture and the plain radiographs appear normal, bone scanning is a useful method for finding a rib fracture. Radionuclide imaging is especially useful in osteoporotic and elderly patients. The majority of these patients will have positive bone scans 48 to 72 hours after the initial injury.

Rib injuries usually are appreciated better on plain radiographs than on computed tomographic (CT) imaging. The exceptions to this would be costochondral displacement or costovertebral dislocation. Sometimes these injuries are visualized on CT scanning but not seen on plain film radiographs. Magnetic resonance imaging (MRI) may show the surrounding soft tissue injuries better than either plain film or CT

examination. Also, osseous edema or bone bruising may only be seen using MRI. STIR sequences on MRI are very sensitive for bony injury but are not specific for fracture. Therefore, because of its cost and lack of specificity, MRI may be utilized in an extreme diagnostic dilemma but is not practical for determining the extent of everyday rib injuries.

It is not uncommon for rib fractures to occur in multiple adjacent ribs. In these situations, bone scans are more sensitive and often will reveal a linear distribution of uptake within multiple adjacent ribs. Many times the plain radiograph will demonstrate one or more but not all of the fractures. This may or may not be clinically significant.

A *flail chest* is described as segmental fractures (fractures in two or more locations on the same rib), most often involving more than one adjacent rib and resulting in an unstable chest wall segment (10) (Fig. 6-7). However, sometimes the second fracture involves a costochon-

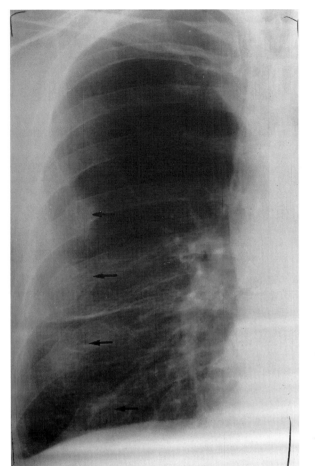

F I G U R E   **6-6**

Multiple healing right-sided rib fractures (*arrows*).

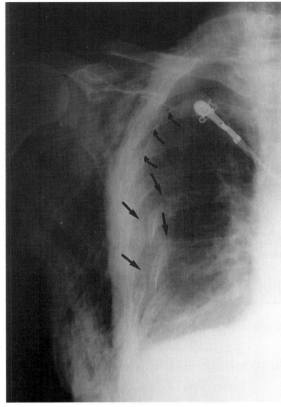

F I G U R E   **6-7**

Flail chest. The patient has multiple right-sided rib fractures. There are at least two fractures noted involving the right seventh, eighth, and probably ninth ribs (*straight black arrows*).Also note a small right apical pneumothorax (*curved black arrows*) with a significant amount of associated subcutaneous emphysema extending into the neck.

dral junction and therefore is not seen radiographically. Alternatively, a sternal fracture can act as the second segmental fracture leading to the unstable flail chest. Unfortunately, the diagnosis of a flail chest sometimes may be obvious only using fluoroscopy to identify the paradoxical movement of the unstable segment.

As stated earlier, acute fractures of the upper ribs, especially when caused by high-speed motor vehicle accidents, are often associated with other intrathoracic injuries (this is not true in first rib fractures caused by muscle contraction). Therefore, secondary signs of lung, pleura, and especially vascular injuries should be sought. Although a fracture of the first rib has been associated with both vascular and bronchial injuries, the need for arteriography remains a clinical de-

cision. A combination of clinical history and evaluation of the secondary signs on the patient's x-rays (including but not limited to the presence of pneumothorax, hemopneumothorax, hemothorax, mediastinal widening, tracheal displacement, and interstitial emphysema of the chest wall) should determine the necessity for additional studies, including arteriography. It is also important to remember that fractures of the lower ribs may be associated with major organ trauma within the abdomen, especially to the liver and spleen (Fig. 6-8). Once again, a combination of clinical information and secondary radiographic signs (such as but not limited to the displacement of the colon and stomach bubble, as well as intraperitoneal air) should determine the necessity for further imaging such as arteriography and CT scanning.

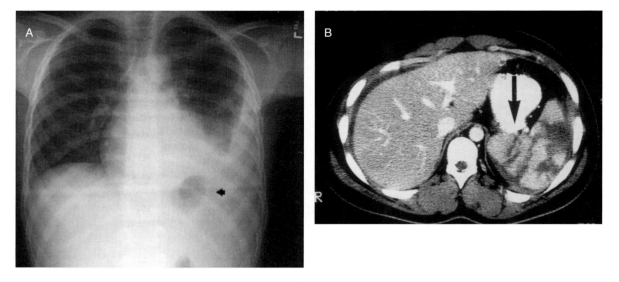

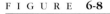

F I G U R E **6-8**

(A) PA chest film demonstrates displacement of the stomach bubble to the right (*black arrow*) in this 8-year-old involved in a sledding accident. Also note the moderate left pleural effusion. (B) CT scan of the abdomen showing a significant rupture of the spleen (*black arrow*).

Stress injuries of the ribs also occur. Radiographically, these are seen most commonly as chronic changes within the ribs such as callus formation. This is usually not seen until the patient has been symptomatic for at least 3 weeks. However, plain radiographs may never be positive despite the presence of a stress fracture. If a stress injury is suspected clinically but not visualized, a bone scan would be a useful method of diagnosis.

Bone scans are performed using technetium-labeled phosphates (Tc-99m MDP). When evaluating an athlete for a rib injury, especially a stress-related injury, the clinician should order a triple-phase bone scan (TPBS). TPBS is not only an anatomic imaging method but also a *physiologic scan*. The pattern of radiotracer uptake on the three different phases helps to estimate the chronicity of a stress fracture (11). Single photon emission computed tomographic (SPECT) scanning is not necessary, nor is it practical due to the anatomy of the bony thorax.

In triple-phase scanning, images are obtained immediately and then every 2 seconds for the first minute after injection of radioisotope. These images are referred to as *dynamic images*. Next, images are taken at 2 through 10 minutes and are referred to as the *blood-pool im-*

ages. Finally, images in multiple different projections are obtained at 3 hours and are referred to synonymously as *delayed, bony,* or *static images*.

Intense uptake in a small area, usually round or oval, seen on all three phases is consistent with an acute stress fracture (Fig. 6-9). It should be noted that uptake on a bone scan is not specific for fractures. Uptake in the blood-pool and delayed images is most consistent with a stress fracture that has been present for 4 to 8 weeks. Uptake only in the delayed images is not consistent with a stress fracture in its early stages. It is more consistent with an old stress fracture (greater than 12 weeks). The bone scan may remain "hot" in the delayed images for up to and sometimes longer than 1 year.

When evaluating x-ray studies for rib fractures, one must be aware that pathologic fractures may occur. Pathologic changes within the ribs may cause an osseous weakness, causing the rib to fracture with only minor athletic trauma.

Implications for Management

Return-to-play decisions always must be individualized to each athlete, taking into account the nature of the sport, the athlete's motivation

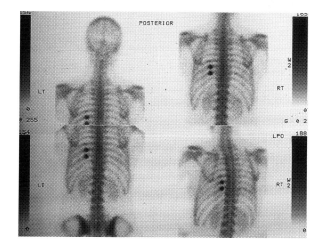

FIGURE **6-9**

These are the delayed static images of a triple-phase bone scan done on an 18-year-old collegiate rower with left midthoracic back pain for 4 weeks. There are two areas of focal radioisotope uptake within the posterior eighth and ninth ribs representing stress fractures.

to compete while injured, and the athlete's willingness to accept the risk that is always present when an athlete participates while injured. The following discussion suggests guidelines for return to play in athletes with rib fractures.

The athlete who competes in a sport classified at or below the strenuous level with an acute traumatic fracture of the middle ribs may be allowed to compete when the symptoms allow. The risk of complication or displacement of the fracture is acceptably low.

The athlete who competes in a contact/collision or limited-contact/impact sport with an acute traumatic fracture of the middle ribs must be protected from further trauma because of the risk of complication. This mandates restricting the athlete from competition until the risk of displacement from further trauma is acceptably low. Some authors have suggested that athletes can return to contact sports at 3 weeks with the protection of a commercial vest or flak jacket (3).

Acute fractures of the upper and lower three ribs carry a higher risk of complication, and therefore, decisions regarding return to play involving these injuries must be made on a case-by-case basis. Acute fractures of the first three ribs caused by external trauma should raise the suspicion for other intrathoracic injury, especially injury to the aorta. Refer to the discussion

of traumatic aortic rupture later in this chapter for details on how to approach such a patient.

Acute traumatic fractures of ribs 9 through 12 should raise suspicion of renal, hepatic, or splenic injury. The absence of blood in the urine can be used as a screen for renal injury if the fracture is nondisplaced. In a displaced fracture near the liver, spleen, or kidneys, a contrast-enhanced CT scan of the abdomen and kidneys is indicated to rule out injury to these organs.

First rib fractures caused by repetitive stress or muscular pull also do not require therapy beyond pain control and relative rest. No acute neurovascular complications have been reported; however, late complications such as Horner's syndrome have been reported. There is a tendency to slow healing, and pseudoarthrosis or nonunion has been reported (7). Often these lesions are asymptomatic. First rib fractures were identified relatively frequently in asymptomatic patients in a large series of screening chest x-rays (1,3). Return to contact sports has not been specifically addressed in the sports medicine literature. Barrett et al reported two cases of first rib fracture in football players (1). In both cases, pain subsided in 3 weeks. One was reported to return to football without problems, but the time to return was not mentioned.

As mentioned earlier, pain from an avulsion

fracture of a floating rib can be alleviated partially by injection of lidocaine and cortisone. If x-rays are negative and the rib-tip syndrome is suspected, a diagnostic and possibly therapeutic injection of anesthetic and corticosteroid should be attempted. If this brings complete relief of the pain but is not lasting, the athlete may be considered for operative intervention, as mentioned earlier.

Stress fractures of the middle ribs can be managed with relative rest through a program of modified activity. No reports of complicated stress fractures of the middle ribs have appeared in the literature, but we are aware of a case of nonunion in a collegiate rower and an anecdotal report of a rower with a pneumothorax from a stress fracture. Certainly complications are rare. Athletes usually respond to 4 to 8 weeks of relative rest. McKenzie has reported a case of an elite rower with a stress fracture of the ninth rib who gradually returned to rowing over 3 weeks and was back to full training with only minimal discomfort by 4 weeks (12).

Sternal Fractures

Fractures of the sternum occur most commonly in motor vehicle accidents when the sternum is struck by the steering wheel. Although previously thought to be rare, one recent series found sternal fractures in 8% of all admissions for blunt chest trauma (13). Sternal fractures in sports are seen most commonly in motor vehicle sports. However, sternal fractures have been reported to be caused by trauma other than motor vehicle accidents. In a retrospective study of 60 sternal fractures, 20% were caused by falls or other non-motor vehicle accidents (14). These authors reported that this subset of patients generally did not have significant associated injuries, while those patients with sternal fractures after motor vehicle accidents frequently had associated injuries. Despite the occurrence of sternal fractures not associated with motor vehicle accidents, reports of sternal fractures in athletes are apparently rare. We are aware of two reports of sternal fractures in athletes, one in a football player that was acute and one in a wrestler that was classified as a stress fracture (15,16).

Clinical Presentation

Buchman et al reported that the most common clinical syndrome associated with sternal frac-tures is pain and tenderness over the sternum without other accompanying visible, palpable, or audible physical signs. Interestingly, other confirmatory physical signs such as ecchymosis, crepitus, or instability were present in only a small minority of patients (14).

Associated injuries frequently seen with sternal fractures are closed head injuries, fractured ribs, flail chest, cardiac injury, aortic injury, and pulmonary contusion.

Indications for Imaging

Any athlete who sustains significant trauma to the sternum and complains of pain and tenderness over the sternum should be evaluated for sternal fracture, especially if he or she was injured participating in a motor vehicle sport such as auto racing or motocross.

Imaging Methods

To interpret any diagnostic image of the sternum properly, it is necessary to understand the anatomy of the sternum, especially the ossification and fusion of its different parts. The adult sternum is broken into three parts, the manubrium, the body, and the xiphoid process (Fig. 6-10). All parts of the sternum except the xiphoid process ossify by the first year of life. The xiphoid process ossifies anywhere from age 5 to 18 years (17). The body of the sternum originates from four sternebrae that fuse in an ascending fashion from early childhood to the middle twenties (Fig. 6-11). The manubrium articulates with the sternal body most commonly through a symphysis. The ends of each bone are lined with hyaline cartilage and then connected by fibrocartilage. This joint ossifies in approximately 10% of adults, becoming a synostosis (18). The xiphoid process fuses with the sternal body in approximately 30% of adults.

Imaging of the sternum in the lateral view is uncomplicated. However, because the position of the sternum is directly anterior to the thoracic spine, visualization of the sternum in an AP or PA view is not possible. Therefore, angulated views are necessary. The angulation depends on the depth of the chest, using less angulation for deep chests than for shallow chests. Pulmonary markings also may interfere with visualization of the sternum, and therefore, imaging with shallow breathing may be necessary. If this technique is used, exposure time should be long

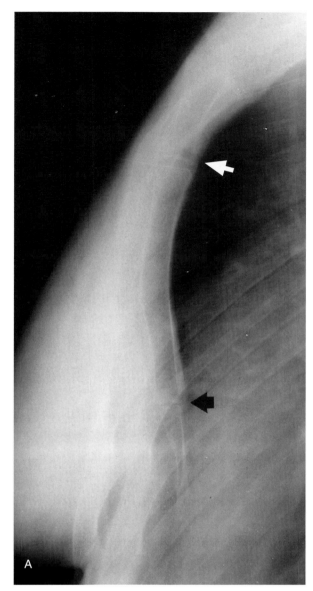

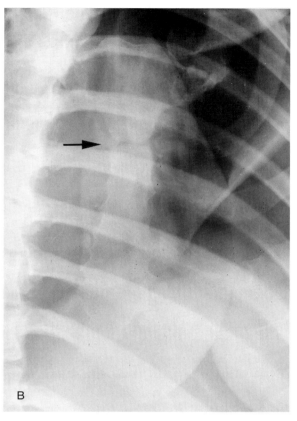

F I G U R E   **6-10**

Sternal images. (A) Lateral view of the sternum. A black arrow points to the manubriosternal joint. The white arrow points to the persistent xiphosternal joint. (B) Oblique view of a normal sternum. The black arrow points to the manubriosternal joint.

enough to cover several phases of shallow respirations. The milliampere (mA) setting also must be low (19).

Sternal fractures, both nondisplaced and displaced, often are visualized on the lateral view (Fig. 6-12). In addition, dislocation at the manubriosternal joint may be seen. Dislocation of the manubriosternal joint usually is seen in patients who suffered a forced flexion injury in the cervical spine and upper thorax. The sternal body most commonly is displaced posteriorly. With frontal trauma, such as a steering wheel injury, a fracture of the body of the sternum with posterior displacement of the inferior fragment

is seen most commonly. This is often associated with a localized retrosternal hematoma. This hematoma usually is confined by the pleura and appears as a rounded mass behind the sternum. This degree of hematoma is important to note on the lateral film, in that sometimes it may give the false appearance of mediastinal widening on the PA or AP chest x-ray (13). However, sternal fracture alone rarely causes sufficient bleeding to widen the mediastinal shadow on the roentgenogram (14). True mediastinal widening on the PA film may be secondary to major vessel injury. Radiographic mediastinal widening occurring with sternal fracture should be con-

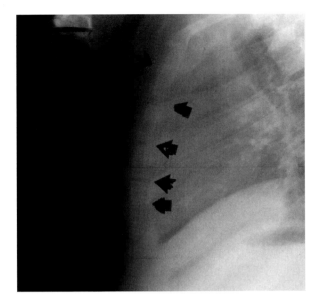

FIGURE 6-11

Normal sternal development. On the left are, in descending order, the manubrium and the four sternebrae that ultimately fuse to form the sternal body. On the right, the black arrows point to, in descending order, the manubriosternal joint, which remains open in 90% of adults; the joint between the first and second sternebrae, which fuses between the ages of 16 and 25 years; the joint between the second and third sternebrae, which fuses near puberty; and the joint between the third and fourth sternebrae, which fuses in early childhood. Not shown is the xiphoid, which has not yet ossified in this infant (it normally ossifies between 5 and 18 years), and the xiphosternal joint, which remains open in 70% of adults.

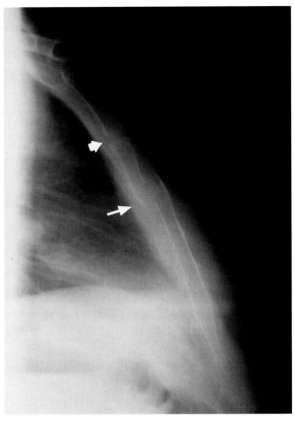

FIGURE 6-12

Sternal fracture. Note a displaced fracture of the upper body of the sternum. There is minimal soft tissue swelling associated with this fracture. The white arrowhead points to the normal manubriosternal joint.

sidered a primary indication for aortography (13).

CT scanning is of little value in axial fractures of the sternum. However, the secondary soft tissue signs of pleural-based hematoma, mediastinal fluid, and pericardial fluid is more obvious with CT scanning (17).

Implications for Management

The majority of sternal fractures, especially simple nondisplaced fractures, heal promptly without stabilization. Rarely, nonunion with pseudoarthrosis develops, which requires operative stabilization (20,21). Fractures that are displaced or comminuted should be considered for immediate operative reduction and internal fixation.

Associated injuries to intrathoracic organs are of far greater significance than the sternal

fracture itself. A study of sternal fractures in the 1960s reported a high incidence of associated injuries and a mortality rate of 25%. However, a more recent study of sternal fractures in hemodynamically stable patients, which is more applicable to primary care sports medicine, reported a mortality rate of only 1.7% (14).

Cardiac injury is so frequent with sternal fractures that it mandates observation in the intensive care unit setting with continuous electrocardiographic (ECG) monitoring. Buckman et al reported abnormal ECGs in 62% of their patients sometime during their hospitalization (14). Harley and Mena reported cardiac impairment in 91% of their patients when evaluated by first-pass biventricular radionuclide angiography. The most common locations of impairment were the right ventricle and the anterior left ventricle. Interestingly, only 4 of their 12 patients had abnormal ECGs at admission, indicating the insensitivity of admission ECG for detecting cardiac impairment (13).

Finally, as mentioned earlier, a widened mediastinum occurring with a sternal fracture is a primary indication for aortography.

Injuries to the Pleura and Lungs

Pneumothorax

There are three general types of pneumothorax: 1) simple, 2) tension, and 3) open or communicating. *Simple pneumothorax* can be spontaneous or traumatic and is defined as air in the pleural space with ipsilateral collapse of the lung without mediastinal shift and without communication through the chest wall. *Tension pneumothorax* develops when air is allowed to enter progressively but not exit the pleural space through a leak in the pleura, tracheobronchial tree, or chest wall. This causes ventilatory and circulatory compromise that can progress rapidly and become fatal. *Communicating pneumothorax* is caused by a penetrating chest wound that remains open.

Clinical Presentation

The athlete with pneumothorax universally will complain of some level of pleuritic chest pain and dyspnea. Physical findings include decreased breath sounds, hyperresonance to percussion, and possibly chest wall crepitus secondary to subcutaneous emphysema.

Spontaneous pneumothorax is seen most commonly between the ages of 20 and 40 years. It is caused by the rupture of small blebs on the visceral pleural surface, usually in the upper lobes. It has been reported to occur in athletes while participating in noncontact sports (22).

Tension pneumothorax can lead to respiratory distress, hypotension, and tachycardia. It can be recognized by distended neck veins, tracheal deviation, absent breath sounds, and hyperresonance to percussion on the involved side.

Indications for Imaging

Spontaneous pneumothorax must be considered in the differential diagnosis of chest pain and dyspnea in any athlete. Traumatic simple pneumothorax should be considered in the athlete who complains of pleuritic chest pain and dyspnea following a blow to the chest. If ten-

sion pneumothorax is suspected clinically, treatment should not be delayed for radiographic confirmation.

Imaging Methods

Radiographically, a pneumothorax, which is air within the pleural cavity, is defined by visualization of the visceral pleural surface as it is displaced from the chest wall (Fig. 6-13). We rely on the air between the pleural surfaces to define this surface of the lung. The air is seen most commonly at the apices of the hemithorax and sometimes at the costophrenic angles. It is best seen with an expiratory erect PA film. In expiration, the lung volume is reduced, making the apparent area of pleural air appear larger. In critically ill patients in the supine position, it is very difficult, often impossible, to diagnose a pneumothorax (23) (Fig. 6-14). The pneumothorax often is difficult to visualize. Lateral decubitus films may be necessary. Sometimes air may only be seen within the costophrenic sulcus. This would be a case where CT demonstration of a pneumothorax may be necessary.

The simple pneumothorax involves air between the pleural surfaces and does not involve mediastinal displacement. In a tension pneumothorax, a ball-valve phenomena exists that allows more air to enter the intrapleural space than to leave. This causes tension and pressure within the hemithorax and displacement of the mediastinum. There is also depression of the ipsilateral diaphragm (see Fig. 6-14).

If air is also seen within the mediastinum, one must consider the presence of a leak within the trachea, bronchi, or possibly the esophagus. Sometimes air may enter the peritoneal cavity.

Great care must be taken when diagnosing a pneumothorax. Artifacts, most commonly skin folds, clothing, and emergency bandages, can have the appearance of a pleural surface overlying the chest (Fig. 6-15). A pleural surface is a very thin line, whereas most of those mentioned above should give a thicker appearance.

Implications for Management

The size of a pneumothorax is an important factor in determining appropriate therapy. Small pneumothoraces occupy 15% or less of the pleural cavity, moderate ones occupy 15% to 60%, and large ones occupy more than 60% (24) (see Fig. 6-13).

All significant closed pneumothoraces (if

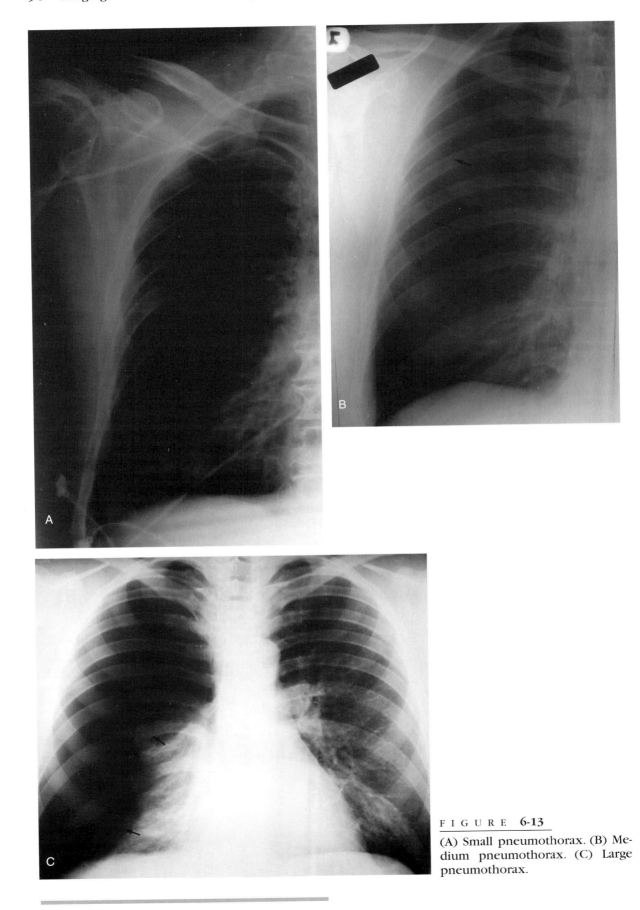

F I G U R E   **6-13**
(A) Small pneumothorax. (B) Medium pneumothorax. (C) Large pneumothorax.

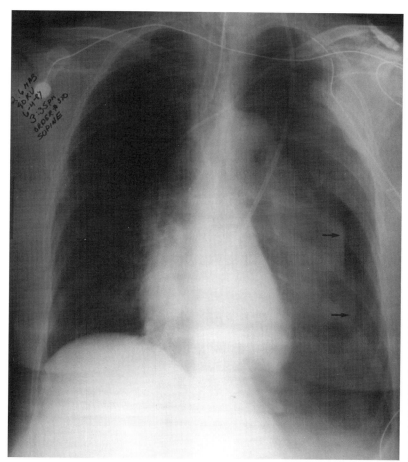

F I G U R E **6-14**

Tension pneumothorax. This is an AP chest x-ray taken in the supine position. The patient has a large pneumothorax. It is difficult to see the pleural air interface (*small black arrows*) because of the patient's supine position. The patient's left tension pneumothorax is indicated by the significant shift of the mediastinum to the right. In addition, there is significant depression of the left hemidiaphragm.

greater than 20%) should be treated with tube thoracostomy drainage (25). Lesser degrees can be followed with serial chest x-rays until they are resorbed.

Fifty percent of all patients who suffer a first episode of spontaneous pneumothorax will develop a recurrence. Recurrent spontaneous pneumothorax requires pleurodesis or parietal pleurectomy. Athletes with a history of spontaneous pneumothorax should not be allowed to scuba dive or pilot aircraft. Should a pneumothorax occur underwater, enlargement of the pneumothorax on ascent may be catastrophic. Similarly, the decrease in atmospheric pressure in an unpressurized aircraft can cause the pneumothorax to expand.

Tension pneumothorax is a life-threatening emergency that requires prompt diagnosis and treatment, usually without the availability of x-ray. It must be decompressed promptly using a large-bore needle (14–16 gauge) attached to a syringe with the plunger in place. The needle is inserted into the pleural space by going through the second intercostal space anteriorly in the midclavicular line. If the diagnosis is correct, the plunger will be pushed under pressure out of the syringe. This procedure will convert a tension pneumothorax to a simple pneumothorax. Tube thoracostomy through the fifth intercostal space at the anterior axillary line provides definitive treatment.

An open chest wound should be covered immediately with any material available and later converted to a sterile occlusive dressing. Some authors recommend fixing the dressing only on three sides and allowing the one side to act as a one-way valve that allows air to escape from the involved hemithorax (26).

Hemothorax

While not seen commonly in sports, hemothorax must be considered in athletes with chest trauma, especially those with rib fractures. In

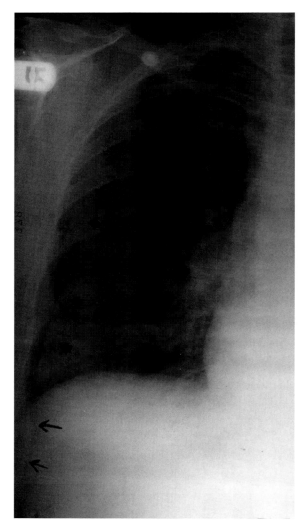

There is a large skin fold along the right lateral chest border (*black arrows*) that extends far below the diaphragm. Therefore, this cannot represent the pleural air interface.

one study hemothorax was found in 13.6% of patients with rib fractures. Interestingly, it was a late finding in 53% of the cases. The risk of hemothorax was directly related to the number of ribs fractured and the degree of displacement (27).

Clinical Presentation

The presentation is very similar to pneumothorax, but the involved area will be dull to percussion rather than hyperresonant. Major hemothorax will result in shock and ventilatory embarrassment.

Indications for Imaging

The presence of physical signs suggestive of a pleural effusion in an athlete with chest trauma is an absolute indication for upright PA and lateral chest x-rays. However, hemothoraces often are discovered during radiographic evaluation for other injuries such as rib fractures.

Due to the possibility of late hemothoraces, a follow-up upright PA chest x-ray should be done 2 and 4 weeks after injury in patients with a *rib injury index* greater than or equal to 4. The index is calculated by multiplying the number of ribs fractured by the grade of displacement. The *grade* of displacement is said to be 1 if there is no displacement, 2 if the displacement is less than half the width of the rib, and 3 if the displacement is greater than half the width of the rib (27).

Imaging Methods

A hemothorax presents on plain radiographs as pleural fluid (Fig. 6-16). Pleural bleeding does not often form a clot, and therefore, it often has the appearance of a free-flowing pleural effusion. Therefore, blunting of the costophrenic angles, the formation of a meniscus along the lateral chest wall, and increased density within overlying lung fields may be signs of a hemothorax. A hemothorax is better seen in an upright chest film than in a supine chest film. This is so because more than a liter of blood in the pleural space can lead to only a slight increase in density over the involved hemithorax on a supine film (25). In contrast, an upright PA chest x-ray will show blunting of the costophrenic angle with as little as 250 cc (24).

Extrapleural bleeding has a more loculated appearance along the edges of the pleural surfaces, which helps to differentiate it from intrapleural bleeding. As with visualization of the free fluid itself, the presence of a hemopneumothorax may only be seen either in an upright or lateral decubitus chest film. To diagnose a pleural effusion, an upright chest film is the study of choice.

Implications for Management

Fibrothorax and empyema are complications of hemothoraces managed with only observation or thoracentesis. These complications have been reported even with small hemothoraces (25). Tube thoracostomy is recommended for any traumatic hemothorax because of its multi-

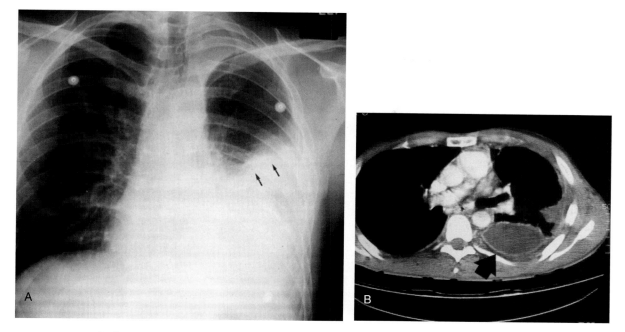

FIGURE **6-16**

Hemothorax. An expiratory semierect AP film of the chest (A) and a
CT examination of the chest (B) were performed in this 38-year-old
with a known posterior rib fracture. There is an associated large fluid
collection that is seen on both the chest film (*black arrows*) and the
CT scan (*black arrowhead*). Blood was found at thorocentesis.

ple benefits: evacuation of the hemothorax, re-
expansion of the lung, reduction of further
bleeding by coaptation of the lung to the chest
wall, and the ability to monitor any further
blood loss.

Operative intervention with open thora-
cotomy is necessary if the initial hemorrhage is
greater than 1500 cc, there is continued blood
loss of 200 cc per hour after the chest has been
cleared initially, or there is a total of 1500 cc
within 24 hours.

Pulmonary Contusion

Pulmonary contusion is the most common lethal
chest injury seen in this country (24). It is frequently associated with flail chest syndrome and
is the most lethal aspect of this condition. Although it is seen rarely in sports medicine, it is
important to be able to recognize radiographically.

Clinical Presentation

Presenting signs and symptoms may include
hemoptysis, ineffective cough, increasing short-
ness of breath, and increased respiratory rate.

Indications for Imaging

Any athlete who sustains severe chest trauma is
at risk for pulmonary contusion and should be
evaluated with PA and lateral chest x-rays.

Imaging Methods

Pulmonary contusions occur within minutes of
the injury, usually can be seen on the initial chest
x-ray, and if they do not become infected, tend
to resolve in 2 to 6 days (25). A pulmonary contusion presents as a nonspecific area of infiltrate
that may resemble an infectious infiltrate (Fig.
6-17). It may be multifocal or present as a large
area of confluence that may not be confined to
lung segments. The CT and plain radiographic
findings are consistent. The contusion often appears early after the patient's injury. An infiltrate
that appears 6 hours after the patient's injury is
less likely to represent a contusion and more
likely to represent an infectious infiltrate (10).

Implications for Management

Pulmonary contusions must be managed carefully in an intensive care setting because of their

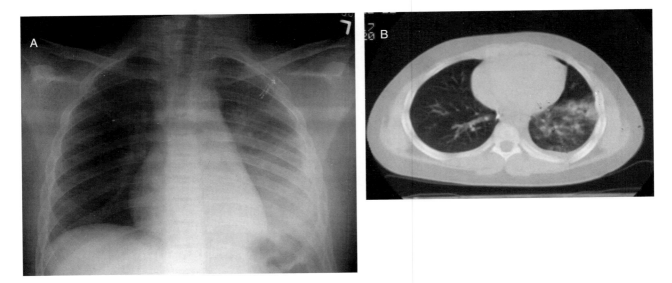

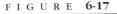

FIGURE   6-17

Pulmonary contusion. Erect chest x-ray (A) and CT scan (B) in this 12-year-old trauma victim. Both the chest film and CT scan demonstrate a diffuse infiltrate within the left lung fields. These findings are consistent with the presence of a pulmonary contusion.

high morbidity and mortality. Associated injuries such as hemothorax, pneumothorax, or traumatic aortic rupture must be excluded. Fluid resuscitation must be used cautiously, and if possible, a fluid restriction of 50 cc per hour should be set. Other therapeutic interventions may be indicated, such as mechanical ventilation with positive end-expiratory pressure (PEEP), diuretics, albumin or plasma to maintain oncotic pressure, and prophylactic antibiotics.

The most common serious complication of pulmonary contusion is infection. Between 50% and 75% of those sustaining a pulmonary contusion will develop pneumonia in the contused segment of lung, and 35% will go on to pulmonary abscess, empyema, or both (25).

Diaphragmatic Rupture

Like many of the injuries discussed in this chapter, diaphragmatic ruptures are seen most commonly in persons involved in motor vehicle accidents; however, there has been a report of a diaphragmatic rupture occurring in a wrestler (27).

Not all diaphragmatic injuries are diagnosed at the time of injury; in fact, it has been reported that the correct diagnosis is made in less than 50% of cases (28). Carter et al described three phases of diaphragmatic injury: 1) *immediate*

phase, extending from the time of injury to 14 days afterward; 2) *interval phase,* any time from day 15 after injury but prior to the obstruction or strangulation; and 3) *obstruction* or *strangulation phase* (29).

Clinical Presentation

In the immediate phase, the symptoms of the diaphragmatic injury often are overshadowed by the symptoms of other associated injuries. The most common symptoms are chest pain and dyspnea. Physical signs include decreased breath sounds, the presence of bowel sounds in the thorax, and a scaphoid abdomen (Gibson's sign). Ninety percent of diaphragmatic tears are left-sided owing to the protective effect of the liver on the right.

Indications for Imaging

In an athlete with chest or abdominal trauma, a chest x-ray is indicated either by the magnitude of trauma or by the presence of the signs and symptoms listed above. The chest x-ray is abnormal in almost all cases and is diagnostic in many cases, especially those where viscera has herniated across the tear in the diaphragm. In one study, the chest x-ray was interpreted as normal in only 3% of cases. It was diagnostic in

41% of cases and read as abnormal in the remaining 56% (30). Therefore, the chest x-ray will either be diagnostic or indicate the need for further studies. There are many options for further study (Table 6-4) but no general consensus on the optimal sequence of their application.

Imaging Methods

This is a difficult plain film diagnosis to make in many cases. Indications of a diaphragmatic rupture on a plain PA chest x-ray include apparent elevation of the hemidiaphragm and/or the presence of a gas-containing structure such as the colon or stomach within the thorax (Fig. 6-18). Since often a non-gas-filled portion of viscera is present through the diaphragmatic hernia, the diagnosis of diaphragmatic hernia is missed (28). This diagnosis should be considered in any patient who has sustained significant abdominal trauma. There are usually other significant associated injuries (31).

CT scanning can be used to make the diagnosis. The diaphragmatic contour is seen to be disrupted, with abdominal contents appearing to be within the chest (Fig. 6-19). Barium swallows and barium enemas also may show you contrast material above the diaphragm. On rare occasions, radionuclide liver scans can be used. In this case, the eventration of a small portion of liver above the diaphragm can be seen.

Implications for Management

All diaphragmatic ruptures should be repaired immediately. Transabdominal repair is usually preferred if there are other suspected injuries to intra-abdominal viscera, which is the case in 75% of patients (25).

Traumatic Rupture of the Aorta

Traumatic rupture of the aorta (TRA) is seen in high-speed motor vehicle accidents, which result in sudden deceleration of the aorta with shearing forces created where the mobile portion of the aorta joins the more fixed portions of the aorta. The three relatively fixed sites are the ligamentum arteriosum (just distal to the origin of the left subclavian artery), the aortic root, and the aortic hiatus in the diaphragm. Between 80% and 90% of TRAs are at the ligamentum arteriosum.

T A B L E   **6-4**

Tests for Identifying Diaphragm Injuries

Test	Advantages	Disadvantages
Chest radiograph	Rapid, safe, minimal equipment needed	False-negative rate 60%
Peritoneal lavage	Safe, rapid, minimal equipment needed; may be used in conjunction with contrast material or a marker	False-negative rate 10% to 25%; does not definitively identify the injury
Liver/spleen scan	Safe, rapid; visualizes the two most commonly injured organs	May not be diagnostic unless herniated; requires more equipment
CT scan	Safe, rapid; identifies associated injuries	Reliability uncertain; requires more equipment
Upper and/or lower gastrointestinal series	Facilities for the test are ubiquitous	May not be diagnostic unless viscera is herniated; difficult and potentially injurious in polytrauma patients
Fluoroscopy	Safe, rapid, easy to perform	Reliability uncertain
Thoracoscopy	Rapid; minimal equipment needed	Requires trained personnel; chest tube needed; reliability unknown
Peritoneography (with air or water-soluble contrast)	Rapid; minimal equipment needed; high accuracy expected	Air may cause pneumothorax; accuracy untested

Reproduced by permission from Troop B, et al. Early recognition of diaphragmatic injuries from blunt trauma. Ann Emerg Med 1985;14:97–101.

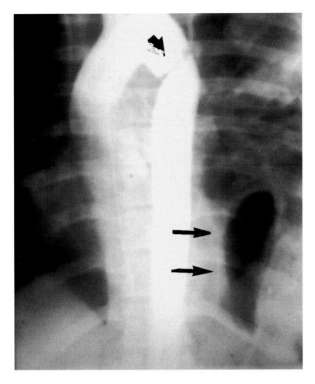

F I G U R E   **6-18**

Aortic transection (*black arrowhead*) and left diaphragmatic hernia (*thin black arrows*) in a posttraumatic patient. Note the herniated bowel loops in the left hemithorax.

It has been estimated that 1 in every 6 to 10 fatal accident victims sustains a TRA. If left untreated, death is instantaneous in 80% to 90%. One-third of the remainder will die within 6 hours, another third in 24 hours, and another third will live 72 hours (26).

Clinical Presentation

The most common symptom is retrosternal or interscapular pain. Less frequently seen are dysphagia, dyspnea, and hoarseness. Clinical findings include acute onset of upper extremity hypertension, decreased femoral pulses, and a harsh murmur heard over the precordium or in the interscapular area (25). Overall, clinical findings are present in less than half of patients, and up to a third have no evidence of external trauma (32).

Indications for Imaging

In their review of imaging of thoracic trauma, Mirvis and Templeton stated, "the diagnosis of

injury to the great arteries of the thorax constitutes one of the most controversial subjects in the field of trauma radiology" (33).

In general, signs and symptoms have not been shown to have predictive value in TRA (33). Therefore, any patient involved in a high-speed (>45 mph) deceleration-type accident should be evaluated carefully for a TRA. The admission chest x-ray is the best screening test for TRA. A standing PA chest x-ray is optimal but often unobtainable in the seriously injured patient. In the bedridden patient, a supine chest x-ray is often overread as positive; therefore, it has been recommended that a "true" erect view be obtained. This view is taken with the patient leaning a few degrees forward beyond the vertical.

Numerous radiographic signs present on the erect chest x-ray have been suggested as indicators of the need for aortography. Older studies focused on mediastinal widening as the primary sign (34,35), whereas more recently other radiographic signs of abnormal mediastinal anatomy have been stressed as more important (32,36). These signs will be discussed below.

One common-sense approach to this controversial issue has been suggested by Mirvis et al: ". . . the inability of the reader to discern the normal anatomy of the superior mediastinum constitutes our indication for aortography" (32). Gundry et al stated it this way: "in a young patient if you think the mediastinum looks widened, you should obtain an aortogram" (34).

Fractures of the first and second ribs as an indication for aortography deserve special mention. Previous teaching held this to be true; however, more recently, there has been a wealth of literature that reveals a lack of sensitivity and specificity for predicting TRA. However, these fractures, when caused by high-speed motor vehicle accidents, should prompt a careful evaluation of other clinical findings that might indicate the need for aortography. Also, as mentioned earlier in the section on rib fractures, most fractures of the first rib seen in sports are due to muscle trauma from either repetitive stress or sudden violent contraction. These injuries are not associated with trauma to the great vessels and should not be considered an indication for aortography.

Imaging Methods

Rupture of the thoracic aorta is an extreme emergency that demands immediate diagnosis. A combination of clinical signs and plain ra-

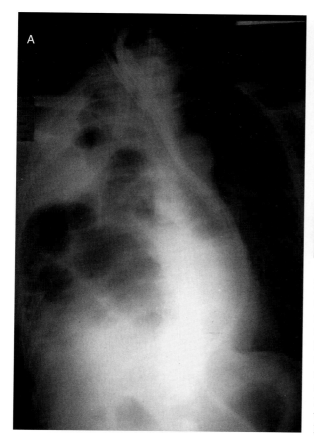

FIGURE **6-19**

(A) Large right-sided post-traumatic diaphragmatic hernia. Note the significant number of bowel loops within the right hemithorax and displacement of the mediastinal structures. (B) Moderate lateral right-sided diaphragmatic hernia. Note the intra-abdominal fat and vascular structures within right hemithorax.

diographic pictures can suggest this diagnosis. CT scanning can help contribute to the diagnosis, but the definitive diagnosis is usually made using aortography.

In a patient with a deceleration injury or significant chest trauma, the presence of mediastinal widening should be taken seriously. Often this is an artifactual appearance, and by placing the patient in the erect position and taking a good PA radiograph, one can eliminate the appearance of mediastinal widening. However, if one does find persistent widening of the mediastinum, which may be associated with deviation of the trachea to the right and/or fluid above the left lung, one should consider the presence of an aortic rupture (10) (Fig. 6-20). Hemothorax is often present. The presence of upper rib fractures will further support the suspicion of a traumatic rupture. Other signs such as blurring of the aortic knob, shifting of the trachea to the right, depression of the left mainstem bronchus, and suspected pleural injury also should raise the suspicion for a thoracic aortic tear (36). If a tear is suspected clinically, then all these radiographic signs should be used

to assist the clinician in deciding who should undergo aortography.

A CT scan may be used in patients in whom the clinical or radiographic signs are indeterminate. CT findings such as free fluid within the thoracic cavity, aortic dissection, or diffuse mediastinal hematomas are seen in patients with aortic tears. In these patients, if the CT is normal, then an aortogram does not need to be performed. False-positive chest films and CT diagnoses are seen commonly in patients with traumatic injuries. There are multiple other causes of bleeding within the mediastinum and chest cavity that can mimic the presence of an aortic rupture. A study from the University of Maryland Medical System, published in 1987, reported eight to nine negative aortograms for each case of traumatic rupture detected (32).

Implications for Management

Once TRA is suspected, a cardiothoracic surgeon should be consulted, because if the aortogram is positive, immediate operative repair is indicated (see Fig. 6-18).

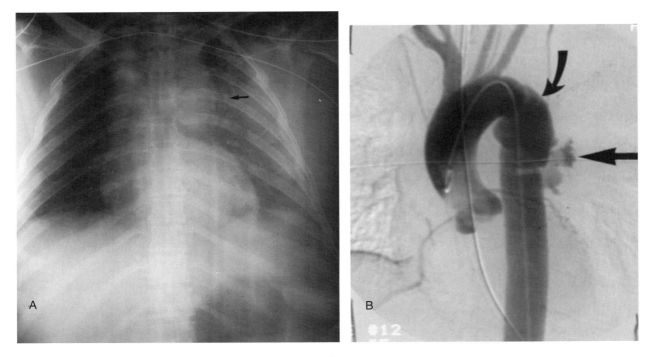

FIGURE 6-20

Traumatic rupture of the aorta. (A) This is a PA film of a post-traumatic patient in the supine position. The black arrow points to bilateral widening of the mediastinum, with obscuration of the normal aortic knob shadows. The increased density within the left hemithorax likely represents a pleural effusion in this supine patient. (B) A single digital subtraction film of an aortic root injection showing a spiral tear of the aortic knob distal to the left subclavian artery (*curved arrow*). There is also evidence of extravasation at the distal end of the tear (*straight arrow*).

Myocardial Injury

Overall, cardiac injuries are rare in sports. However, there is a case report of a patient with a cardiac contusion resulting from "spearing" in football (16). The patient also had sustained a sternal fracture. Furthermore, much attention recently has been given to commotio cordis, which has been said to be "the most common cause of sudden death in youth baseball" (37). This condition is a fatal injury caused by the impact of a baseball or other sport missile on the chest of an athlete. The cause of death is thought to be arrhythmic. Such deaths have been reported following a blow to the chest from a stick, a pitched ball, a softball, and a punch during a boxing match (38). This injury can be classified as a cardiac concussion, which is the first level of a continuum of traumatic cardiac injury from concussion to contusion to rupture.

Although the most severe form of traumatic cardiac injury, cardiac rupture, almost always results in sudden death, the intermediate form, cardiac contusion, can vary from a benign condition to a life-threatening condition. The reported incidence of cardiac contusion varies from 16% to 76% of patients admitted with blunt chest injury (38). The variability is partly due to the lack of a consistent definition of the terms *concussion* and *contusion*. In patients with blunt anterior chest trauma, three criteria are used to classify myocardial injury: 1) reversible changes on the ECG, 2) elevation of the MB isoenzyme of creatine phosphokinase above the normal range, and 3) abnormal wall motion as detected by echocardiography or gated radionuclide angiography. All authors classify patients with ECG changes only as myocardial concussion and patients with abnormal wall motion as myocardial contusion. The variability lies in whether patients with normal wall motion and elevated creatine phosphokinase MB fraction are classified as concussion or contusion.

Clinical Presentation

Patients with commotio cordis collapse and die immediately or shortly after being struck in the chest. Most other patients with blunt cardiac injury will have other signs of thoracic trauma such as rib fractures, sternal fractures, flail segments, abrasions, or palpable crepitus. Some patients will experience pain specifically from the cardiac contusion, which is retrosternal and anginal in quality.

Indications for Imaging

Imaging with either echocardiogram or ECG gated first-pass radionuclide angiography (RNA) is indicated in patients with suspected myocardial contusion who are hemodynamically unstable. The need for either of these studies in hemodynamically stable patients is less clear. In two studies, RNA was not predictive of cardiac complications (39,40). In a third study, the authors concluded that echocardiography and RNA added little clinically to diagnoses and management (41). A persistently abnormal ECG is one indication for either echocardiography or RNA in a hemodynamically stable patient. Abnormal ECG patterns reported in myocardial contusion are ST-T wave abnormalities, right bundle branch block, intraventricular conduction delay, atrial dysrhythmias, premature ventricular contractions, and myocardial infarction patterns (39,41).

Imaging Methods

Two-dimensional echocardiography and RNA are considered the best tests to confirm the diagnosis of myocardial contusion. Abnormalities are found predominately in the right ventricle in both studies.

Abnormalities found on RNA in myocardial contusion include depressed global right ventricular ejection fraction (<40%), depressed global left ventricular ejection fraction (<50%), and segmental wall motion abnormalities of both the right and left ventricles (39,40).

Abnormalities found on echocardiography include generalized right ventricular dilatation, localized myocardial thinning, segmental wall motion abnormalities, thrombi, pericardial effu-

sion, valvular rupture, and right ventricular intramyocardial hematoma (42,43) (Fig. 6-21).

Echocardiography has an advantage over RNA because, unlike RNA, it is able to detect cardiac valve dysfunction, papillary muscle dysfunction, abnormalities of the aortic root, mural thrombus, and pericardial effusions.

Implications for Management

If myocardial contusion is suspected, the patient should be observed in a monitored bed with creatine phosphokinase MB fraction determinations every 8 hours. The majority of authors recommend 24 hours of observation to rule out cardiac injury. However, in one study of hemodynamically stable patients, all complications were seen in patients who had abnormal ECGs on admission. The authors concluded that hemodynamically stable patients with normal ECGs on admission could be discharged safely

F I G U R E **6-21**

Case 1. Apical four-chamber view showing ventricular cavities. In the right ventricular apex, there is a huge hyperrefractile thrombus (*T***) (***arrows***). Associated features include dilated right ventricle and akinetic free wall (***RA,*** right atrium; ***RV,*** right ventricle; ***LV,*** left ventricle; ***LA,*** left atrium; ***VS,*** ventricular septum; ***S,*** superior; ***L,*** left; ***I,*** inferior, ***R,*** right). (Reproduced by permission from King RM, et al. Cardiac contusion: a new diagnostic approach utilizing two-dimensional echocardiography. J Trauma 1983;23:610–614.)**

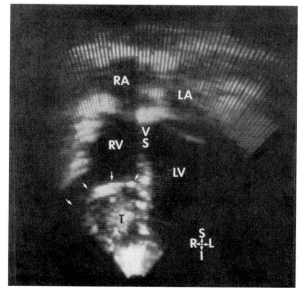

if no problems developed after monitoring for 6 to 12 hours (39). Patients with dysrhythmias should be monitored until their rhythm returns to normal.

The risk of anesthesia and surgery in patients with myocardial contusions is not well defined. Some studies have reported a high incidence of dysrhythmias and hypotension, while others reported no complications (39,41). However, the risk with myocardial contusion seems less than the risk with myocardial infarction. McSwain, in his review of chest injuries published in 1992, said, "neither contusion nor concussion [is] a deterrent to operative management of trauma" (26).

The indications for anticoagulation in myocardial contusion with or without thrombi have not been well studied.

REFERENCES

1. Barrett GR, Shelton WR, Miles JW. First rib fractures in football players. Am J Sports Med 1988; 16:674–678.

2. Mikawa Y, Kobori M. Stress fracture of the first rib in a weightlifter. Arch Orthop Trauma Surg 1991;110:121–122.

3. Miles JW, Barrett GR. Rib fractures in athletes. Sports Med 1991;12:66–69.

4. Tullos HS, Erwin WD, Woods GW, et al. Unusual lesions of the pitching arm. Clin Orthop 1972;88: 169–182.

5. McBeath AA, Keene JS. The rib-tip syndrome. J Bone Joint Surg 1975;57A:795–797.

6. Holden DL, Jackson DW. Stress fracture of the ribs in female rowers. Am J Sports Med 1985;13: 342–348.

7. Gurtler R, Pavlov H, Torg JS. Stress fracture of the ipsilateral first rib in a pitcher. Am J Sports Med 1985;13:277–279.

8. DeLuca SA, Rhea JT, O'Malley T. Radiographic evaluation of rib fractures. AJR 1982;138:91–92.

9. Thompson BM, Finger W, Tonsfeldt D, et al. Rib radiographs for trauma: useful or wasteful? Ann Emerg Med 1986;15:261–265.

10. Rodgers L. Radiology of skeletal trauma. 2nd ed. New York: Churchill-Livingstone, 1992.

11. Martire JR. Differentiating stress fracture from periostitis: the finer points of bone scans. Phys Sportsmed 1994;22:71–81.

12. McKenzie DC. Stress fracture of the rib in an elite oarsman. Int J Sports Med 1989;10:220–222.

13. Harley DP, Mena I. Cardiac and vascular sequelae of sternal fractures. J Trauma 1986;26:553–555.

14. Buckman R, Trooskin SZ, Flancbaum L, Chandler J. The significance of stable patients with sternal fractures. Surg Gynecol Obstet 1987;164:261–265.

15. Keating TM. Stress fracture of the sternum in a wrestler. Am J Sports Med 1987;15:92–93.

16. Rose KD, Stone F, Fuenning SI, et al. Cardiac contusion resulting from "spearing" in football. Arch Intern Med 1966;118:129–131.

17. Stark P, Jaramillo D. CT of the sternum. AJR 1986; 147:72–77.

18. Grant JCB. An atlas of anatomy. 6th ed. Baltimore: Williams & Wilkins, 1972.

19. Ballinger P. Radiographic physicians and radiologic procedures. 7th ed. St. Louis: Mosby–Year Book, 1991.

20. Mayba II. Sternal injuries. Orthoped Rev 1986; 15:35–43.

21. Mayba II. Non-union of fractures of the sternum. J Bone Joint Surg 1985;67-A:1091–1093.

22. Chester VBE, Murphy M. Pneumothorax in an athlete. Brit J Sports Med 1982;16:254–255.

23. Tocino I, Miller M, Fairfax W. Distribution of neumothorax in the supine and semirecumbent critically ill adult. AJR 1985;144:901–905.

24. Hammond SG. Chest injuries in the trauma patient. Nurs Clin N Am 1990;25:35–43.

25. Jones KW. Thoracic trauma. Surg Clin N Am 1980;60:957–981.

26. McSwain, NE. Blunt and penetrating chest injuries. World J Surg 1992;16:924–929.

27. McCormack DL, Bliss WR. Rupture of the diaphragm in a wrestling match. J Iowa Med Soc 1983;October:406–408.

28. Ball T, McCrory R, Smith JO, Clements JL Jr. Traumatic diaphragmatic hernia: errors in diagnosis. AJR 1982;138:633–637.

29. Carter BN, Giuseffi J, Felson B. Traumatic diaphragmatic hernia. AJR 1951;65:56–72.

30. Troop B, Myers RM, Nikileshwer AN. Early recognition of diaphragmatic injuries from blunt trauma. Ann Emerg Med 1985;14:97–101.

31. Griswald F, Warden H, Gardner R. Acute diaphragmatic rupture caused by blunt trauma. Am J Surg 1972;124:359–362.

32. Mirvis SE, Bidwell JK, Buddemeyer EU, et al. Imaging diagnosis of traumatic aortic rupture: a review and experience at a major trauma center. Invest Radiol 1987;22:187–196.

33. Mirvis SE, Templeton PA. Imaging of thoracic trauma. Sem Thoracic Cardiovasc Surg 1992;4: 177–186.

34. Gundry SR, Williams S, Burney RE, et al. Indications for aortography in blunt thoracic trauma: a reassessment. J Trauma 1982;22:664–671.

35. Gundry SR, Burney RE, Mackenzie JR, et al. Assessment of mediastinal widening associated with traumatic rupture of the aorta. J Trauma 1983;24:293–299.

36. Mirvis SE, Bidwell JK, Buddemeyer EU, et al. Value of chest radiography in excluding traumatic aortic rupture. Radiology 1987;163:487–493.

37. Abrunzo TJ. Commotio cordis: the single most common cause of traumatic death in youth baseball. Am J Dis Child 1991;145:1279–1282.

38. Green ED, Simson LR Jr, Kellerman HH, et al. Cardiac concussion following softball blow to the chest. Ann Emerg Med 1980;9:155–157.

39. Dubrow TJ, Mihalka J, Eisenhauer DM, et al. Myocardial contusion in the stable patient: what level of care is appropriate? Surgery 1989;106: 267–274.

40. Fenner JE, Knopp R, Lee B, et al. The use of gated radionuclide angiography in the diagnosis of cardiac contusion. Ann Emerg Med 1984;13: 688–694.

41. Fabian TC, Mangiante EC, Patterson CR, et al. Myocardial contusion in blunt trauma: clinical characteristics, means of diagnosis, and implications for patient management. J Trauma 1988;28: 50–57.

42. King RM, Mucha P Jr, Seward JB, et al. Cardiac contusion: a new diagnostic approach utilizing two-dimensional echocardiography. J Trauma 1983;23:610–614.

43. Miller FA, Seward JB, Gerish BJ, et al. Two-dimensional echocardiographic findings in cardiac trauma. Am J Cardiol 1982;50:1022–1027.

CHAPTER 7

Imaging of the Shoulder

BRIAN HALPERN
SHELDON KAPLAN

*S*houlder and upper arm injuries are commonplace in athletics today. While such injuries are not as prevalent as knee injuries, racquet and throwing sports have generated a large patient population with sometimes perplexing shoulder complaints.

Generalized shoulder pain frequently develops from overuse. Contact injuries also produce an array of shoulder problems. To determine the diagnosis, the examiner always must begin with the history and physical examination. Mechanism of injury and location of pain, weakness, or instability on testing all narrow the differential diagnosis. Imaging of the affected area then helps confirm the findings, isolates the problem, and aids in directing the treatment plan.

Numerous imaging modalities have become available for evaluating shoulder: plain x-ray, tomography, computed tomographic (CT) scanning, arthrography, ultrasound, magnetic resonance imaging (MRI), kinematic MRI, planar and single photon emission computed tomographic (SPECT) bone scanning, and other studies. The choice of imaging techniques for diagnostic confirmation is often difficult for the sports medicine physician. He or she must be cognizant of radiation exposure, accessibility, cost, benefit, risk, and the overall sensitivity and specificity of the imaging technique utilized. Beyond this, the physician must be able to interpret these studies and utilize this information to develop an appropriate treatment plan. This is achieved more easily with a good working knowledge of the various injuries affecting the shoulder and upper arm.

Optimal evaluation of shoulder injuries requires a thorough knowledge of regional anatomy. The shoulder girdle is comprised of the sternoclavicular joint, the acromioclavicular joint, the glenohumeral joint, the subacromial space, and the scapulothoracic articulation. Movement about all these articulations allows for the complexity of the throwing motion (1,2).

The sternoclavicular joint supports the anteromedial clavicle. The articulation is between the proximal clavicle and the superolateral portion of the manubrium (2). The posterior capsule of the joint is much stronger than the anterior capsule, predisposing to more frequent anterior dislocations. In athletes 22 years of age or younger, epiphyseal separation of the medial clavicle needs to be considered when sternoclavicular injuries occur. Posterior dislocations may cause trauma to the underlying structures of the mediastinum, necessitating a high index of suspicion when entertaining this diagnosis. More selective imaging techniques therefore may be warranted in this situation.

The acromioclavicular joint is situated between the lateral end of the clavicle and the medial surface of the acromion. It is associated with an intra-articular meniscus that may be incomplete. The acromioclavicular ligament provides superior support, but the major stabilizing structures are the coracoclavicular ligaments (the conoid and trapezoid). The degree of acromioclavicular separation may be assessed by determining the relative displacement of the acromion from the clavicle radiographically. X-rays are also useful for identifying a fracture component.

The glenohumeral joint is a synovial ball-and-socket joint in which a one-third spherical humeral head sits in the shallow glenoid fossa.

To improve the containment of the humeral head, the glenoid labrum attaches peripherally around the margin of the glenoid. Thickenings of the capsule form the glenohumeral ligaments: the superior, middle, and inferior (3). MRI and CT arthrography afford visualization of these structures with specific attention to possible Bankart lesions (anteroinferior labral and inferior glenohumeral capsular detachment from the glenoid) in patients with glenohumeral instability.

The muscles of the shoulder girdle that comprise the rotator cuff are the subscapularis anteriorly, the supraspinatus, the infraspinatus, and the teres minor posteriorly. The anatomic detail displayed by MRI has advanced diagnostic acumen with reference to injuries of these structures.

The subacromial space lies between the acromial arch and the rotator cuff. The supraspinatus muscle and the biceps tendon lie adjacent to each other in this area. This space allows free movement between the rotator cuff below and the coracoacromial ligament and acromion above, enabling the wide functional mobility of the shoulder girdle.

The scapulothoracic articulation contributes significantly to shoulder function. Abduction occurs with glenohumeral and scapulothoracic movement in a 3:2 ratio. The scapula is stabilized by multiple muscles (rhomboid; serratus anterior; upper, middle, and lower trapezius; and levatores scapulae). Dysfunction of this group can lead to shoulder pain in the throwing athlete. Imaging of the shoulder joint always should begin with plain radiography. A minimum of three to four views should be obtained. The age of the patient, history of trauma, and mechanism of injury help determine which views to obtain. Even experts continue to vary as to their specific recommendations. In general, the four views obtained are an anteroposterior (AP) internal rotation view, an AP external rotation view, an axillary view, and a scapular Y view. The AP internal and external rotation views can be replaced by a true AP shoulder view (at right angles to the scapular plane) in internal and external rotation.

In the true AP internal rotation view (Fig. 7-1), the proximal humerus assumes a symmetric, light-bulb shape. The lesser tuberosity is seen medially. The greater tuberosity is identified by the increased density overlying the neck of the humerus (4). This view is useful for visualizing the acromioclavicular joint, humeral head, and tuberosities.

In the AP external rotation view, the humeral head appears club shaped (Fig. 7-2). The bicipi-

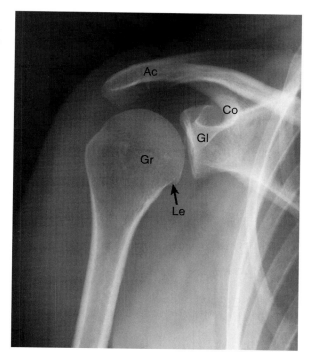

F I G U R E   7-1

True AP internal rotation view of the shoulder. Please note the following features: (*Ac*) acromion process, (*Gl*) glenoid, (*Gr*) greater tuberosity of the humerus, (*Le*) lesser tuberosity, and (*Co*) coracoid process.

tal groove may be identified as a space between thin, parallel bands of sclerotic bone (4). Alignment, arthritic changes, and calcium deposition are better demonstrated than in internal rotation. Calcification may indicate calcific tendonitis, intra-articular loose bodies, or chondrocalcinosis. Osteophytes are seen more frequently at the medial head-neck junction of the humerus, indicating degenerative joint disease.

The true AP view affords a better look at the glenohumeral joint, since there is no bony overlap between the humeral head and the glenoid. This allows a better assessment of fractures of the glenoid or humeral head and osteoarthritic changes (Fig. 7-3).

In the axillary view, the glenohumeral joint is visualized in another plane. Bony Bankart lesions may be demonstrated by a fracture or ectopic bone at the inferior glenoid rim. This view also helps assess glenoid version (normal is 6 to 7 degrees of retroversion relative to the scapular plane) (5), humeral head compression fractures, and the position of the humeral head relative to the glenoid (6). There are many formats to performing the axillary view: the supine axillary

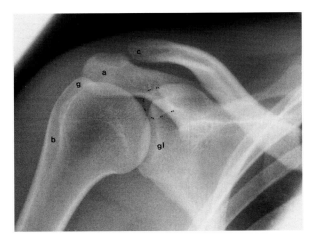

F I G U R E   **7-2**

AP external rotation view of the shoulder: (*a*) acromian process, (*c*) distal clavicle, (*gl*) glenoid, (*g*) greater tuberosity of the humerus, and (*b*) bicipital groove. The coracoid process is outlined.

view (Fig. 7-4) and the West Point axillary view (Fig. 7-5) being the most common.

The scapular Y view (true scapular lateral view) is important following a traumatic event to identify an anterior or posterior dislocation (Fig. 7-6). The scapula assumes the shape of the letter Y, with the letter's arms formed by the scapular spine and coracoid process and its tail by the body of the scapula. The humeral head

should line up with the glenoid fossa at the junction of the arms and tail of the Y (4).

The following discussion outlines simple and complex injuries of the shoulder with subsequent assessment through appropriate imaging.

Acromioclavicular Joint Injuries

Acromioclavicular (AC) joint injuries are mostly traumatic, usually from a direct force to the point of the shoulder with the arm in the adducted position. X-rays of the AC joint using routine shoulder technique often will be overpenetrated (too dark), and small fractures may be overlooked. Plain x-rays are taken with an AP and 15-degree cranial angulation view. If utilizing comparison views, both AC joints ideally should be imaged simultaneously on one large cassette (Fig. 7-7). A true scapular lateral view adds another plane in which to visualize the AC joint (7). This radiograph with a normal side comparison helps identify anteroposterior displacement of the clavicle (see Fig. 7-6). Additionally, stress views (with 5- to 15-lb weights) help demonstrate the integrity of the coracoclavicular ligaments. The weights should be hanging from the wrist to encourage complete muscle relaxation. Although helpful, diagnosis can be obtained without the costs of these weighted stress views.

F I G U R E   **7-3**

(A) True AP external rotation view. Note the lack of overlap of the humeral head on the glenoid (*h*, humeral head; *g*, glenoid; *j*, glenohumeral joint space). This view is obtained using a 45-degree posterior oblique tube angle. (B) Imaging technique for routine AP and true AP shoulder views. (B: Reproduced by permission from Curtis R. Injuries of the proximal humerus. In: Orthopaedic sports medicine, Vol. 1. Philadelphia: Saunders. 1994:672.)

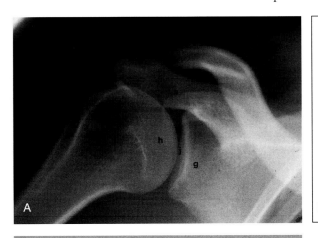

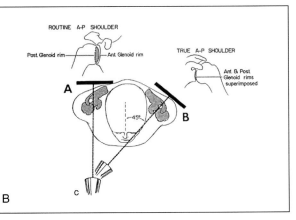

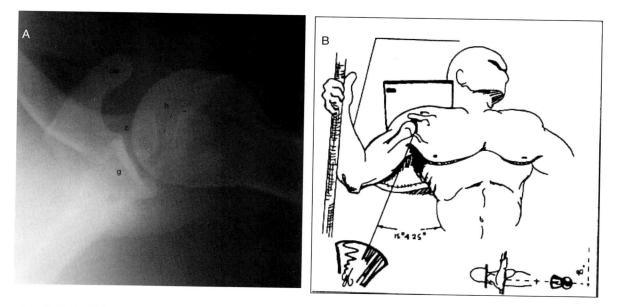

FIGURE 7-4

(A) Routine supine axillary view: (*h*) humeral head, (*g*) glenoid, (*c*) distal clavicle, (*co*) coracoid. The acromion process is outlined. (B) Routine supine axillary view. Demonstrates the glenohumeral joint in craniocaudad orientation. Useful for evaluation of the glenohumeral joint alignment, the glenoid margins, and the acromion. The patient is supine with the arm in neutral rotation and 45 degrees of abduction. The film cassette is placed perpendicular to the table against the top of the shoulder. The x-ray beam is horizontal to the axilla at an angle of 15 to 25 degrees from the sagittal plane. (B: Reproduced by permission from Curtis R. Injuries of the proximal humerus. In: Orthopaedic sports medicine, Vol. 1. Philadelphia: Saunders. 1994.)

Instability of the AC joint can be approached through a classification system from grade I to grade VI (Fig. 7-8):

Grade I: Acromioclavicular ligament partially torn, normal x-rays.

Grade II: Acromioclavicular ligament disruption and stretching of the coracoclavicular ligament, decrease in horizontal stability of the AC joint, slight relative upward migration of the clavicle, potential widening of the AC joint (Fig. 7-9).

Grade III: Complete disruption of the acromioclavicular and coracoclavicular ligaments, acromion displaced downward relative to the clavicle and unstable in both horizontal and vertical planes, plain radiographs demonstrating a coracoclavicular distance of greater than 1.3 cm or a coracoclavicular interval that is more than 25% greater than that of the uninvolved shoulder (Fig. 7-10).

Grade IV: Clavicle is grossly displaced posteriorly into or through the trapezius muscle, best seen using the scapular Y view (Fig. 7-11).

Grade V: Severe vertical separation of the clavicle from the scapula, coracoclavicular interval exceeds 100% of that of the uninvolved shoulder.

Grade VI: Clavicle dislocated inferiorly into the subacromial or subcoracoid position.

Plain radiography continues to be the most readily available and cost-effective method for routine investigation of the AC joint injuries described above (7).

The information gleaned from these plane radiographs allows grading of these injuries. Understanding of grade determines the treatment plan. Grade I and II injuries are treated nonoperatively. Extensive bracing and splinting can be attempted for 3 to 6 weeks, but most authors recommend a sling for symptomatic relief, followed by early rehabilitation and return to sport. With the diagnosis of grade III separa-

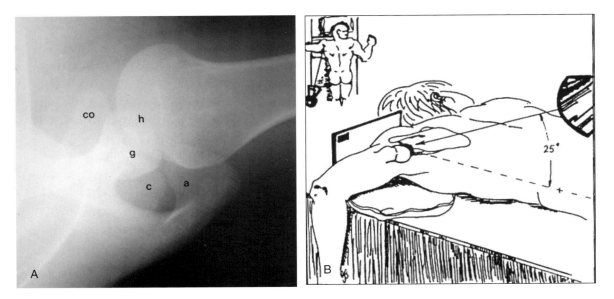

F I G U R E   **7-5**

(A) Westpoint axillary view (*h,* humeral head; *g,* glenoid; *c,* distal clavicle; *a,* acromion; *co,* coracoid). (B) Imaging technique for the Westpoint axillary view. The anteroinferior glenoid margin is visualized without structure superimposition. Specifically used for detecting osseous Bankart lesion. Patient is in prone position with shoulder propped over a pillow. The arm is in internal rotation and hanging down from the edge of the table. The x-ray beam is angled downward 25 degrees from the horizontal plane and 25 degrees from the sagittal plane of the body. (B: Reproduced by permission from Curtis R. Injuries of the proximal humerus. In: Orthopaedic sports medicine, Vol. 1. Philadelphia: Saunders. 1994:101.)

tions, three main treatment options are available: 1) sling and early rehabilitation, 2) closed reduction with application of sling and harness, and 3) operative reduction. Many authors recently have recommended short-term immobilization followed by early motion. There has been little, if any, deficit in strength or function documented in patients treated nonoperatively (7), with the possible exception of the dominant arm in a high-performance thrower.

Clavicle Fractures

Clavicle fractures are very common, especially in childhood. They are frequently the result of direct trauma. Classification includes distal, middle, and proximal third fractures.

Distal third fractures may present as an AC separation. For this reason, routine AC views, as just discussed, would be appropriate. Additional clavicular shaft images also may be helpful with an AP view and a 45-degree cephalic-tilt AP view. These fractures can be classified as type 1, minimal displacement; type 2, displaced sec-

ondary to a fracture medial to the coracoclavicular ligaments (Fig. 7-12); and type 3, articular surface fracture (8). Type 1 fractures can be treated symptomatically with a sling and early rehabilitation. Type 2 fractures sometimes can be splinted to healing, but many times operative reduction and internal fixation are necessary. Poor reduction often leads to a bony nonunion. Type 3 fractures also can be treated with just a sling. However, a late complication of this injury is distal clavicular osteolysis (Fig. 7-13), sometimes requiring treatment with a lateral clavicle excision.

Fractures of the shaft in the middle third, diagnosed by AP clavicular images, usually can be managed with a well-padded figure 8 splint worn for 4 to 8 weeks (Fig. 7-14). It is unusual for these fractures to go on to nonunion. Gentle range-of-motion exercises can begin as the pain subsides and increased as union progresses.

Fractures of the proximal third are treated with a supporting sling unless displaced or associated with a fracture-dislocation of the sternoclavicular joint (Fig. 7-15). These may be visualized with clavicular shaft images, as

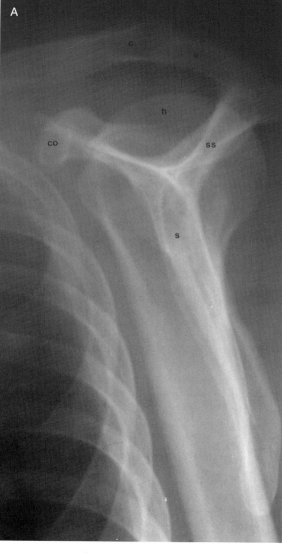

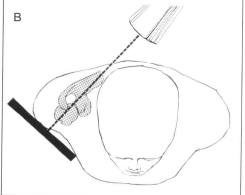

FIGURE **7-6**

(A) True scapular lateral (Y) view (*a,* acromion; *c,* distal clavicle; *h,* humeral head; *co,* coracoid process; *ss,* scapular spine; *s,* scapular body). Note that the humeral head, when normally positioned, is centered over the branch point of the scapular Y on this view. (B) Imaging technique for scapular Y view. The cassette is placed lateral to the affected shoulder and the x-ray beam is directed along the scapular spine. (B: Reproduced by permission from Rockwood CA, Matsen DD, eds. The shoulder. Philadelphia: Saunders. 1990.)

FIGURE **7-7**

Bilateral AP view of acromioclavicular joints (*a,* acromion process; *cl,* distal clavicle; *c,* coracoid process). The arrow indicates the location of the acromioclavicular joint. The arrowhead points to the region of the coracoclavicular ligaments.

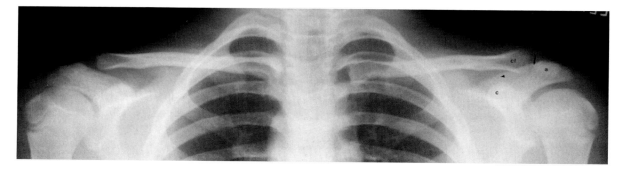

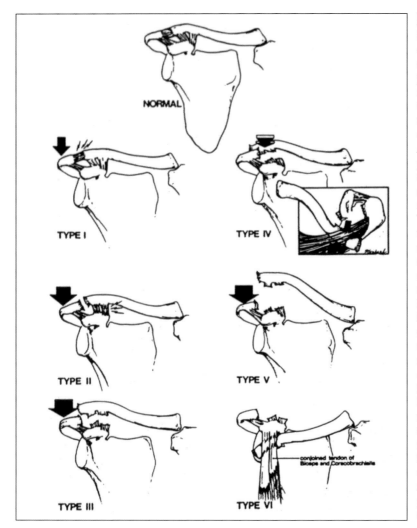

F I G U R E **7-8**

Schematic drawings of the classification of ligamentous injuries that can occur to the acromioclavicular joint. (*Type I*) In a type I injury, a mild force applied to the point of the shoulder does not disrupt either the acromioclavicular or the coracoclavicular ligament. (*Type II*) A moderate to heavy force applied to the point of the shoulder disrupts the acromioclavicular ligaments, but the coraclavicular ligaments remain intact. (*Type III*) When a severe force is applied to the point of the shoulder, both the acromioclavicular and the coracoclavicular ligaments are disrupted. (*Type IV*) In a type IV injury, not only are the ligaments disrupted, but the distal end of the clavicle is also displaced posteriorly into or through the trapezius muscle. (*Type V*) A violent force applied to the point of the shoulder not only ruptures the acromioclavicular and coracoclavicular ligaments but also disrupts the muscle attachments and creates a major separation between the clavicle and the acromion. (*Type VI*) This is an inferior dislocation of the distal clavicle in which the clavicle is inferior to the coracoid process and posterior to the biceps and coracobrachialis tendons. The acromioclavicular and coracoclavicular ligaments also have been disrupted. (Reproduced by permission from Rockwood CA, Green DP, eds. Fractures in adults. 2nd ed. Philadelphia: JB Lippincott, 1984:871.)

described above; additional sternoclavicular views, to be discussed later, also may be helpful.

Scapular Fractures

Scapular fractures are usually the result of severe trauma, most commonly involving the scapular body and neck. Significant associated injuries may be seen in up to 90% of patients with scapular fractures (9). A true AP view of the scapula, or sometimes a standard AP view, combined with an axillary or true scapular lateral view demonstrates most scapular body or spine fractures, glenoid neck fractures, and acromion fractures (9) (Figs. 7-16 and 7-17). A true AP view of the scapula is obtained in a manner similar to a true AP view of the shoulder, by obliquing the patient approximately 40 degrees to the x-ray plate. CT scanning is useful for evaluation of glenoid fractures, which are many times associated with glenohumeral instability. Other suspected scapular fractures that are radiographically occult may be well demonstrated by CT.

Most extra-articular fractures are managed nonoperatively, with a sling followed by an exercise regimen, whereas the converse applies to the intra-articular fractures.

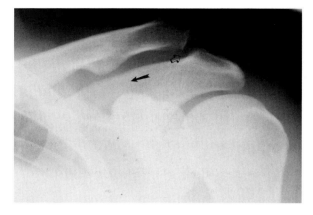

FIGURE **7-9**

Grade II acromioclavicular ligament sprain. The open arrow indicates disruption of the acromioclavicular ligament with separation of the joint. The black arrow indicates the region of the coracoclavicular ligaments. The coracoclavicular ligaments remain intact, as evidenced by a normal coracoclavicular interval.

Sternoclavicular Joint Injuries

Sternoclavicular joint dislocations/subluxations are almost always the result of trauma. Anterior dislocations are more common, the medial end of the clavicle being displaced anteriorly or anterosuperiorly with respect to the anterior margins of the sternum (Fig. 7-18). Posterior dislocations are less frequent but more severe because of possible injury to the underlying structures (trachea, great vessels, esophagus, and other mediastinal structures) (2).

Traumatic injuries are graded I, intact ligaments and stable joint; II, subluxation of the sternoclavicular joint with partial disruption of ligaments and capsule; and III, dislocation with complete ligamentous and capsular disruption (10).

AP or PA views of the chest or sternoclavicular joint (Fig. 7-19) may suggest an abnormality when one end of the clavicle appears to be displaced compared with the normal side. It is sometimes difficult to differentiate between an anterior and posterior dislocation. In this situation, a 40-degree cephalic-tilt view may be utilized (11) (Fig. 7-20). The cephalic-tilt view causes differential displacements of the clavicles depending on their distance from the x-ray plate and tube. A cephalic tilt is performed if the x-ray is AP, but a caudal tilt is employed if the x-ray is PA. Tomograms can help distinguish fractures from dislocations and determine the anterior or posterior direction as well. CT scanning and MRI create cross-sectional tomographic images that

FIGURE **7-10**

(A) Grade III acromioclavicular ligament sprain. The double-headed arrow indicates the torn ends of the acromioclavicular ligament. Separation of the AC joint is evident. The arrows indicate the torn ends of the coracoclavicular ligament. Note the increase in coracoclavicular interval (*A* to *B*). (B) Grade III acromioclavicular ligament sprain. Note the separation of the acromioclavicular joint and the increased coracoclavicular interval (*arrows*).

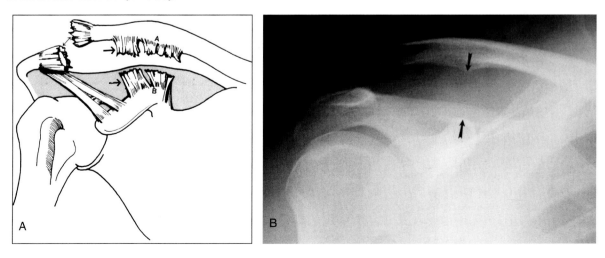

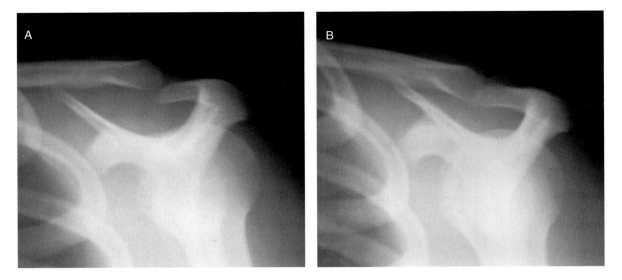

F I G U R E   **7-11**

(A) Grade IV AC ligament sprain (posterior dislocation) (*arrow*). The clavicle is displaced posteriorly. (B) Other side in the same patient suggests a normal acromioclavicular joint (*arrow*).

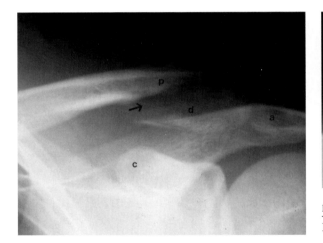

F I G U R E   **7-12**

Type II fracture of the distal third of the clavicle (*p* and *d,* proximal and distal clavicular fragments). The arrow points to the fracture (*a,* acromion; *c,* coracoid).

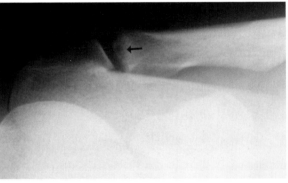

F I G U R E   **7-13**

Distal clavicular osteolysis. Lytic defects (*arrow*).

allow evaluation of bone but additionally visualize injury to the great vessels, trachea, and esophagus that may occur secondary to posterior dislocation.

In patients with posterior dislocations, it is vital to rule out underlying mediastinal structural injury before reduction is attempted, unless

the patient is hemodynamically compromised. Cross-sectional imaging (CT or MRI) is useful for evaluating these structures. In the rare instance of progressive respiratory and/or vascular compromise from a posterior dislocation, reduction can be attempted before imaging is obtained. This reduction is performed by using a towel clip to pull the medial clavicle anteriorly. Anterior dislocation may be reduced without cross-sectional mediastinal imaging because there is significantly less risk of concomitant injuries than with posterior dislocations (11).

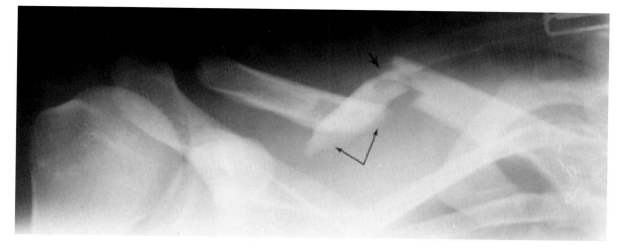

FIGURE **7-14**

Fracture of the middle third of the clavicle in two locations, both severely angulated.

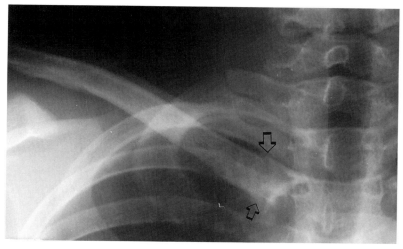

FIGURE **7-15**

Fracture of the proximal third of the clavicle. Open arrows indicate the location of the nondisplaced fracture.

Glenohumeral Instability

Shoulder subluxations and dislocations are other common contact injuries of the shoulder. Subluxation occurs with abnormal translation of the humeral head in the glenoid without complete separation of the articular surfaces. With a dislocation, the articular surfaces become completely separated, and the humeral head loses contact with the glenoid and can lodge along the sides of the joint (1). Subluxation may be so transient that the athlete only feels a sudden pain and the arm "goes dead" (12). Subluxation may occur without contact, particularly in the throwing athlete as a result of the microtrauma associated with repetitive use (6).

Instability may occur anteriorly, posteriorly, inferiorly, or even multidirectionally. On physical examination, the patient with the more common anterior dislocation is unable to rotate the arm internally and cannot touch the opposite shoulder with the hand of the involved arm. With the less common posterior dislocation, the arm is locked in internal rotation (13).

Imaging should begin with three views that comprise the "trauma series": true AP view (see Figs. 7-1 and 7-3), true scapular lateral view (Y view; see Fig. 7-6), and an axillary view (6) (see Fig. 7-5).

Additional complementary views may be used when needed. These include the Stryker notch view and the apical oblique projection.

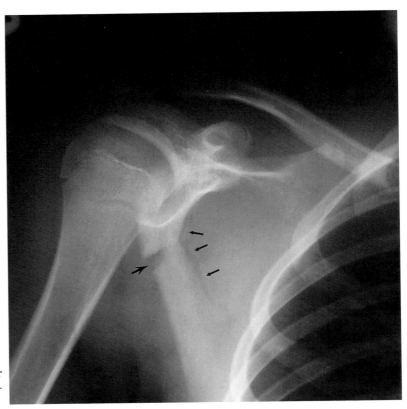

F I G U R E   **7-16**

Standard AP view of the shoulder demonstrates scapular body fracture (*arrows*).

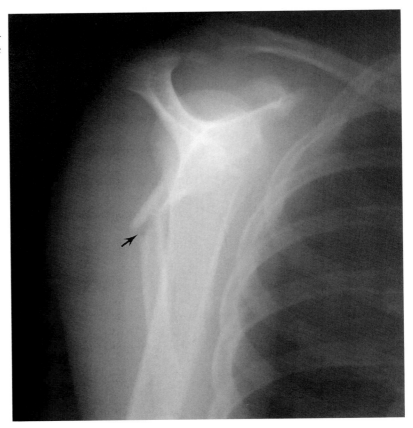

F I G U R E   **7-17**

True scapular lateral view demonstrates scapular body fracture (*arrow*).

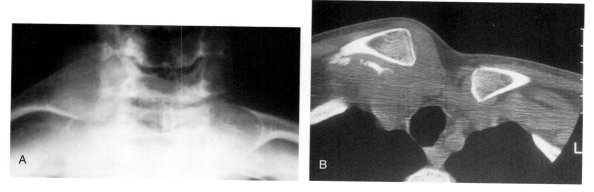

F I G U R E   **7-18**

Anterior dislocation of the right sternoclavicular join. (A) The plain film was obtained with the patient supine and the x-ray tube angled toward the head, accounting for the projection of the right clavicular head superior to that of the left clavicle. (B) The axial CT demonstrates anterior dislocation of the head of the right clavicle in the same patient.

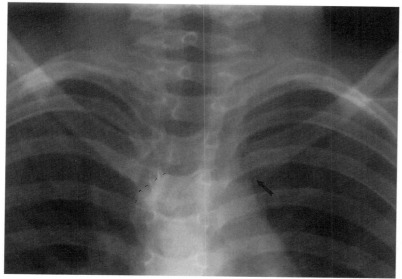
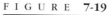

F I G U R E   **7-19**

AP view of the sternoclavicular joints. Arrow indicates the SC joint. Dotted line shows the location of the manubrial articular surface.

The Stryker notch view (Fig. 7-21) helps demonstrate Hill-Sachs lesions (the "notch in the posterior lateral humeral head") (6) (see also Fig. 7-23B).

Further evaluation incorporates MRI, defining the soft tissue pathology noted in many patients with shoulder instabilities. MRI is useful for identifying labral and capsular lesions in the acute and chronic settings. However, one must first have knowledge of the normal anatomy as depicted by MRI.

The anterior labrum is a triangular shape in cross section, whereas the posterior labrum is frequently more rounded. Superiorly, the cartilaginous labrum is contiguous with the long head of the biceps. The normal labrum on MRI demonstrates a homogeneously dark appearance with well-defined outlines (14) (Fig. 7-22).

Evaluation of patients with anterior instability may demonstrate fraying or tearing of the anteroinferior labrum (Fig. 7-23). Less often associated with acute dislocation, tears of the superior labrum have been demonstrated to occur in throwers. This is thought to occur more from repetitive injury than from acute traumatic events (6). Also, superior labral injuries extend-

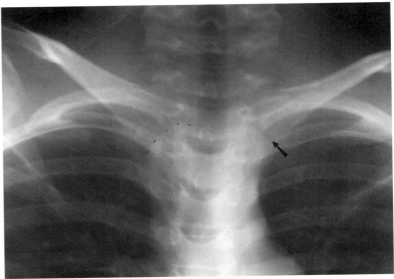

FIGURE 7-20

Forty-degree cephalic-tilt view of sternoclavicular joints. Arrow indicates the SC joint. Dotted line shows the location of the manubrial articular surface.

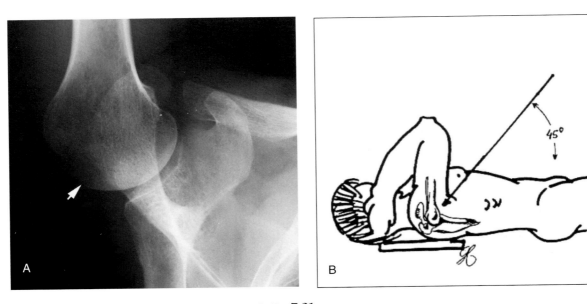

FIGURE 7-21

(A) Stryker notch view. The arrow indicates the expected location of a Hill-Sach's defect at the posterosuperior aspect of the humeral head. This particular humeral head is normal. (B) Imaging technique for Stryker notch view. Posterosuperior aspect of the humeral head is tangentially projected. Specifically useful for demonstrating Hill-Sach's defects. The patient is supine, the arm is elevated 90 degrees, and the elbow is flexed so that the palm of the hand is on the ear or resting on the side of the head. The humerus is parallel to the sagittal plane of the body. The x-ray beam is directed to the axilla 45 degrees from the horizontal plane. A variation of the view may be obtained with a 10-degree cephalad angulation of the beam. (B: Reproduced by permission from Curtis R. Injuries to the proximal humerus. In: Orthopaedic sports medicine, Vol. 1. Philadelphia: Saunders. 1994:103.)

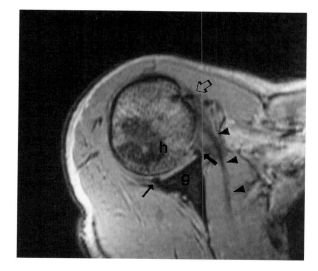

F I G U R E   **7-22**

Normal axial gradient-echo MRI image through the midlevel of the glenohumeral joint. Intact anterior and posterior glenoid labra are indicated by thicker and thinner black arrows, respectively. Note the homogeneous signal intensity of the labra and well-defined contour (*h* and *g*, humeral head and glenoid). The open arrow indicates the location of the biceps tendon. The arrowheads demonstrate the normal position of the subscapularis tendon.

ing from posterior to anterior (SLAP lesions) are seen from falls on outstretched arms or from traction injuries (6). These lesions occur in the region of the insertion of the biceps tendon. SLAP lesions have been classified into four types (37) (Fig. 7-24A). Many of these labral tears fail to heal in an aggressive rehabilitation program and need to progress to arthroscopy for definitive treatment (see Fig. 7-24B). Many times debridement has been shown to afford temporary relief, whereas repair of the lesion demonstrates greater success (15).

The capsule arises along the periphery of the glenoid labrum. Anteriorly, the capsule comprises three distinct areas of fibrous thickening forming capsular ligaments (superior glenohumeral, middle glenohumeral, and inferior glenohumeral ligaments (6) (see Fig. 7-24C). The superior glenohumeral ligament originates from the anterosuperior labrum, anterior to the biceps tendon, and inserts superiorly onto the lesser tuberosity near the bicipital grove. The middle glenohumeral ligament begins adjacent to the superior glenohumeral ligament and attaches on the lesser tuberosity proximate to the subscapularis tendon. The inferior glenohumeral ligament

extends from the anteroinferior labrum to insert just inferior to the middle glenohumeral ligament. The inferior glenohumeral ligament complex functions as the primary static stabilizer against anterior or posterior instability (6). Glenohumeral ligament imaging by MRI appears as homogeneous intermediate to dark zones of capsular thickening, similar in appearance to tendons (14). It is particularly important that these images be obtained with high resolution using small fields of view and thin sections.

MRI has taken a leading role in imaging of the labrum, capsule, and ligamentous structures of the glenohumeral joint. Axial imaging specifically provides a good cross-sectional view of the anterior and posterior labra (see Fig. 7-22). Labral tears are demonstrated by linear bands of increased signal intensity contiguous with a free labral margin (14) (see Fig. 7-23). Labral detachments are identified by the absence of a normal labrum at the margin of the bony glenoid or by a detached fragment surrounded by an effusion on T2-weighted images (14). MRI and MR arthrography appear more sensitive than CT arthrography in detecting the presence of a tear or detachment (35). Patients with anterior or posterior instability also may have more subtle subscapularis tendon tears demonstrated well by MRI (Fig. 7-25) with retraction of the tendon.

Treatment of acute dislocations consists of many, varied closed reduction methods (16). Following the reduction, 3 to 4 weeks of immobilization in a sling succeeded by an intensive rehabilitation program of muscular strengthening exercises, emphasizing internal rotators and adductors, the rotator cuff, and scapular stabilizers, is recommended. Some authors recommend operative stabilization for a first-time dislocation, but long-term follow-up is still limited. Most physicians would agree that one should surgically stabilize a shoulder that already has had three dislocations. In older patients, immobilization should be of shorter duration. An associated rotator cuff tear also should be considered. MRI is very useful for defining or excluding a rotator cuff tear in the patient over 40 years of age who is not progressing well after dislocation.

Posterior dislocations account for only 2% to 4% of all shoulder dislocations (6). Radiographically, the diagnosis is difficult to make on an AP view alone. Normally, the head of the humerus is superimposed on the glenoid in a smooth-bordered ellipse. Distortion of this ellipse may indicate a posterior dislocation (Fig. 7-26).

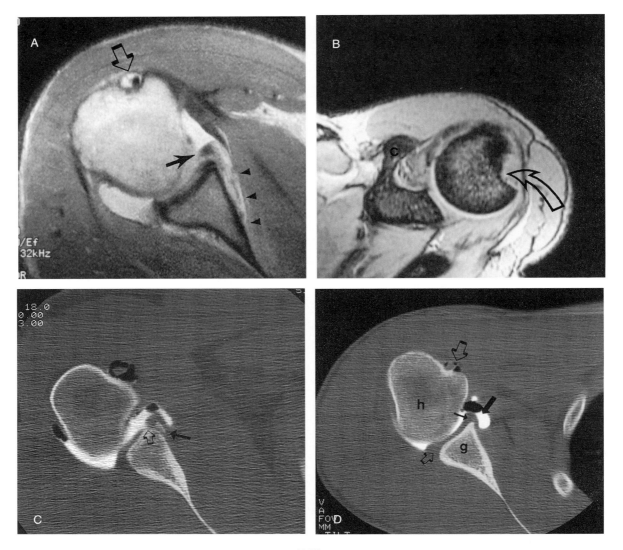

FIGURE 7-23

(A) MRI of anteroinferior glenoid labral avulsion. Proton-density image through the inferior glenohumeral joint demonstrates detachment of the anterior cartilaginous labrum from the underlying glenoid (*arrow*). Note the stripping of the capsule from the anterior surface of the glenoid process (*arrowheads*). The capsule now inserts far medially on the scapular (most inferior arrowhead), a sign of glenohumeral instability. The biceps tendon is seen within its groove, surrounded by fluid within the tendon sheath (*open arrow*). (B) A large Hill-Sach's notch in the glenohumeral head (*curved arrow*). Note that this notch is at the level of the coracoid process (*c*), the expected level of a Hill-Sach's lesion. (C and D) CT arthrograms of glenohumeral instability compared with normal. Image C demonstrates a traumatic cleft in the articular cartilage of the anterior inferior labrum (*open arrow*), along with a bony Bankart fracture (*arrow*). Compare this with image D, a double-contrast CT arthrogram at approximately the same level in a normal shoulder. The thin and small open arrows demonstrate normal-appearing anterior and posterior glenoid labra, respectively. The thick black arrow shows iodinated contrast material and air within the joint space. The large open arrow demonstrates air surrounding the tendon of the long head of the biceps within its sheath. This sheath normally communicates with the glenohumeral joint.

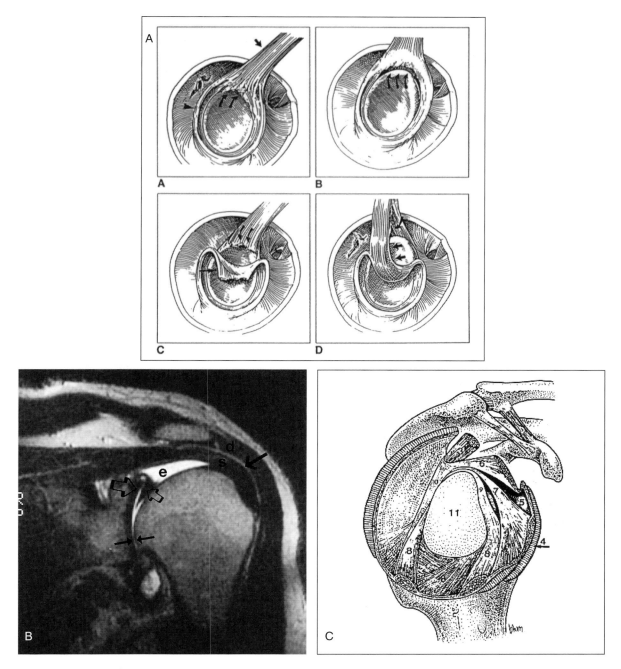

FIGURE 7-24

(A) Types of SLAP lesions. (*A*) Type I SLAP lesion. Diagram shows intact biceps tendon (*straight arrow*), glenoid labrum (*arrowhead*), and fraying of free edge of superior part of glenoid labrum (*curved arrows*). (*B*) Type II SLAP lesion. Diagram shows avulsion of labral-biceps anchor from superior portion of glenoid fossa (*arrows*). (*C*) Type III SLAP lesion. Diagram shows bucket-handle tear of superior portion of glenoid fossa (*straight arrow*) and intact labral-biceps anchor (*curved arrows*). (*D*) Type IV SLAP lesion. Diagram shows bucket-handle tear of superior portion of glenoid fossa (*straight arrows*) with extension of tears into the proximal biceps tendon (*curved arrow*). (Reprinted by permission from Cartland J, et al. MR imaging in the evaluation of SLAP injuries of the shoulder. AJR 1992;159:787–792.) (B) Superior labral tear. The small open arrow indicates the cartilaginous superior glenoid labrum; the large open arrow points to the glenoid. Situated between these two structures is a fine linear focus of high signal intensity representing fluid beneath the detached labrum. On this T2-weighted image note the loss of glenohumeral joint space between arrows (*e*, joint effusion; *s*, suspraspinatus tendon; *d*, deltoid). Large arrow points to the normal subdeltoid fat plane. (C) Anatomy of the glenohumeral ligaments viewed from the side with humeral head removed. (Key: *3*, biceps tendon, long head; *4*, subscapularis muscle and tendon; *5*, subscapularis recess; *6*, superior glenohumeral ligament; *7*, middle glenohumeral ligament; *8*, anterior band axillary pouch and posterior band of the inferior glenohumeral ligament complex; *9*, anterior labrum; *10*, posterior labrum; *11*, glenoid fossa.) (Reproduced by permission from Coumas JM, Waite RJ, Goss TP, et al. CT and MR evaluation of the labral capsular ligamentous complex of the shoulder. AJR 1992;158:591.)

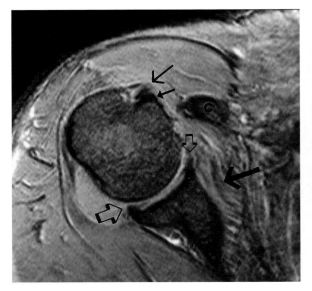

F I G U R E   **7-25**

Subscapularis tendon rupture. This is a single slice from an axial gradient-echo sequence. The thick black arrow indicates the wavy appearance of the completely torn subscapularis tendon. The smallest black arrow points to the normal insertion site of the subscapularis tendon onto the humeral head, just proximal to the bicipital groove. The biceps tendons within the bicipital groove is indicated by the thin black arrow. The small and large open arrows, respectively, indicate the intact anterior and posterior glenoid labra (*C*, coracoid process). Note the intracapsular effusion posterior to the glenohumeral joint, on which the large open arrow is superimposed.

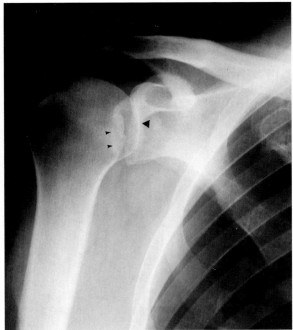

F I G U R E   **7-26**

Posterior dislocation of the glenohumeral joint. The small arrowheads demonstrate a trough line in the medial aspect of the humeral head secondary to impaction fracture against the posterior glenoid. The medial border of the humeral head is indicated by the large arrowhead. It overlaps the rim of the glenoid.

Normally, the humeral head fills most of the glenoid. With a posterior dislocation, the glenoid may appear vacant. X-ray may demonstrate a positive *rim sign;* the space between the anterior rim of the glenoid and the humeral head is greater than 6 mm, suggesting a posterior dislocation (6). The scapular Y view and an axillary view make the diagnosis much simpler. Lesser tuberosity fractures are commonly associated with posterior dislocations, the presence of which should suggest possible posterior dislocation (6).

Following reduction for posterior dislocations, the arm is immobilized in 0 degrees of abduction and in slight extension for 4 to 6 weeks for younger patients and 2 to 3 weeks for older patients. An aggressive rehabilitation program with emphasis on external rotator strengthening is then instituted (6).

Rotator Cuff Problems

The supraspinatus muscle functions primarily as a stabilizer of the glenohumeral joint by providing a compressive force. This action, coupled with deltoid function, allows for the fulcrum effect at the joint and results in abduction (17). The other cuff muscles also provide some humeral head depression but function more as internal and external rotators.

Pathology of the rotator cuff varies from complete tears, seen usually in an older population, to impingement problems, seen commonly in those participating in overhead sports. Primary impingement is thought to result from narrowing of the subacromial space due to edema of the cuff or bony encroachment from the overlying coracoacromial arch (17). Impingement also may occur secondary to eccentric overload of the cuff or glenohumeral instability, which results in failure. In addition, overuse and fatigue of the scapular stabilizers can lead to scapular lag and secondary impingement. Acute trauma can lead to secondary impingement as well.

In summary, the five causes of impingement are 1) bony impingement due to outlet obstruction (the Neer classification), 2) overuse and fatigue of the scapular stabilizers leading to scapular lag and secondary impingement, 3) eccentric overload from repetitive use leading to degeneration and tearing, 4) instability, and 5) acute trauma (17).

Plain radiographic imaging for patients with cuff pathology begins with a true AP film, an axillary view, and an outlet view. The outlet view (a lateral film in the scapular plane with the beam tilted 10 degrees caudad) helps visualize the coracoacromial arch and assess acromial shape and slope (Fig. 7-27). Flat, curved, or hooked acromions can be identified using this view. This has significance, whereby variation in the shape or slope of the acromion may be related to cuff disorders (18). The type III (hooked) acromion has been shown to have a high association with rotator cuff tears (25,30) (Fig. 7-28). In addition, advanced rotator cuff disease often demonstrates increased sclerosis and cystic changes in the greater tuberosity, osteophyte formation on the acromion, and an

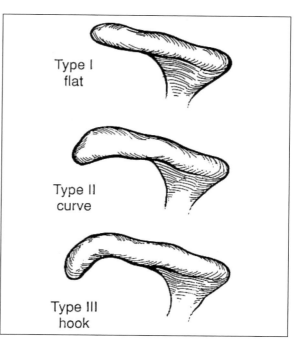

F I G U R E 7-28

Types of acromion processes. (*Top*) Type I, the flat acromion process. (*Middle*) Type II, the curved acromion process. (*Bottom*) Type III, the hooked acromion process. (Redrawn by permission from Rockwood CA, Lyons FR. Shoulder impingement syndrome: diagnosis, radiographic evaluation and treatment with a modified Neer acromioplasty. J Bone Joint Surg 1993;75A:409–424.)

F I G U R E 7-27

Supraspinatus outlet view allows evaluation of the acromioclavicular joint and subacromial arch, specifically geared toward detecting the presence of bony spurs that may impinge on the supraspinatus tendon (*O*, supraspinatus outlet; *a*, acromion; *c*, clavicle).

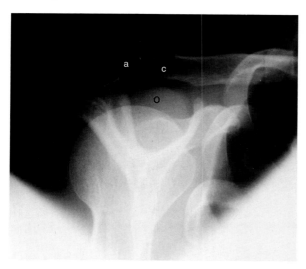

acromiohumeral interval of less than 7 mm (18) (Fig. 7-29).

Plain radiographic imaging for cuff pathology also helps evaluate glenohumeral arthritis (Fig. 7-30) and calcific tendonitis (Fig. 7-31). When calcification in the tendon becomes painful, it causes a reaction in the overlying bursa, which may itself become inflamed (36). Common symptoms include severe shoulder pain that occurs suddenly and inhibits any movement of the shoulder. In these cases, steroid and anesthetic injections into the bursa are indicated to decrease the inflammatory response (36). Once the acute symptoms are relieved, the patient can progress to range-of-motion, flexibility, and strengthening exercises.

For more definitive evaluation, MRI is fast becoming the investigative tool of choice to visualize rotator cuff pathology. Sensitivities have ranged from 69% to 100%, with specificities of 84% to 100% (19). Sensitivity and specificity can approach 100% with MR arthrography using a

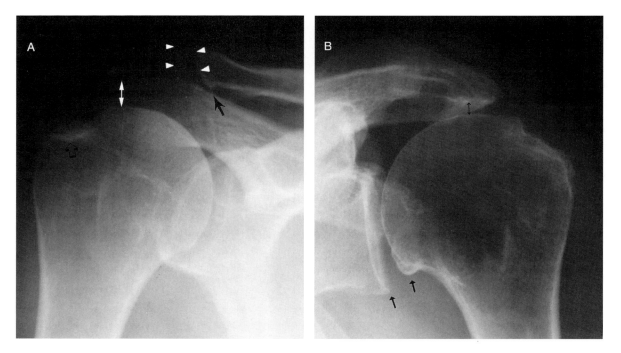

FIGURE   7-29

Plain film evidence of rotator cuff disease. (A) Acromioclavicular arthritis (*white arrowheads*), as evidenced by irregularity and sclerosis of the articular surfaces of both the acromion and the clavicle. The black arrow points to a spur along the undersurface of the distal clavicle. The open arrow indicates sclerosis of the greater tuberosity of the humerus. The acromiohumeral interval is normal in this case (*double-headed white arrow*). (B) Diminished glenohumeral interval (*double-headed arrow*) and glenohumeral arthritis with spur (*arrows*).

FIGURE   7-30

Glenohumeral arthritis, as evidenced by markedly diminished glenohumeral joint space, flattening of the articular surface of the humeral head, and sclerosis along both sides of the joint (*arrowheads*).

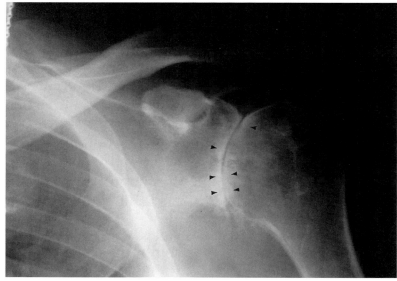

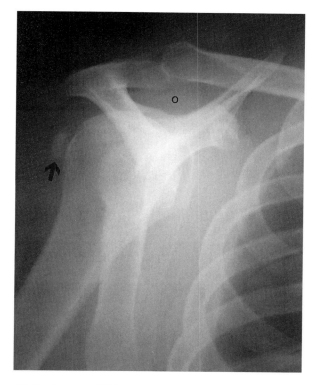

F I G U R E   **7-31**

Calcific tendonitis. Supraspinatus outlet view (*O, outlet*). The calcification indicated by the black arrow represents calcific tendonitis of the infraspinatus tendon.

minute amount of intra-articular gadolinium DTPA in saline and imaging with fat-suppression T1-weighted sequences (31). MRI can detect size, location, and characteristics of cuff pathology. However, MRI cannot be used for all patients. It is time-consuming, very costly, and requires absolute lack of patient motion during each scan sequence. Between 1% and 10% of patients are unable to comply due to pain or claustrophobia.

The normal cuff tendons are characterized by smooth, sharp outlines with a homogeneously dark appearance on T1-weighted, proton-density, and T2-weighted images that blend into the normal intermediate signal of muscle at the musculotendinous junction (14) (Fig. 7-32).

The rotator cuff is best visualized with oblique coronal and oblique sagittal images. The oblique coronal views are obtained parallel to the course of the supraspinatus muscle and tendon, demonstrating the relationship of the supraspinatus to the anteroinferior aspect of the acromion and to the acromioclavicular joint and

allowing appreciation of cuff impingement, tears, and tendonosis (32) (see Fig. 7-32).

MRI in cuff tendonosis demonstrates an increased signal intensity within the supraspinatus tendon near its insertion. However, the diagnosis of supraspinatus tendonosis in the absence of a tear is sometimes problematic. There are several reports in the literature of asymptomatic volunteers who have had MRIs showing increased signal intensity within the substance of the supraspinatus tendon on T1-weighted and proton-density images without clinical evidence for tears. Various explanations have been offered. Some believe that age-related degeneration of the tendon is responsible for the abnormal signal. Others postulate the presence of connective tissue interposed between two separate muscle bundles just prior to the musculotendinous junction, creating the "abnormal" signal. Still others suggest that there is a "magic angle" of orientation of the curving supraspinatus tendon within the magnetic field, which is most evident at 55 degrees. At this angle, the tendons, because of properties of their collagenous structure, become intermediate in signal intensity on T1-weighted and proton-density images (34,43,44). It therefore seems appropriate to make a diagnosis of tendonosis when there is truly enlargement of the tendon as well as abnormal signal on T1-weighted and proton-density images (42) (Fig. 7-33). However, the tendon does not become bright on the T2-weighted image. If it does, tear of the tendon is suspected.

Since the supraspinatus more frequently exhibits tendonosis, so it is more commonly the sight of single tendon cuff tears than the infraspinatus or teres minor alone. The oblique sagittal view offers a perpendicular look at the supraspinatus muscle and tendons, helping again to assess these tears, as well as acromial shape and muscle atrophy (32). Selective atrophy of the infraspinatus muscle may suggest the unusual suprascapular nerve injury sometimes caused by a spinoglenoid notch ganglion, often visualized by MRI (Fig. 7-34). Muscle atrophy also may be present with long-standing cuff tears. Increased signal can be seen within the muscle belly on T1-weighted images (Fig. 7-35).

In the more acute setting of a rotator cuff tear, the tendon demonstrates bright signal on T1-weighted images that increases significantly on T2-weighted images (Fig. 7-36). This increased signal on T2-weighted images is actually fluid (effusion, hemorrhage) filling the defect

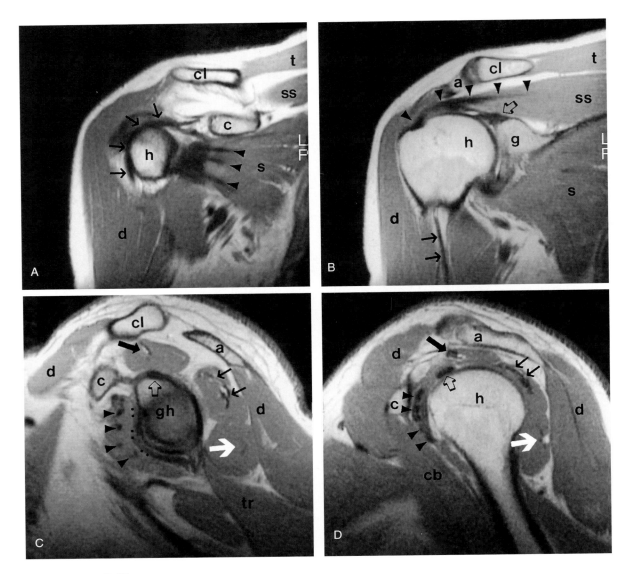

F I G U R E   **7-32**

(A) Normal oblique coronal proton-density image through the anterior aspect of the humeral head (*h*, humeral head; *c*, coracoid process; *cl*, clavicle; *d*, deltoid; *ss*, supraspinatus; *t*, trapezius; *s*, subscapularis). Arrowheads indicate slips of the subscapularis masculotendinous junction. Arrows point to the long head of the biceps tendon as it passes from the bicipital groove over the top of the humeral head, ultimately headed for its attachment onto the superior glenoid labrum. (B) Normal oblique proton-density image through the midhumeral head (*g*, glenoid; *h*, humeral head; *cl*, clavicle; *a*, acromion; *s*, subscapularis; *ss*, supraspinatus; *t*, trapezius; *d*, deltoid). Arrowheads demonstrate a normal-appearing supraspinatus tendon with homogeneously low signal intensity through its course. The most medial arrowhead indicates the origin of the musculotendinous junction. The most lateral arrowhead points to the insertion of the supraspinatus tendon onto the greater tuberosity. Note the normal fat (high signal) between the acromio-clavicular joint and the underlying supraspinatus musculotendinous junction. The open arrow indicates a normal-appearing superior glenoid labrum. Double arrows point to the long head of the biceps tendon. (C) Oblique sagittal proton-density MRI through the glenohumeral joint, parallel to it. The muscles and tendons of the rotator cuff are indicated as follows: *black arrow*, supraspinatus; *double arrows*, infraspinatus; *white arrow*, teres minor; *arrowheads*, subscapularis. The open arrow indicates the tendon of the long head of the biceps. The middle glenohumeral ligament is outlined (*d*, deltoid; *tr*, long head of the triceps; *c*, coracoid; *cl*, clavicle; *a*, acromion; *gh*, glenohumeral joint). (D) Oblique sagittal proton density MRI through the *black arrow*, humeral head supraspinatus; *double arrows*, infraspinatus; *white arrow*, teres minor; *arrowheads*, subscapularis; *open arrow*, long head of biceps; *d*, deltoid; *cb*, coracobrachialis; *c*, coracoid; *a*, acromion; *h*, humeral head.

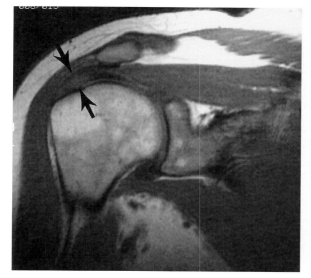

Supraspinatous tendinopathy. There is abnormal, diffusely increased signal intensity within the supraspinatus tendon on this T1-weighted oblique coronal image. Note the increased width of the tendon consistent with edema (between arrows).

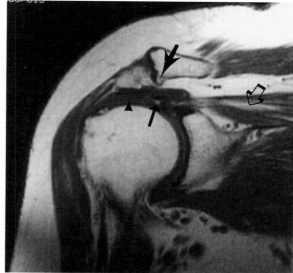

F I G U R E 7-35

Fatty infiltration of the supraspinatus. The open arrow points to high signal within the belly of the supraspinatus muscle in this patient who has a chronic rotator cuff tear with retraction. The torn end is indicated by the small arrow. The arrowhead points to fluid within the joint space, communicating with the subacromial/subdeltoid bursa. The signal of fluid on T1-weighted images is intermediate dark gray, as seen here. Marked spurring of the acromioclavicular joint is evident (*large arrow*).

F I G U R E 7-34

Spinoglenoid notch ganglion. The arrow indicates the location of the ganglion cyst on this T2-weighted image. Atrophy of the infraspinatus tendon was not exhibited in this patient.

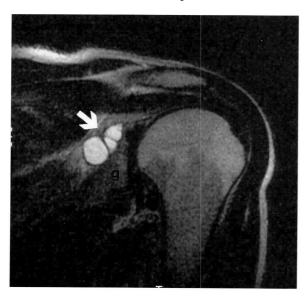

and helps to differentiate a tear from tendonosis. The supraspinatus tendon is involved most frequently. Tears may be partial thickness on either the articular or bursal surface, intrasubstance, or full thickness. Full-thickness tears extend from the articular to the bursal surface.

Absence of a normal peribursal fat plane may be suggestive of severe tendonosis or a cuff tear. Fluid within the subacromial bursa also suggests a rotator cuff tear versus inflammatory bursitis. MRI accuracy for complete cuff tears approaches that of plain arthrography and is superior for partial tears (19).

Plain arthrography is not useful for the diagnosis of rotator cuff tendonosis. However, it may approach 90% accuracy for identification of full-thickness rotator cuff tears. The critical finding is identification of contrast material in the subacromial bursa (14) (Fig. 7-37). Plain arthrography, however, is not as good for partial tears (20).

Magnetic resonance arthrography (MRA) offers a technique to improve the sensitivity and specificity of conventional MRI for identifying

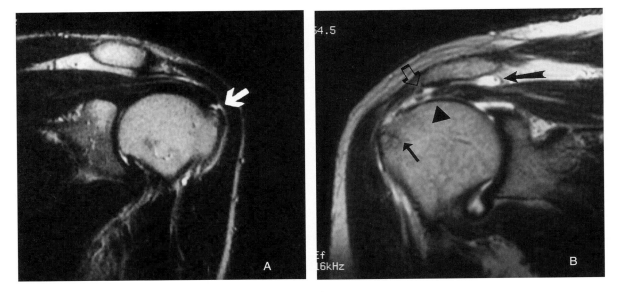

F I G U R E   **7-36**

(A) Supraspinatus tendon tear. This patient has a high-grade partial-versus a full-thickness tear of the supraspinatus tendon distally at its insertion onto the greater tuberosity. The tear extends to at least the bursal surface of the tendon. Note the high signal within the tear on this T2-weighted image. (B) Full-thickness tear with retraction of the supraspinatus tendon. The arrowhead indicates the end of the retracted tendon. Degenerative sclerosis of the greater tuberosity is indicated by the small arrow. Fluid is seen within the subacromial bursa (*large arrow*) secondary to communication with the joint space. The open arrow points to a subacromial spur which may abraid the tendon, predisposing to a tear.

shoulder pathology (see Fig. 7-37C). With the addition of contrast material, cuff pathology can be identified more accurately, as documented by some studies. This is enabled by the contrast medium entering the defect in the rotator cuff, revealing the extent of the tear. However, MRA does not detect bursal surface tears reliably, since the contrast material is injected intra-articularly (27). Adding fat suppression to MRA seems to improve the sensitivity and specificity of differentiating partial- from full-thickness tears (31).

Sonography also may be utilized to evaluate the rotator cuff. Sonographic signs of a cuff tear include focal discontinuity, abnormal morphology, focal or diffused echogenicity, and fluid in the subacromium bursa (21).

All these imaging techniques generate varying costs. Fees can vary as much as 78% in the same locale, as demonstrated in a recent study (33) (Table 7-1).

The less expensive studies may give us limited information with less specificity and sensitivity, yet they can be utilized effectively when clinically appropriate. Consideration must be given to the probable pathology—bony, rotator cuff, or capsular labral—and treatment options. This will help direct the most cost-effective imaging workup.

Treatment for rotator cuff problems should begin conservatively, except in the instance of an obvious new complete tear. Anti-inflammatory medications, rest, and strengthening and flexibility exercises, with emphasis on the scapular-stabilizing muscle groups, are important elements of conservative treatment.

Injuries to the Proximal Humerus

Fracture of the proximal humerus represents 4% to 5% of all fractures (22). The most com-

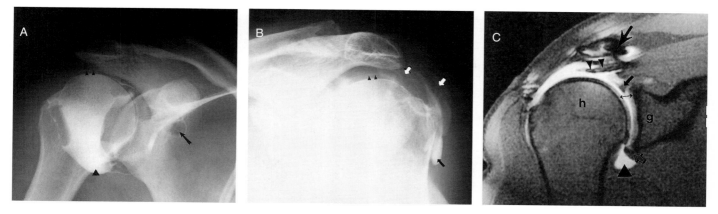

F I G U R E   **7-37**

(A) Normal double-contrast arthrogram. Contrast and air are contained within the confines of the glenohumeral joint. The superior aspect of the capsule outlines the undersurface of the intact supraspinatus tendon (*arrowheads*). The axillary recess is demonstrated (*large arrowhead*). The arrow indicates double contrast within the subscapularis recess, a normal finding. (B) Full-thickness tear of rotator cuff. This arthrogram demonstrates a full-thickness tear of the rotator cuff. The confines of the capsule are seen along the undersurface of the supraspinatus tendon (*arrowheads*). Extravasated contrast material is evident within the subacromial/subdeltoid bursa (*white arrows*). Contrast material is seen within the sheath of the long head of the biceps tendon (*black arrow*) within the bicipital groove. This is a normal finding. (C) MR arthrogram. This study was performed in a patient who had two previous operations for rotator cuff tears. This is a T1-weighted fat-saturation image in the oblique coronal plane obtained after intra-articular injection of a minute amount of gadolinium DTPA diluted in saline. Arrowheads point to the retracted, full-thickness tear of the supraspinatus tendon. Susceptibility artifact secondary to surgical clips or metallic drillings from previous surgery can be seen (*large arrow*). Superior and inferior glenoid labra are well defined (*small arrow* and *open arrow*, respectively). The normal articular cartilage is nicely seen along the glenoid and humeral cortices (*double-headed arrow*). The axillary recess is filled with contrast material (*large arrowhead*) (*h*, humeral head; *g*, glenoid).

T A B L E   **7-1**

Shoulder Imaging Fees

Imaging Study	Professional Fees (dollars)	Technical Fees (dollars)	Total Charge (dollars)
Radiography, complete series	29	78	107
Shoulder arthrography	121	172	293
Shoulder arthrography with CT	165	480	635
Shoulder MR imaging	250	988	1,238
Shoulder US	74	109	183

Note: These fees represent an average of the fees from two different hospitals in the same metropolitan area. The actual fees from the two hospitals varied by as much as 78%.

Reproduced by permission from Stiles R, Otte M. Imaging of the shoulder. Radiology 1993; 188:603–613.

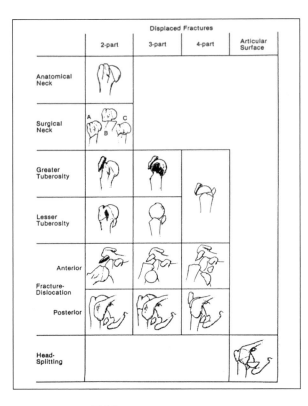

FIGURE **7-38**

The Neer four-segment classification. A fragment is considered displaced when greater than 1-cm displacement or 45-degree angulation is present. A fracture-dislocation is present only if the articular segment is no longer in contact with the glenoid. (Reproduced by permission from Neer CS, Displaced proximal humeral fractures: I. Classification and evaluation. J Bone Joint Surg 1970;52A:1077–1089.)

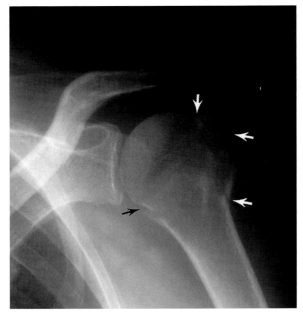

FIGURE **7-39**

Proximal humeral fracture. Greater tuberosity (*white arrows*) and surgical neck fractures (*black arrow*) without significant displacement.

mon classification system for fracture of the proximal humerus is the Neer classification. This is a four-segment classification (articular segments, greater tuberosity, lesser tuberosity, and humeral shaft). To identify these segments, the "trauma series" is again utilized (true AP view, lateral view of the scapular plane, axillary view). When any of the segments is displaced more than 1 cm or angulated more than 45 degrees, the fracture is considered displaced (22).

The following delineates the classification (Fig. 7-38):

One-part or minimally displaced fracture (80% of all fractures): Not displaced greater than 1 cm or angulated greater than 45 degrees.

Two-part fracture: One fragment is displaced in reference to the other three segments. The segments are the anatomic head, lesser tuberosity, greater tuberosity, and shaft.

Three-part fracture: Two fragments displaced in relation to each other.

Four-part fracture: All four fracture fragments are displaced.

CT scanning is often helpful for complete evaluation of these fractures.

Treatment involves a short period of immobilization, followed by an aggressive range-of-motion program for the minimally or nondisplaced fracture (Figs. 7-39 and 7-40). Bony union usually occurs in 6 to 8 weeks, but pendulum exercises and isometrics can be used early in the first week. With the ensuing weeks and stable x-rays, a more aggressive rehabilitation program begins. Two-, three-, and four-part fractures often need surgical intervention.

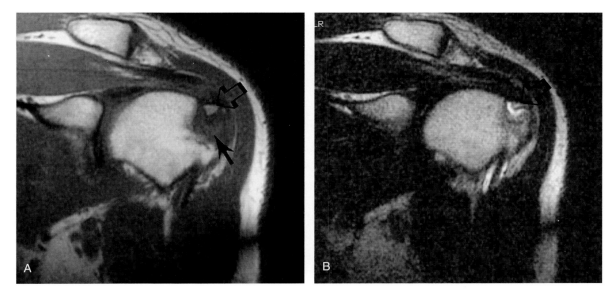

F I G U R E **7-40**

Greater tuberosity fracture. MRI in oblique coronal. T1-weighted (A) and T2-weighted (B) images show a minimally displaced fracture of the humeral greater tuberosity, the fragment indicated by the open arrows. The gray intermediate signal seen within the bone on the T1-weighted image (*arrow*) indicates bone edema and contusion.

REFERENCES

1. Halpern B, Incremona B. Injuries to the shoulder and elbow. Boca Raton: CRC Press, 1994.

2. Halpern B. Upper extremity injuries: The shoulder, toe, elbow, arm. Philadelphia: Hanley & Belfus, 1988.

3. Halpern B. Injuries to the shoulder and elbow: office evaluation and treatment. In: Office management of sports injuries and athletic problems. Philadelphia: Hanley and Belfus, 1988:186–198.

4. Cone R. Reading shoulder films. Hosp Med 1986;83–112.

5. Tibone J, et al. The shoulder: functional anatomy, biomechanics and kinesiology. In: Orthopaedic sports medicine: principles and practice. vol. 1. Philadelphia: Saunders, 1994:580–622.

6. Pagnani M, Galinat B, Warren R. Glenohumeral instability. In: Orthopaedic sports medicine: principles and practice. vol. 1. Philadelphia: Saunders, 1994:580–622.

7. Williams G, Rockwood C. Injuries to the acromioclavicular joint. In Orthopaedic sports medicine: principles and practice. vol. 1. Philadelphia: Saunders, 1994:481–512.

8. Young D, Rockwood C. Fracture of the clavicle. In: Orthopaedic sports medicine: principles and practice. vol. 1. 532–540.

9. Williams G, Rockwood C. Fractures of the scapula. In: Orthopaedic sports medicine: principles and practice. vol. 1. Philadelphia: Saunders, 1994:546–559.

10. Neer C, Rockwood C. Fractures and dislocations of the shoulder. In: Rockwood C, Green D, eds. Fractures in adults. Philadelphia: JB Lippincott, 1984:675–985.

11. Williams G, Rockwood C. Injuries to the sternoclavicular joint. In: Orthopaedic sports medicine: principles and practice. vol. 1. Philadelphia: Saunders, 512–532.

12. Rowe CR, Zarins B. Recurrent transient subluxation of the shoulder. J Bone Joint Surg 1981; 63A:863–872.

13. Rowe CR, Zarins B. Chronic unreduced dislocations of the shoulder. J Bone Joint Surg 1982; 64A:494–505.

14. Cone R. Imaging the glenohumeral joint. In: Orthopaedic sports medicine: principles and practice. vol. 1. Philadelphia: Saunders, 1994: 717–770.

15. Altchek DW, Warren RF, Wickiewicz TL, Ortiz G. Arthroscopic labral debridement. Am J Sports Med 1992;20:702–706.

16. Rowe CR. Acute and recurrent anterior dislocations of the shoulder. Orthop Clin North Am 1980;11:253.

17. Hawkins R, Mohtadi N. Rotator cuff problems in athletes. In: Orthopaedic sports medicine: principles and practice. vol. 1. Philadelphia: Saunders, 1994:623–656.

18. Norwood L, Barrack R, Jacobson K. Clinical presentation of complete tears of the rotator cuff. J Bone Joint Surg 1989;71A:499–505.

19. Iannotti J, et al. Magnetic resonance imaging of the shoulder. J Bone Joint Surg 1991;73A:17–28.

20. Stiles R, Otte M. Imaging of the shoulder. Radiology 1993;188:603–613.

21. Collins RA, et al. Ultrasonography of the shoulder. Orthop Clin North Am 1987;18:351–360.

22. Curtis R. Injuries of the proximal humerus region. In: Orthopaedic sports medicine: principles and practice. vol. 1. Philadelphia: Saunders, 1994:664–716.

23. Rafii M, Minkoff J, DeStefano V. Diagnostic imaging of the shoulder. In: The upper extremity in sports medicine. St Louis: CV Mosby, 1990:91–158.

24. Skyhar M, Warren R, Altchek D. Instability of the shoulder. In: The upper extremity in sports medicine. St. Louis: CV Mosby, 1990:181–212.

25. Marion DS, Bigliani LU. The clinical significance of variations in acromial morphology. Orthop Trans 1987;11:234.

26. Miniaci A, Fowler P. Impingement in the athlete. Clin Sports Med 1993;12:91–110.

27. Karzel R, Synder S. Magnetic resonance arthrography of the shoulder. Clin Sports Med 1993;12:123–136.

28. Aaron J. A practical guide to diagnostic imaging of the upper extremity. Hand Clin 1993;9:347–358.

29. Engebresten L, Craig E. Radiologic features of shoulder instability. Clin Orthop 291:29–44.

30. Epstein R, et al. Hooked acromion: prevalence on MR images of painful shoulders. Radiology 1993;187:479–481.

31. Palmer W, et al. Rotator cuff: evaluation with fat-suppressed MR arthrography. Radiology 1993;188:683–687.

32. Magnetic resonance imaging of the shoulder. Curr Prob Diagn Radiol 1992;7–27.

33. Stiles R, Otte M. Imaging of the shoulder. Radiology 1993;188:603–613.

34. Neumann C, et al. MR imaging of the shoulder. AJR 1992;158:1281–1287.

35. Chandnani V, et al. Glenoid labral tears: prospective evaluation with MR imaging, MR arthrography, plus CT arthrography. AJR 1993;161:1229–1235.

36. Simon WH. Soft tissue disorders of the shoulder. Orthop Clin North Am 1975;6:521.

37. Cartland J, et al. MR imaging in the evaluation of SLAP injuries of the shoulder: findings in 10 patients. AJR 1992;159:787–792.

38. Rodosky M, Harner C, Fu F. The rule of the long head of the biceps muscle and superior glenoid labrum in anterior stability of the shoulder. Am J Sports Med 1994;22:121–130.

39. Gerscovich E, Greenspan A. Magnetic resonance imaging in the diagnosis of suprascapular nerve syndrome. Can Assoc Radiol J 1993;44:307–309.

40. Sidor M, et al. The Neer classification system for proximal humeral fractures. J Bone Joint Surg 1993;75A:1745–1750.

41. Tyson LL, Crues JV III. Pathogenesis of rotator cuff disorders: magnetic resonance imaging characteristics. MRI Clin North Am 1993;1:37–46.

42. Stoller DW, Fritz RC. Magnetic resonance imaging of impingement and rotator cuff tears. MRI Clin North Am 1993;1:47–63.

43. Erickson SJ, Cox HJ, Hyde JS, et al. Effect of tendon orientation on MR imaging signal intensity: a manifestation of the "magic angle" phenomenon. Radiology 1991;181:389–392.

44. Davis SJ, Fereri LM, Bradley WG, et al. Effect of arm rotation on MR imaging of the rotator cuff. Radiology 1991;181:265–268.

CHAPTER 8

The Elbow

RICHARD J. BORGATTI, JR.

Anatomy

Bones

The elbow can be considered to be a simple hinge joint. Actually, the elbow joint consists of two articulations, one of which is a true hinge joint formed by the trochlea of the distal humerus and the proximal ulna. The other articulation is a rotating ball joint formed by the capitellum of the distal humerus and the proximal radius. Both articulations are contained in a single synovial compartment (Fig. 8-1).

Ligaments

Sports-related injuries often involve the soft tissues surrounding the elbow. Recent attention has been focused on the soft tissue stabilizers of the elbow joint. The primary medial stabilizer of the elbow joint that guards against valgus stress is the medial collateral ligament complex. This complex consists of three parts. The anterior bundle is a well-delineated structure that originates on the undersurface of the medial epicondyle and inserts on the medial aspect of the coronoid process of the ulna (1). The anterior bundle acts as the major stabilizer of the medial aspect of the elbow, particularly with the elbow in extension. The second portion of the medial ligament complex is the posterior bundle, which originates more posterior on the medial epicondyle than the anterior bundle and inserts along the medial aspect of the semilunar notch of the proximal ulna. The posterior bundle assists the anterior bundle in stabilizing the joint

in flexion. The third portion of the ligament complex is the transverse bundle, which contributes little to stability of the elbow joint. On the lateral side of the elbow the ligaments are not as well defined either anatomically or functionally. There appears to be a common origin of the radial collateral ligament complex on the lateral epicondyle with a proper radial collateral ligament that inserts on the annular ligament. Another branch called the *lateral ulnar collateral ligament* inserts on the supinator tubercle of the ulna (2,3) (Fig. 8-2).

Nerves

One of the two palpable nerves of the body is found in the cubital tunnel of the elbow. The ulnar nerve is superficial and subject to blunt trauma. It courses behind the medial epicondyle on its route from the posterior aspect of the arm to the volar aspect of the forearm. The ulnar nerve is held in the cubital tunnel by a retinaculum extending from the medial epicondyle to the olecranon. The radial nerve also courses from the posterior aspect of the arm to the volar-radial aspect of the forearm at the elbow joint. This nerve divides into two branches at the elbow joint. The superficial branch provides sensation to the radial aspect of the forearm. The deep or motor branch dives deep around the radial neck and through the supinator muscle to become the posterior interosseous nerve, which is the motor nerve to the extensor muscles of the forearm. The median nerve remains anterior and volar throughout its course over the anterior elbow.

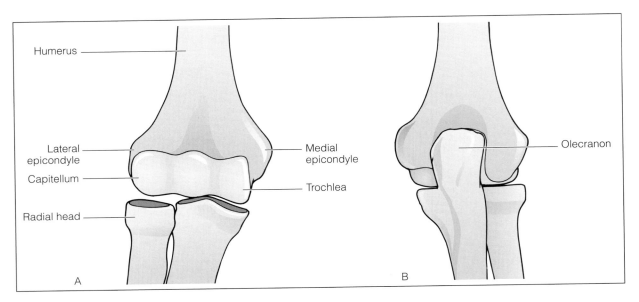

F I G U R E   **8-1**

(A) Anterior view and (B) posterior view of bony anatomy of the elbow. (Redrawn by permission from Hoppenfeld S, deBoer P. Surgical exposures in orthopaedics. Philadelphia: JB Lippincott, 1984.)

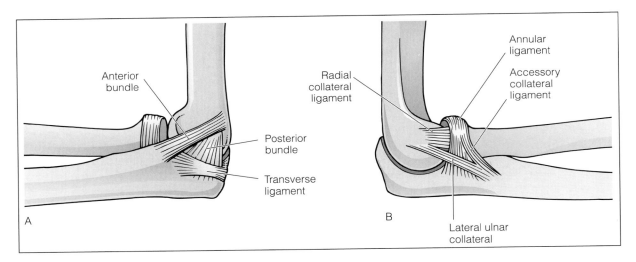

F I G U R E   **8-2**

Artist's rendition of the ligaments of the elbow. (A) The medial collateral ligament complex with the distinction between the anterior and posterior bundles demonstrated. (B) The lateral complex. Note that on the lateral side of the elbow the ligaments extend from the humerus to both the annular ligament of the radial head and the proximal ulna. (Reproduced by permission from Morrey BF, ed. The elbow and its disorders. 2nd ed. Philadelphia: WB Saunders, 1993.)

Bursae

Eight bursae have been described in the elbow. Clinically, however, the olecranon bursa is by far the most common bursa involved in sports injuries. This bursa is located subcutaneously over the posterior aspect of the olecranon. Owing to its superficial location, it is often subjected to repeated trauma.

Growth Plates

Radiographic evaluation of the immature elbow is sometimes difficult because of the multiple centers of ossification and growth plates found in the pediatric population. Centers of ossification appear at different ages and then fuse at different stages of maturity. The earliest center of ossification to appear on plain radiographs is the capitellar ossification center, which appears around 1 year of age and fuses to the humerus at about 12 years of age. The last center to appear is the lateral epicondylar ossification center at age 10, and this fuses to the humerus around age 13 (4) (Fig. 8-3).

Muscles

The major muscles of the elbow can be described by their function. Flexion occurs through contraction of the brachialis primarily and the biceps to a lessor degree. The biceps is the major supinator of the forearm, inserting on the bicipital tuberosity of the radius. The supinator muscle is a weak supinator, but its function is not affected by elbow position, as is the biceps muscle. Extension is accomplished by the triceps, which inserts on the olecranon. The medial head is the most active. The pronator teres functions as the main pronator of the forearm.

Imaging Modalities

Plain Radiographs

Routine films of the elbow consist of an anteroposterior (AP) view with the elbow in full extension and a true lateral view with the elbow at 90 degrees of flexion. In children, AP and lateral views of the contralateral elbow are usually recommended. The forearm should be fully supinated in both views. On the AP view, both epicondyles, the olecranon fossa, and the radial head are well visualized (Fig. 8-4). On the lateral view, the olecranon, capitellum, radial head, and fat pads are well visualized. The anterior fat pad may be visible on the lateral view in a normal elbow. Displacement of the anterior fat pad indicates a collection of intra-articular fluid or blood, as in the case of an intra-articular fracture. The posterior fat pad is usually not visible on a lateral radiograph of a normal elbow. An intra-articular fluid collection will delineate the fat pad and may be the only radiographic abnormality in an occult radial head fracture. Special views may be indicated when routine views are not revealing. In the case of a suspected radial head fracture, the radial head view may visualize the fracture (Fig. 8-5A). The elbow is placed on the film cassette in the same manner as a routine lateral view. The beam is angled 45 degrees toward the shoulder, which avoids the superimposition of the radius on the ulna (see Fig. 8-5B). The reverse axial or cubital tunnel view is helpful in evaluating ulnar nerve disorders and visualizes the olecranon process clearly (Fig. 8-6). This view is obtained by positioning as for an AP view but with the elbow maximally flexed and the

FIGURE **8-3**

Growth centers of the elbow. (*A* = age at which the growth center appears; *F* = age at which the center fuses to the proximal humerus.)

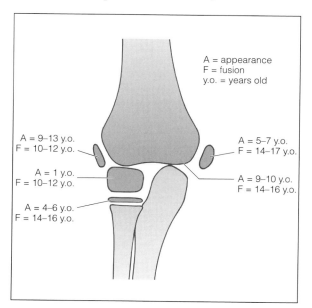

A = appearance
F = fusion
y.o. = years old

A = 9–13 y.o.
F = 10–12 y.o.

A = 1 y.o.
F = 10–12 y.o.

A = 4–6 y.o.
F = 14–16 y.o.

A = 5–7 y.o.
F = 14–17 y.o.

A = 9–10 y.o.
F = 14–16 y.o.

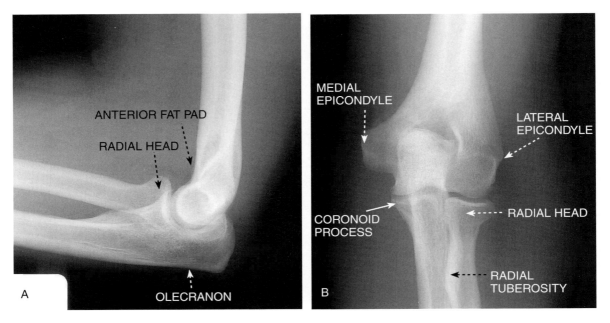

FIGURE 8-4

Radiographic appearance of a normal elbow. (A) Lateral view. (B) AP view.

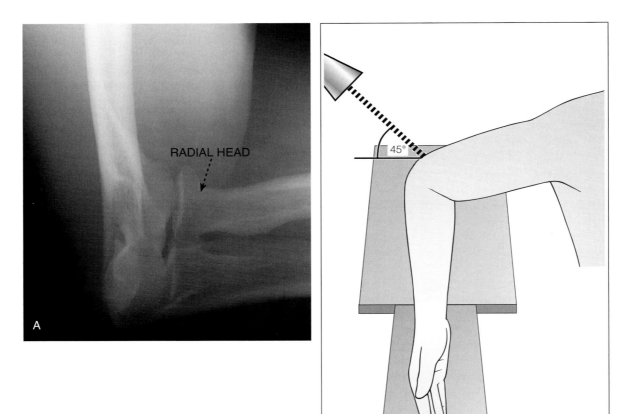

FIGURE 8-5

(A) Radial oblique view of a normal elbow. (B) Diagram of method of obtaining the radial oblique view.

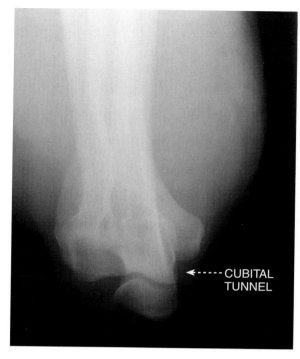

CUBITAL TUNNEL

FIGURE   **8-6**

Reverse axial or cubital tunnel view taken with the elbow maximally flexed and the beam directed as an AP view of the distal humerus.

beam directed perpendicular to the cassette and the distal humerus.

Stress Views

Valgus and varus stress views are helpful in assessing the competence of the collateral liga-

ments. An increase in the joint space of greater then 1 mm compared with the unstressed AP view is considered abnormal (2). A difference of 0.5 mm in the medial joint space between the affected and unaffected elbow on the stress views indicates disruption of the medial collateral ligament complex (5). In patients in whom pain and swelling make stressing the elbow difficult, injection of local anesthesia or use of the gravity stress views may be helpful. The gravity stress test is performed with the patient supine on the x-ray table with the shoulder abducted 90 degrees and the forearm in supination. An AP view in this position stresses the medial collateral ligament (6) (Fig. 8-7).

Arthrography

Arthrography is useful in detecting loose bodies and capsular tears in the elbow. This study is most useful when combined with computed tomographic (CT) images. Cartilaginous loose bodies can be delineated when not visible on plain films (Fig. 8-8). Capsular rents can be detected by leaks of contrast material, as in the case of collateral ligament tears (2,7).

Bone Scintigraphy

Bone scanning can be useful in delineating bony lesion where plain radiographs are not revealing. Early lesions of osteochondritis dissecans can be demonstrated on bone scans (8,9). Plain radiographs are usually sufficient to demonstrate lesions of the capitellum. Bone

FIGURE   **8-7**

The gravity stress test performed with the patient supine and the forearm in full supination. (Reprinted with permission from Woods GW, Tullos HS. Elbow instability and medial epicondyle fractures. Am J Sports Med 1977;5:23–30.)

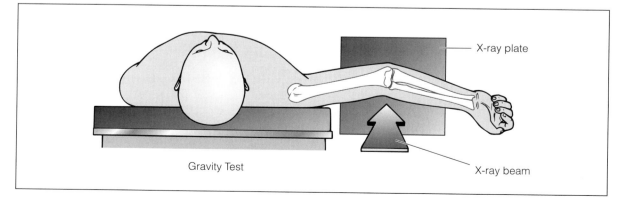

X-ray plate

Gravity Test

X-ray beam

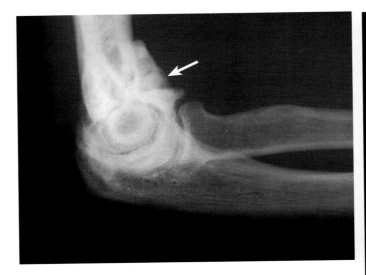

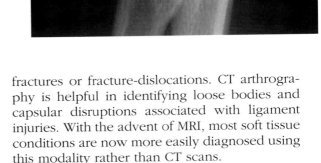

F I G U R E   **8-8**

Elbow arthrogram with contrast material outlining two loose bodies in the coronoid fossa (*white arrow*).

scintigraphy is useful in diagnosing osteomy-elitis, especially in the early stages (10). While very sensitive, scintigraphy is not specific and will be abnormal in other noninfectious diseases such as trauma, gout, or arthritis. Triple-phase scans can distinguish soft tissue infections from bony involvement because late-phase scans are specific for osseous abnormalities. Magnetic res-onance imaging (MRI) has been shown to be both sensitive and specific in the evaluation of musculoskeletal infections (11). MRI cannot dif-ferentiate between edema and bacterially in-duced cellulitis. The efficacy of MRI in the diag-nosis and treatment of osteomyelitis has yet to be determined (12).

CT Scan

CT scan modalities include plain axial tomo-grams, contrast-enhanced studies including CT arthrography, and three-dimensional recon-structions. Plain CT and three-dimensional re-constructions are most useful in fracture man-agement, particularly in complex intra-articular

fractures or fracture-dislocations. CT arthrogra-phy is helpful in identifying loose bodies and capsular disruptions associated with ligament injuries. With the advent of MRI, most soft tissue conditions are now more easily diagnosed using this modality rather than CT scans.

Magnetic Resonance Imaging

MRI has become a major diagnostic tool in the elbow. It is particularly useful in diagnosing soft tissue injuries and abnormalities. Since MRI can detect physiologic changes in tissues, differenti-ation between acute and chronic injuries some-times can be determined. Specific conditions in which MRI can be useful are tendon ruptures such as distal biceps ruptures, medial and lateral collateral ligament tears, osteochondritis of the capitellum, osteochondral defects and associ-ated loose bodies, and occult intra-articular frac-tures such as in the radial head. Epiphyseal in-juries in children are also well identified by MRI; however, because of the time needed for a com-plete study and the poor tolerance for patient movement, MRI is not always practical in such cases. Sedation is often required for an accurate study in young children.

MRI Techniques

Protocols for elbow MRI are not completely standardized and vary somewhat with the manufacturer of the scanner and software. Wrist or knee coils as well as paired surface coils may be used. Images are taken as T1-weighted scans with short TR and TE parameters in three planes: axial, coronal, and sagittal. On the T1-weighted axial views, the coronoid fossa is well delineated and is a common location for loose bodies (Fig. 8-9). Also seen are the proximal radioulnar joint and the olecranon. On T1-weighted coronal views, the distal humerus including the trochlea and capitellum are seen (Fig. 8-10). Sagittal T1-weighted views are useful in identifying the distal biceps tendon and the anterior and posterior fat pads (Fig. 8-11). T1-weighted images generally outline anatomy well but are not particularly useful in identifying

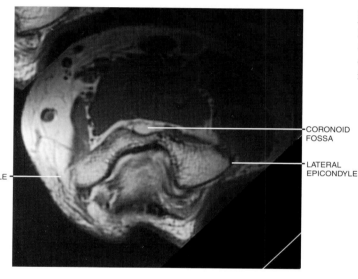

FIGURE **8-9**

MRI of a normal elbow. Axial view demonstrates the coronoid fossa, a common location for loose bodies.

FIGURE **8-10**

(A) Coronal view of a normal elbow demonstrating the olecranon fossa and medial epicondyle. The ulnar nerve can be seen in the cubital tunnel. (B) A second slice done anterior to A shows the medial capsule, trochlea, and capitellum.

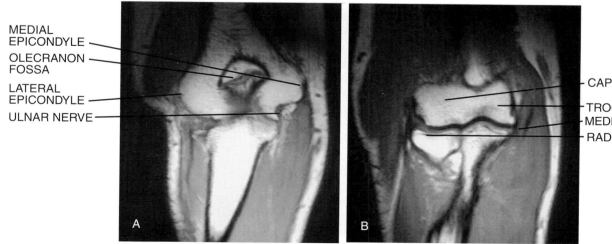

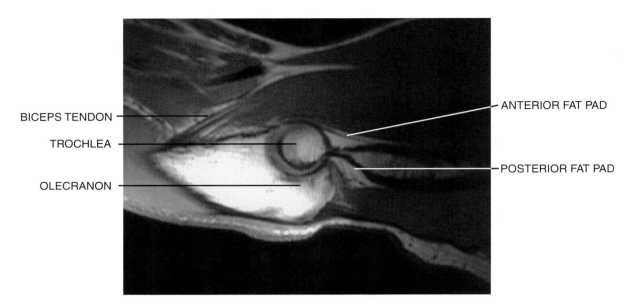

BICEPS TENDON

TROCHLEA

OLECRANON

ANTERIOR FAT PAD

POSTERIOR FAT PAD

FIGURE **8-11**

Sagittal view of a normal elbow. The anterior and posterior fat pads as well as the biceps tendon can be seen.

abnormalities such as swelling, tendonopathies, or hemorrhage. Abnormalities can be identified by the lack of a normal anatomic structure, as in the case of a ruptured distal biceps tendon. T2-weighted images are taken in the coronal and sagittal planes. T2-weighted coronal images can identify medial and lateral collateral ligament tears as well as inflammatory processes such as medial epicondylitis and tennis elbow or lateral epicondylitis. T2-weighted sagittal images can be used to diagnose distal biceps ruptures (13). STIR (short tau inversion ratio) images are intermediate parameter studies that are useful in identifying articular surface defects, hematomas, and effusions. Proton density weighting is useful when fluid or edema is present, as in tendonitis, acute tendon ruptures, or fluid-filled cysts. These images are generated using TR > 2 sec and TE < 20 msec.

Specific Conditions

Acute Traumatic Conditions

Fractures

Many elbow fractures occur as a consequence of participating in sports. Plain radiographs are usually adequate for diagnosing most elbow fractures. In children, comparison views of the normal elbow are often helpful. As mentioned earlier, knowledge of the appearance and fusion of growth centers is also useful (see Fig. 8-3). Oblique views are necessary to fully appreciate angulation in radial neck fractures and displacement in radial head fractures (Fig. 8-12). Occult radial head fractures may not be visible on plain films. The displacement of the anterior fat pad and visualization of the posterior fat pad indicate intra-articular fluid and is presumptive evidence of a radial head fracture (Fig. 8-13). Some authors have questioned the validity of the fat pad sign, particularly when there are no clinical signs of a lateral elbow injury (14). In questionable cases, radial oblique views can demonstrate fractures not seen on routine views (Fig. 8-14). Follow-up radiographs taken 7 to 10 days after injury also may show the fracture line. Minimally displaced radial head fractures that do not block pronation or supination are treated with brief immobilization for comfort and early motion. Displaced fragments of significant size may block pronation and supination and require open reduction or excision.

Two unusual fractures of the olecranon occur in throwing athletes. Stress fractures of the olecranon can result from repetitive throwing and demonstrate a lucency with sclerotic margins on plain radiographs. In young throwers a similar condition results from a traumatic episode to

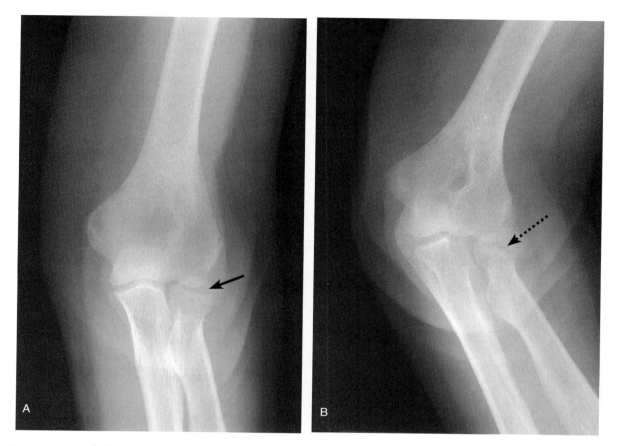

F I G U R E   **8-12**

(A) Arrow showing location of a subtle radial head fracture. (B) Externally rotated oblique view readily demonstrates the fracture and displacement.

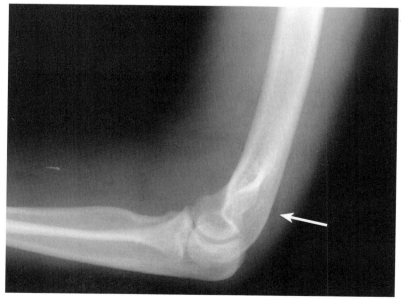

F I G U R E   **8-13**

Lateral radiograph taken the day of injury. Arrow indicates visualization of the posterior fat pad.

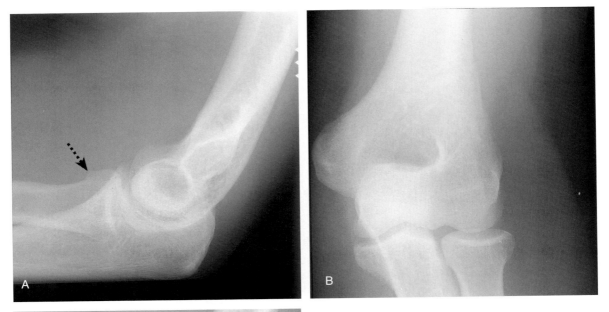

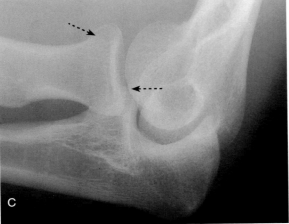

F I G U R E **8-14**

(A and B) Routine film was suspicious for a radial head fracture. (C) Radial oblique view improves visualization of the extent of the fracture.

the olecranon ossification center. Plain radiographs demonstrate asymmetry of the ossification center when compared with the normal elbow with sclerotic edges of the fragments. Open reduction and internal fixation with bone grafting are recommended because nonunions can occur with nonoperative treatment (15) (Fig. 8-15).

Soft Tissue Injuries

Acute soft tissue injuries about the elbow can be classified according to the structures involved. These injuries include damage to tendons, ligaments, and neurovascular structures.

Ligament Injuries Acute disruption of the collateral ligaments of the elbow most often occurs in conjunction with a dislocation of the elbow. In this situation, the diagnosis is made by plain radiographs. The direction of the dislocation indicates the ligaments involved. Posterolateral dislocations are the most common, and the lateral collateral ligament complex is torn. Posteromedial dislocations involve a tear of the medial collateral ligament complex (Fig. 8-16). The treatment is directed at reducing the dislocation and starting early motion. Recurrent instability, while possible, rarely occurs, and the ligaments generally heal satisfactorily (16). Further evaluation of the competency of the ligaments is

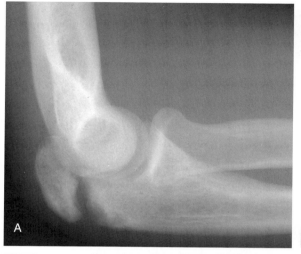

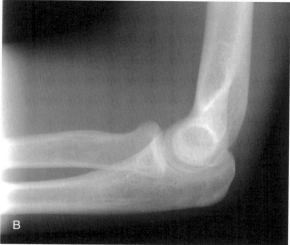

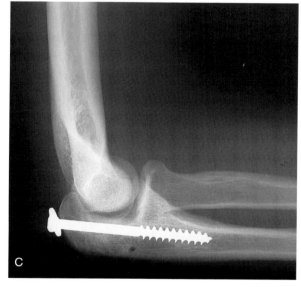

FIGURE **8-15**

(A) Lateral radiograph of the affected elbow of a 15-year-old quarterback who sustained a traumatic injury. (B) Comparison view of opposite elbow. (C) Appearance after open reduction, bone grafting, and internal fixation.

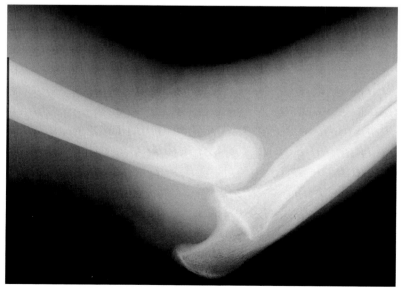

FIGURE **8-16**

Lateral radiograph demonstrating a posterior dislocation of the elbow.

only necessary if chronic instability becomes symptomatic. In some patients, however, posterolateral rotatory instability of the elbow results from an incompetent lateral collateral ligament complex. A history of a complete elbow dislocation is the most common factor in chronic lateral instability. The exact incidence of this entity following an elbow dislocation is not known. The diagnosis of posterolateral rotary instability of the elbow is made on physical examination utilizing the lateral pivot shift maneuver as described by Morrey et al. (Fig. 8-17). Once the diagnosis is made, patients usually continue to be symptomatic, and surgical intervention involving lateral ligament reconstruction is considered.

Acute disruption of the medial collateral ligament complex occurs occasionally. The diagnosis is made by physical examination for medial instability by stressing the elbow at 15 to 30 degrees of flexion. Stress views also may be helpful (5). A short period of immobilization followed by a formal rehabilitation program and gradual return to sports is usually successful. Highly competitive throwers may selectively undergo acute repair with good results.

F I G U R E   **8-17**

The lateral pivot-shift test of the elbow is performed with the patient supine and the shoulder forward flexed and in maximal external rotation. Axial compression, valgus stress, and supination produce apprehension in the conscious patient and subluxation of the radial head under anesthesia. (Reproduced by permission from Morrey BF, ed. The elbow and its disorders. 2nd ed. Philadelphia: WB Saunders, 1993.)

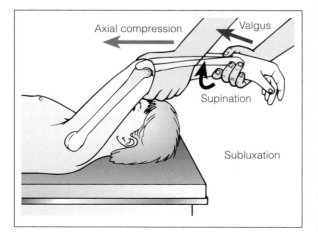

Primary repair of the damaged structures is required (17).

Tendon Ruptures Acute tendon ruptures in the elbow involve the biceps tendon primarily and less frequently the triceps tendon. It is more common for the long head of the biceps to rupture at the shoulder. In less than 10% of cases does the rupture occur at the distal insertion (18). Tendon rupture has a consistent mechanism of injury where a heavy weight lands on the forearm with the elbow flexed around 90 degrees. Patients are all male, and the dominant extremity is involved in 80% of the cases. The diagnosis usually can be made on physical examination, where a visible and palpable defect can be appreciated in the distal biceps when the elbow is actively flexed against resistance. When the examination is difficult or swelling obscures the defect, additional studies may be needed. While irregularities of the biceps tuberosity can be seen occasionally on plain films, an avulsion fracture is not common. MRI delineates the defect in the tendon and shows the retracted muscle on T2-weighted sagittal scans. Hemorrhage and edema are well demonstrated on proton density–weighted sequences (Fig. 8-18). In active patients, primary repair of the tendon back to the biceps tuberosity is recommended within 7 to 10 days (19,20).

Triceps ruptures are even less common than distal biceps ruptures. The mechanism of injury is a fall on a partially flexed elbow, although direct blows have been described (21). Triceps avulsions also have been seen in association with radial head fractures (22,23). A palpable defect with an inability to extend the elbow against resistance is diagnostic. Plain films may demonstrate an avulsion fracture of the olecranon. In patients in whom a partial rupture is suspected or in whom the clinical examination is unrevealing, T2-weighted MRI images taken in the sagittal plane identify the tear (Fig. 8-19). Primary repair for the acute complete rupture is recommended. Nonoperative treatment of partial tendon tears has been successful.

Overuse Syndromes

Because of the unusual magnitude of forces directed to the elbow during throwing and racquet sports, the elbow is subject to a variety of overuse syndromes involving both bony and soft tissue structures. Repetitive stress can lead

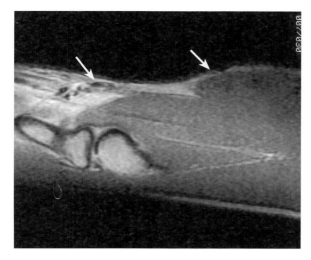

F I G U R E   **8-18**

Proton density–weighted sagittal MRI of the elbow demonstrating a ruptured distal biceps tendon. Left arrow shows the edematous biceps tendon. The right arrow indicates the retracted biceps muscle.

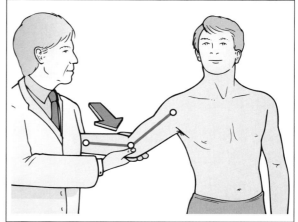

F I G U R E   **8-20**

Method for clinical assessment of medial collateral ligament laxity. Valgus stress is applied in both extension and 30 degrees of flexion while palpating the ligament. (Reproduced by permission from Conway JE, Jobe FW, Glousman RE, Pink M. Medial instability of the elbow in throwing athletes. J Bone Joint Surg 1992;74A:67–83.)

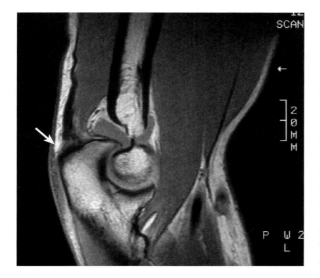

F I G U R E   **8-19**

Acute partial triceps tendon tear at its insertion on the proximal ulna as seen on a proton density–weighted saggital MRI of the elbow.

to ligamentous laxity, osteochondral fragmentation, and tendonopathy.

Medial Collateral Ligament Laxity As mentioned previously, acute tears of the medial collateral ligament (MCL) that occur with an elbow dislocation heal readily, and recurrent instability

is rare. Repetitive valgus stresses on the medial soft tissue structures can cause incompetence of the medial collateral complex due to excessive tensile forces. This mechanism most commonly leads to chronic medial elbow instability in the adult thrower. Clinically, these patients often have vague complaints of medial elbow pain that occurs during and after exercise. On careful questioning, most can recall an acute episode of medial elbow pain. Symptoms are generally relieved by rest but recur upon resuming throwing. Physical examination is directed toward determining the competence of the MCL. This is tested with the elbow in full extension and at 30 degrees of flexion (Fig. 8-20). The amount of laxity is sometimes subtle, and stress radiographs are useful (Fig. 8-21). Comparison views of the opposite elbow are taken, and any widening of the ulnar-humeral space on the medial side is indicative of MCL laxity (5). Localized tenderness is used to help distinguish MCL symptoms from medial epicondylitis. The MCL can be palpated with valgus stress applied to the elbow when flexed beyond 90 degrees (the milking test) (24). Tenderness over the ligament and not the medial epicondyle indicates MCL pathology. Symptoms can be due to subtle laxity in the MCL. In these cases, MRI is useful in

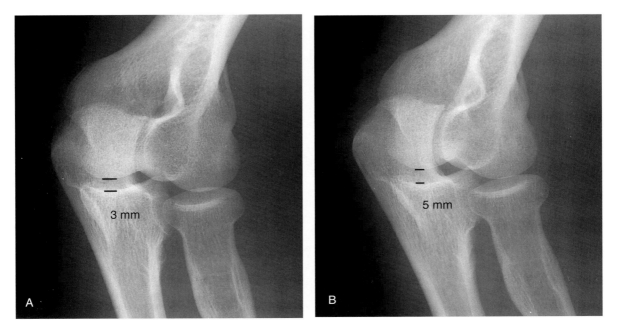

FIGURE **8-21**

Stress views of the elbow. (A) Nonstressed view shows the ulna-humerus space to be 3 mm. (B) Valgus stress is applied, and now the space increases to 5 mm, indicating laxity of the MCL complex.

identifying capsular disruptions and fluid within the MCL complex on T2-weighted sagittal images (25). Treatment is directed at reducing repetitive stress with rest, anti-inflammatory agents, and a rehabilitation program. Acute repair is sometimes indicated to reconstruct significantly unstable MCL complexes in highly competitive athletes (26). Late surgery for chronic instability consists of MCL complex reconstruction using the palmaris longus or another suitable tendon graft. The majority of patients are able to return to sports once stability has been restored (26).

Osteochondritis Dissecans The elbow is the most common site for osteochondritis dissecans, which is the fragmentation of articular cartilage and the underlying bone at the superficial surface of a diarthrodial joint (27). Capitellar abnormalities are seen in children and adolescents who complain of lateral elbow pain. They are usually male, and the dominant arm is almost always involved. In 1927, Panner described an affliction of the capitellum he likened to Legg-Calvé-Perthes disease (28). This condition, which also has been called *osteochondrosis of the capitellum*, appears to be avascular necrosis of the capitellum. It is seen between the ages of

7 and 9 years. Radiographs demonstrate what appears to be fragmentation of the capitellum. This is due to areas of sclerosis and resorption of avascular bone. The overlying cartilage is usually intact, and unlike osteochondritis dissecans, the production of loose bodies does not occur. The condition responds to rest, and residual deformities are rare (29).

Osteochondritis dissecans differs from Panner's disease in age of onset and prognosis. Patients with osteochondritis of the capitellum are 13 to 16 years old with lateral elbow pain aggravated by activity (30). Unlike Panner's disease, where the entire capitellum appears to be involved, the abnormalities are usually subchondral and localized in osteochondritis dissecans, with a predilection for the anterolateral aspect of the capitellum. Radiographs demonstrate subchondral lucency with sclerosis around the defect (Fig. 8-22). Loose bodies may be present, particularly in patients with long-standing symptoms. Treatment depends on the presence of free or partially detached fragments of the capitellum. This is not always easy to determine from plain radiographs. Tomograms may be helpful; however, what appear to be free fragments may have intact articular cartilage overlying them not demonstrable with tomograms.

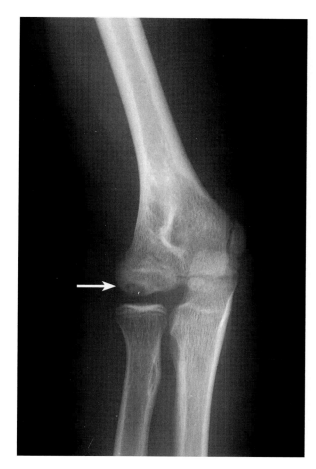

FIGURE **8-22**

AP radiograph showing a lucency in the capitellum in a Little Leaguer's elbow, confirming the diagnosis of osteochondritis dissecans of the capitellum (ODC).

The addition of contrast material may outline the articular surface and aide in determining its integrity. Before the use of MRI, CT scans were useful in visualizing the fragment, particularly with contrast material in the joint. MRI appears to be useful in showing the extent of capitellar involvement and also can demonstrate fragmentation (Fig. 8-23). Occasionally, arthroscopy may be required to determine the integrity of the articular surface of the capitellum.

Treatment depends on the integrity of the articular surface. If the cartilage is intact and there are no free fragments, treatment is symptomatic and consists of rest, immobilization in severe cases, and nonsteroidal anti-inflammatory medication. Return to sports is usually allowed when symptoms have subsided, although a change in position may be suggested (e.g.,

pitcher to second base). Partially detached fragments either may be removed or an attempt may be made to repair them (31). A review of the literature fails to reveal specific guidelines. It seems logical that size may be an appropriate factor in determining which lesions should be removed and which should be repaired. Loose fragments should be removed. Some controversy remains regarding the defect left in the capitellum. Drilling, debridement, and grafting of the defect have been advocated but do not clearly improve results (32).

Valgus Extension Overload *Valgus extension overload* is the term used to describe impingement of the posteromedial olecranon on the olecranon fossa. This produces pain between the acceleration phase and follow-through phase of throwing. Osteophytes form on the posteromedial aspect of the olecranon and may become loose bodies (Fig. 8-24). These can be seen on plain radiographs, although an oblique AP view better demonstrates the osteophytes. Excision of the osteophytes and removal of the loose bodies, either arthroscopically or by a posterolateral approach, restore the ability to throw (33).

Lateral Epicondylitis Tennis elbow, or lateral epicondylitis, is due to repetitive and excessive tensile forces in the extensor tendons of the forearm as they insert on the lateral epicondyle. This is in contrast to the compressive loads responsible for osteochondritis described above. Wrist flexion and elbow extension, such as occurs during a tennis serve, produce stretching of these muscle attachments, particularly in the extensor carpi radialis brevis. These so-called microtears produce an incomplete healing response that results in degeneration and shortening of the muscle attachment at the lateral epicondyle. In chronic cases, histologic changes occur in the muscle origin (34). The diagnosis usually can be made by physical examination, where tenderness is elicited by direct palpation of the lateral epicondyle. Pain at the lateral epicondyle with resisted wrist dorsiflexion is also indicative of lateral epicondylitis. Relief of pain with injection of local anesthetic agents into the origin of the extensor muscle is also diagnostic. Plain x-rays are usually normal. In chronic cases, calcification of the soft tissues as they insert on the lateral epicondyle can be seen (Fig. 8-25). While MRI can demonstrate abnormalities at the lateral epicondyle and in the origin of the ECRB, this test is usually not necessary to make the diagnosis (Fig. 8-26). Treatment consists of discontinuing the

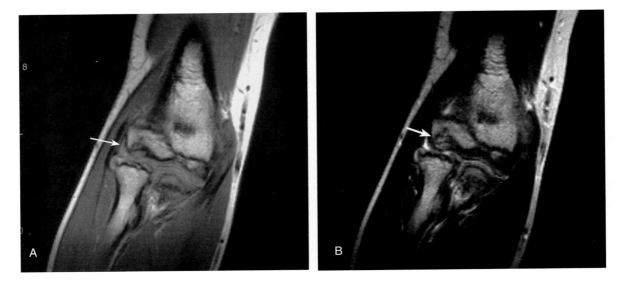

FIGURE **8-23**

(A) Proton density–weighted coronal MRI of the elbow. The lesion in the capitellum is well demonstrated. (B) On the T2-weighted sequence, the fragment does not appear to be separated.

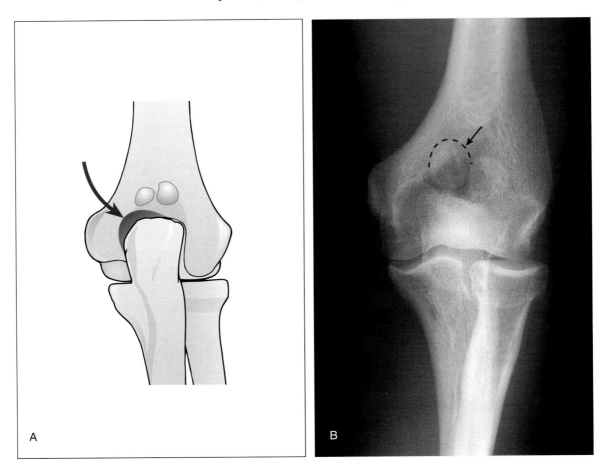

FIGURE **8-24**

(A) Drawing of typical location of osteophytes secondary to chronic valgus extension overload. (B) Radiograph showing osteophyte and loose bodies.

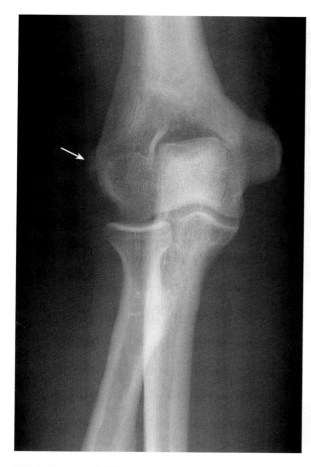

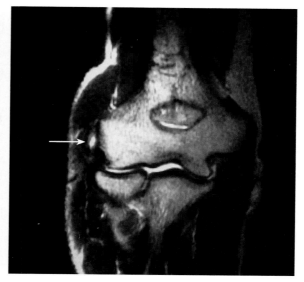

FIGURE   **8-26**

T2-weighted coronal MRI showing increased signal at the insertion of the ECRB on the lateral epicondyle in a patient with chronic lateral elbow pain, confirming the diagnosis of lateral epicondylitis.

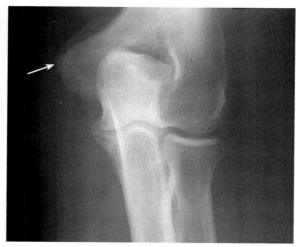

FIGURE   **8-25**

AP radiograph shows calcification of the soft tissues at the lateral epicondyle in a patient with chronic lateral epicondylitis.

repetitive stress, gentle stretching, and rehabilitation of forearm flexors and extensors. Counterforce bracing appears effective in allowing return to sports and prevention of recurrence. Judicious use of injectable steroids can be curative. Surgical treatment is reserved for patients who fail to respond to these measures. The surgical procedure consists of removal of the degenerative tissue in the extensor carpi radialis origin and release of the contracted muscle attachments in selected patients.

Medial Epicondylitis Sometimes called *golfer's elbow,* medial epicondylitis is caused by the same mechanism that results in lateral tennis elbow. Repetitive stretching and microtears in the origin of the pronator teres and flexor carpi radialis produce similar pathologic changes in these tissues. Differentiating this condition from pain produced by chronic laxity of the MCL can

FIGURE   **8-27**

AP radiograph with calcification of the soft tissues medial to the medial epicondyle in a patient with chronic medial epicondylitis.

be difficult. In medial epicondylitis the elbow is stable by examination, the tenderness is directly over medial epicondyle and not the MCL, and ulnar nerve involvement is more common (35). Plain radiographs are usually normal in both conditions. In chronic cases, soft tissue calcifications about the medial epicondyle can be seen (Fig. 8-27). Localized injection of anesthetic

FIGURE **8-28**

Tc-99m bone scan shows diffuse uptake in the entire elbow, more consistent with degenerative joint disease. In medial epicondylitis, the bone scan may be normal or show uptake confined to the medial side of the elbow.

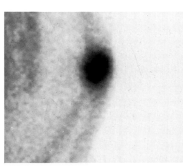

agents into the muscle attachments at the medial epicondyle may relieve pain and confirm the diagnosis. Bone scintigraphy may help localize pain or distinguish this condition from degenerative joint disease, but this is not usually necessary (Fig. 8-28). As in lateral epicondylitis, MRI does demonstrate low-intensity-signal changes at the medial epicondyle on T2-weighted images (36). The diagnosis, however, is made most often on clinical examination. Treatment consists of activity modification, flexor muscle stretching, and conditioning, with the occasional use of injectable steroids. Surgical treatment is similar to that for lateral epicondylitis, where the abnormal tissue is removed. The location of the pathologic tissue is usually at the interval between the pronator teres and the flexor carpi radialis. Care must be taken to preserve the common flexor origin and medial capsule to avoid iatrogenic medial instability.

Loose Bodies Intra-articular loose bodies may be cartilaginous, osseous, or both. They may be free floating or pedunculated. As long as they are in contact with synovial fluid, loose bodies continue to grow larger (37). Loose bodies are either traumatic or degenerative in origin. Osteochondral fractures may involve small fragments initially and years later produce symptoms when they become larger loose bodies. Repetitive hyperextension overload of the elbow causes impingement of an olecranon osteophyte that may break off and become a loose body (33). Clinical signs of loose bodies consist of intermittent pain and locking of the elbow. Osteochondral and osseous loose bodies are seen on plain radiographs, although CT scans and tomograms are used to determine the exact locations of loose bodies (Fig. 8-29). Cartilaginous loose bodies are harder to diagnose. In a patient with true locking and a normal x-ray, special studies are needed to identify loose bodies. CT arthrography demon-

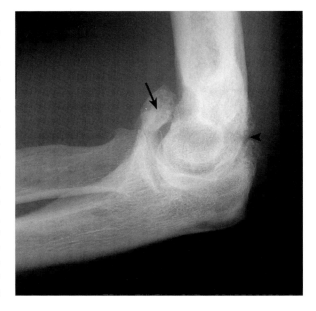

FIGURE **8-29**

Large loose body located in the radial fossa of the elbow (*arrow*). Also note a second loose body in the olecranon fossa (*arrowhead*).

strates the true size of osteochondral loose bodies. Small cartilaginous loose bodies may be obscured by contrast material. T1-weighted MRI images demonstrate loose bodies as intermediate signal densities. As small joint coils improve, MRI may become the modality of choice for demonstrating loose bodies that cannot be identified by conventional means. Symptomatic loose bodies should be removed.

Cubital Tunnel Syndrome and Other Ulnar Nerve Lesions Ulnar nerve symptoms can accompany many elbow disorders. Medial epicondylitis has been found to involve ulnar nerve symptoms in as many as 60% of cases (35).

Repetitive valgus stress can cause a myriad of problems on the medial aspect of the elbow that may involve the ulnar nerve. Thickening of the cubital tunnel retinaculum can cause entrapment of the ulnar nerve (38). Laxity of the MCL complex produces a traction neuritis of the ulnar nerve. Hypermobility of the ulnar nerve where the cubital tunnel retinaculum is incompetent produces ulnar nerve symptoms, particularly during valgus stress activities such as throwing. Diagnostic evaluations should center on determining whether there are any associated conditions that may be responsible for irritating the ulnar nerve. Therefore, diagnostic modalities, as mentioned earlier in this chapter, may be required, such as valgus stress films if instability is suspected and cubital tunnel views to rule out calcification or spur formation causing impingement of the ulnar nerve (Fig. 8-30). Radiographs including oblique views of the ulna more proximal to the elbow joint should be taken to check for a supracondylar styloid process that causes tethering of the ulnar nerve proximal to the intermuscular septum (Fig. 8-31). In primary cubital tunnel syndrome there are no secondary lesions such as instability associated with ulnar nerve symptoms. Imaging modalities in primary cubital tunnel syndrome are typically normal and are used only to rule out associated lesion if they are suspected. Electromyographic and nerve conduction velocity studies confirm ulnar nerve abnormalities. However, these studies can be normal, particularly in patients with intermittent symptoms. In the absence of associated condi-

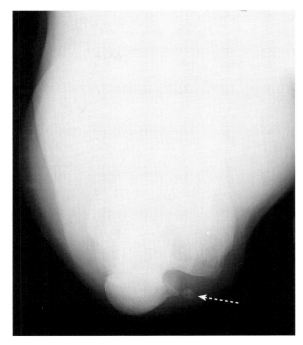

F I G U R E **8-30**

Cubital tunnel view or the reverse axial view is taken with the elbow maximally flexed and done in the AP projection through the distal humerus. Calcifications and osteophytes involving the cubital tunnel are best seen utilizing this technique.

tions, treatment is directed toward decompressing the ulnar nerve either by transferring the nerve anterior to the medial epicondyle or by an oblique osteotomy of the medial epicondyle

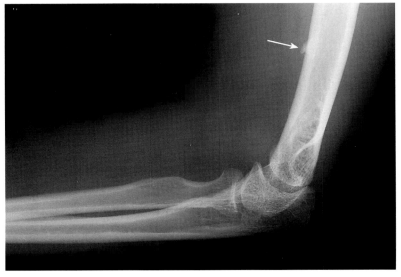

F I G U R E **8-31**

Lateral elbow projection demonstrating a supracondylar process that may produce ulnar nerve compression proximal to the cubital tunnel.

while preserving the MCL (26). Associated conditions such as instability should be corrected along with ulnar nerve surgery.

REFERENCES

1. O'Driscoll SW, Jaloszynski R, Morrey BF. Origin of the attachment of the medial ulnar collateral ligament. J Hand Surg 1992;17:164–168.

2. Morrey BF, ed. The elbow and its disorders. 2nd ed. Philadelphia: WB Saunders, 1993.

3. Morrey BF, An KN. Functional anatomy of the elbow ligaments. Clin Orthop 1985;201:84–90.

4. Brodeur AE, Silberstein MJ, Graviss ER. Radiology of the pediatric elbow. Boston: GK Hall, 1981.

5. Rijke AM, Goitz HT, Andrews JR, Berr SS. Stress radiography of the medial elbow ligaments. Radiology 1994;191:213–216.

6. Woods GW, Tullos HS. Elbow instability and medial epicondyle fractures. Am J Sports Med 1977;5:23–30.

7. Mink JH, Eckhardt JJ, Grant TT. Arthrography in recurrent dislocation of the elbow. AJR 1981; 136:1242–1244.

8. Mesgarzadeh M, Sapega AA, Bonakdarpour A. Osteochondritis dissecans: analysis of mechanical stability with radiography, scintigraphy, and MR imaging. Radiology 1987;165:770–780.

9. Newberg AH. The radiographic evaluation of shoulder and elbow pain in the athlete. Clin Sports Med 1987;6:785–809.

10. Gilday DL, Paul DJ, Paterson J, et al. Diagnosis of osteomyelitis in children by combined blood pool and bone imaging. Radiology 1975;117: 331–335.

11. Tang JSH, Gold RH, Bassett LW, et al. Musculoskeletal infection of the extremities: evaluation with MR imaging. Radiology 1988;166:205–209.

12. Frymoyer JW, ed. Orthopedic knowledge update 4, Chap. 13, AAOS, 1994:155–168.

13. Stoller DW, ed. Magnetic resonance imaging in orthopaedics and sports medicine. Philadelphia: Lippincott–Raven, 1994.

14. Quinton DN, Finlay D, Butterworth R. The elbow fat pad sign: brief report. J Bone Joint Surg 1987; 69B:844–845.

15. Kovach J, Baker BE, Mosher JF. Fracture separation of the olecranon ossification center in adults. Am J Sports Med 1985;13:105–111.

16. Josefsson PO, Gentz C, Johnell O, Wendenberg B. Surgical versus nonsurgical treatment of ligamentous injuries following dislocation of the elbow joint: a prospective, randomized study. J Bone Joint Surg 1987;69A:605–608.

17. Norwood LA, Shook JA, Andrews JR. Acute medial elbow ruptures. Am J Sports Med 1981;9: 16–19.

18. Agins HJ, Chess JL, Hoekstra DV, Teitge RA. Rupture of the distal insertion of the biceps brachii tendon. Clin Orthop 1988;234:34–38.

19. Baker BE, Bierwagon D. Rupture of the distal tendon of the biceps brachii. J Bone Joint Surg 1985;67A:414.

20. Morrey BF, Askew LJ, Dobyns JH. Rupture of the distal biceps tendon: biomechanical assessment of different treatment options. J Bone Joint Surg 1985;67A:418–421.

21. Anderson KJ, LeCoco JF. Rupture of the triceps tendon. J Bone Joint Surg 1957;39A:444–446.

22. Farrar EL, Lippert FG. Avulsion of the triceps tendon. Clin Orthop 1981;161:242–246.

23. Levy M, Goldberg I, Meur I. Fracture of the head of the radius with a tear or avulsion of the triceps tendon: a new syndrome? J Bone Joint Surg 1982;64B:70–72.

24. Veltri D, O'Brien SJ, Field LD, et al. The milking maneuver: a new test to evaluate the MCL of the elbow in the throwing athlete. Presented at the meeting of the American Shoulder and Elbow Surgeons, New Orleans, LA, 1994.

25. Murphy BJ. MR imaging of the elbow. Radiology 1992;184:525–529.

26. Conway JE, Jobe FW, Glousman RE. Medial instability of the elbow in throwing athletes. J Bone Joint Surg 1992;74A:67–83.

27. Pappas AM. Osteochondrosis dissecans. Clin Orthop 1981;158:59–69.

28. Panner HJ. A peculiar affliction of the capitellum humeri resembling Calvé-Perthes disease of the hip. Acta Radiol 1927;8:617.

29. Pappas AM. Elbow problems associated with baseball during childhood and adolescence. Clin Orthop 1982;164:30–41.

30. Lindholm TS, Osterman K, Vankka E. Osteochondritis dissecans of elbow, ankle and hip: a comparison survey. Clin Orthop 1980;148:245–254.

31. Andrews JR. Bony injuries about the elbow in the throwing athlete. In: Stauffer ES, ed. American Academy of Orthopaedic Surgeons instruc-

tional course lectures. Vol 34. St Louis: CV Mosby, 1985.

32. McManama GB, Michel LJ, Berry MV, Sohn RS. The surgical treatment of osteochondritis of the capitellum. Am J Sports Med 1985;13:11–21.

33. Wilson FD, Andrews JR, Blackburn TA, McCluskey G. Valgus extension overload in the pitching elbow. Am J Sports Med 1983;11:83–88.

34. Nirschl RP, Pettrone FA. Tennis elbow: the surgical treatment of lateral epicondylitis. J Bone Joint Surg 1979;61A:832–839.

35. Nirschl RP. Soft-tissue injuries about the elbow. Clin Sports Med 1986;5:637–652.

36. Herzog RJ. Magnetic resonance imaging of the elbow. Magn Reson Q 1993;9:188–201.

37. Milgram JW. The development of loose bodies in human joints. Clin Orthop 1977;124:295–304.

38. Osborne GV. The surgical treatment of tardy ulnar neuritis. J Bone Joint Surg 1957;39B:782.

CHAPTER 9

Radiology of Hand and Wrist Disorders

JOHN M. HENDERSON

General Considerations

The hand is a finely engineered terminal appendage designed for grasping/holding tasks with evolutionary modifications that allow for thumb opposition and abduction away from the middle (long) finger. Exquisitely orchestrated sequences of flexion, such as throwing a baseball or grasping a racket, depend on maintaining the integrity of this region. Mechanisms of injury include axial loading, distraction/tensile force, torque, angular force, and extremes of the normally intended ranges of motion. The thumb and the fifth (little) finger have the greatest ranges of motion and so can accept the greatest latitude in deformities. The middle three fingers, the index, long, and ring fingers, are not so forgiving and must maintain their original anatomic position. Shortening, rotation, and angular deformities out of the plane of flexion/extension are complications of bony trauma. The mechanical advantages inherent to the hand, such as the cam contour of the metacarpal heads and the gliding movement of the carpus, must be kept in mind when assessing any imaging modality.

The jargon used in the description of hand x-rays can be confusing. Generally speaking, if the athlete's physician uses a systematic approach in describing the bony architecture, a mental picture of the trauma can be made by another physician listening on a distant telephone connection. To help the physician become fluent with this region, Figure 9-1 is provided.

The wrist is composed of the distal radioulnar joint as it articulates with the carpal bones, which are arranged in two rows: the proximal (scaphoid, lunate, triquetrum, pisiform) and the distal (trapezium, trapezoid, capitate, hamate) carpal rows. These bones are arranged to have palmar concavity. The articular surface of the radius part of the wrist joint is inclined palmarward and ulnarward to allow a tighter grasp.

The wrist, hand, and fingers are graceful appendages that, on x-ray, even appear naturally functional, with each bone situated in a comfortable posture with its neighbor. This alignment is critical to assess. If the x-ray image does not look gracefully situated, the clinician should suspect some covert pathology. Figure 9-2 depicts a couple of these relationships. The soft tissue shadows are minimal and, when widened, give additional clues about suspected pathology. A fusiform bulge or skewed soft-tissue stripe should be the cause for heightened awareness.

Terminology

X-rays usually are taken in at least two planes at 90 degrees to each other: posteroanterior (PA) and lateral (LAT) views. For the hand, the lateral view has confounded many physicians because of the overlapping shadows. These views are

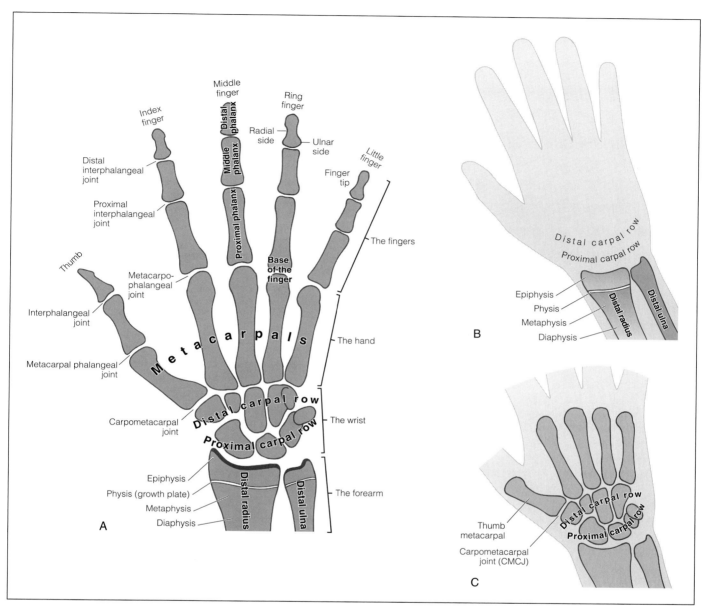

F I G U R E **9-1**

Hand and wrist terminology. (A) Hand and wrist terminology involves common names as well as technical anatomic names. Current usage includes both anatomic and common (lay) terms. Several key groups of terms should be considered to become fluent with this region. (B) The distal forearm is made up of the distal radius and ulna that join to make the distal radioulnar joint. The growth plate is the physis. The epiphysis is distal to the physis, whereas the metaphysis is proximal to the physis. The diaphysis is proximal to the metaphysis. The radiocarpal joint is a main wrist joint involving the articulations of the radius and the scaphoid and lunate. (C) The carpus, or wrist, is composed of two rows of carpal bones: the proximal and distal carpal rows. The articulations with the metacarpals are termed *carpometacarpal joints* (CMCJs). The thumb CMC is a convenient way to describe the joints involving the trapezius, trapezoid, and first metacarpal. (*Continued on next page.*)

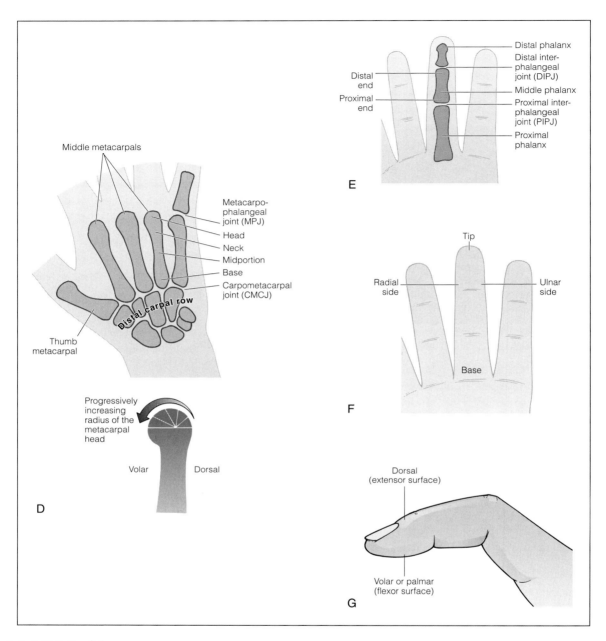

F I G U R E   **9-1**

(*Continued*) (D) The metacarpals are named after the fingers, that is, the "thumb metacarpal" and the "middle metacarpal." The meta-carpal has a base, midportion, neck, and head. The radius of the metacarpal head increases from the dorsal to the volar side (*bottom*). The distal metacarpal joint, called the *metacarpophalangeal joint* (MPJ), is the base of the finger. (E) Each finger has a proximal, middle, and distal phalanx. These articulate by the proximal interphalangeal joint (PIPJ) and the distal interphalangeal joint (DIPJ). Each phalanx has a proximal and distal end, so a complicated phrase could include the "proximal end of the distal phalanx." (F) The most distal end of the digit is the fingertip. The most proximal end of the finger is the base of the finger. The "thumb side" of the finger is the radial side; the "little finger side" of the finger is the ulnar side. (G) The anterior aspect of the finger is the volar aspect, palmar aspect, or flexor aspect. The posterior aspect of the finger is the dorsal aspect, dorsum, or extensor aspect. In describing a tiny avulsion fracture, the location might be described as "volar aspect of the radial side of the proximal end of the distal phalanx." (This is analogous to using eight-digit map coordinates to precisely locate an object on a map.)

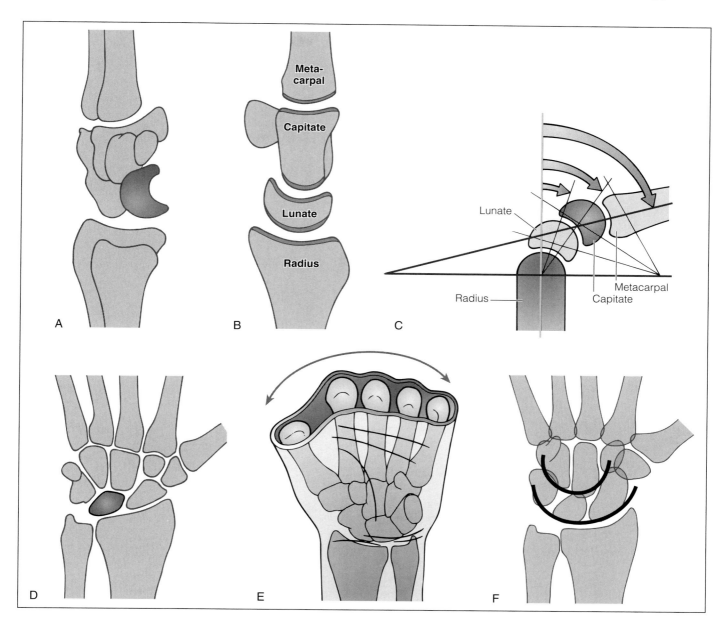

F I G U R E   **9-2**

X-ray alignment. If the x-ray does not look graceful, some covert injury must be suspected. The architecture of this region includes small, irregularly shaped bones fitting closely together to create smooth, curved lines with a few overlapping densities. (A–C) Lunate dislocation appearing as a "spilled teacup." Normally, the concave articular surface of the radius juxtaposes the convex surface of the lunate, which, in turn, has a concave surface that articulates with distal carpal bones. In a lunate dislocation, these well-fit relationships are disrupted. (D) The quadrilateral shape of the lunate after reduction. The carpus is densely packed, but the individual bones have a fairly uniform intercarpal space like a stained glass window. Any carpal disruption changes the orientation and intercarpal articulations. (E) The transverse metacarpal arch. The metacarpal bones are arranged as "rays" that provide an archlike contour at rest and with grasping. The transverse carpal arch provides strength and support. After sustaining a fracture of the metacarpal neck, the head of that metacarpal falls forward (palmarward), flattening the arch and decreasing grasp strength. (F) The smooth curves of the proximal and distal margins of the scaphoid, lunate, and triquetrum.

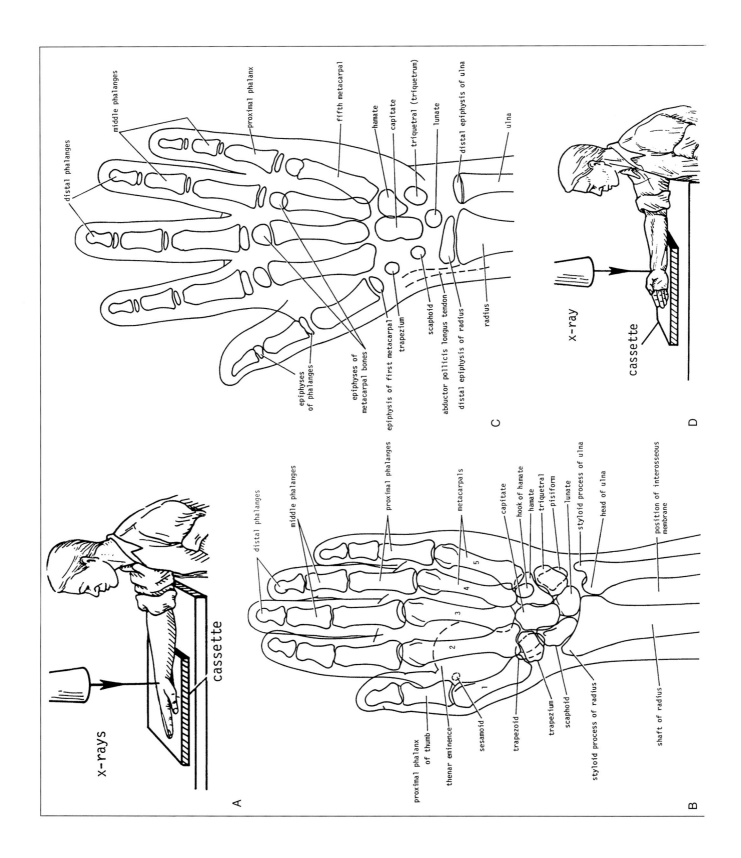

middle phalanges

distal phalanges

proximal phalanx

fifth metacarpal

hamate

capitate

triquetral (triquetrum)

lunate

distal epiphysis of ulna

ulna

epiphyses of phalanges

epiphyses of metacarpal bones

epiphysis of first metacarpal

trapezium

scaphoid

abductor pollicis longus tendon

distal epiphysis of radius

radius

x-ray

cassette

C

D

x-rays

cassette

A

distal phalanges

middle phalanges

proximal phalanges

metacarpals

capitate

hook of hamate

hamate

triquetral

pisiform

lunate

styloid process of ulna

head of ulna

position of interosseous membrane

proximal phalanx of thumb

thenar eminence

sesamoid

trapezoid

trapezium

scaphoid

styloid process of radius

shaft of radius

B

160

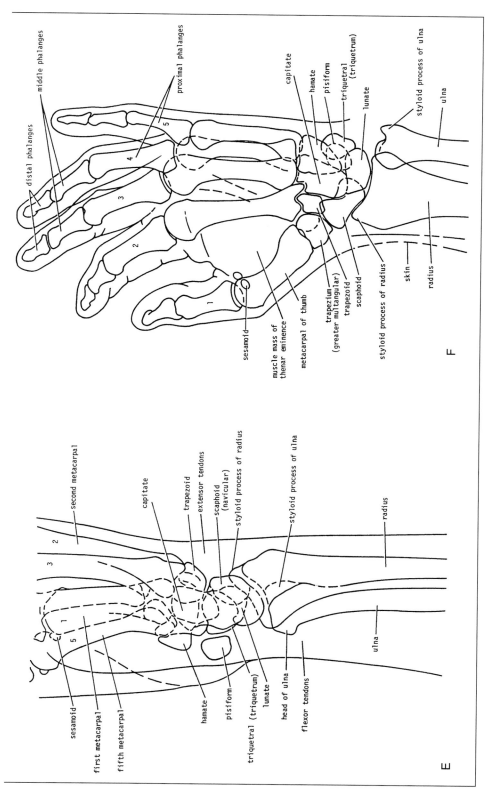

distal phalanges

middle phalanges

proximal phalanges

5

4

3

2

1

sesamoid

muscle mass of
thenar eminence

metacarpal of thumb

trapezium
(greater multangular)

trapezoid

scaphoid

styloid process of radius

skin

radius

capitate

hamate

pisiform

triquetral
(triquetrum)

lunate

styloid process of ulna

ulna

F

second metacarpal

3

2

capitate

trapezoid

extensor tendons

scaphoid
(navicular)

styloid process of radius

styloid process of ulna

radius

sesamoid

first metacarpal

fifth metacarpal

hamate

pisiform

triquetral (triquetrum)

lunate

head of ulna

flexor tendons

ulna

1

5

E

FIGURE 9-3

X-ray views. The common views of hand x-rays include PA and lateral views. The view is named for the direction of shooting the x-ray beam. The anatomic part closest to the x-ray cassette holding the film will be sharpest in contrast and have the least magnification. (A–C) Posteroanterior views. The hand rests pronated with the palm of the hand on the cassette. The configuration of the scaphoid can be assessed as well as the spaces between the various carpal bones. The anteroposterior view can accentuate the width of the scapholunate gap. PA views in radial and ulnar deviation can help assess carpal motion. (D, E) Lateral views. The hand rests with the ulnar side on the cassette. The scapholunate angle can be measured on this view. Lateral views in full flexion and extension can help assess carpal motion.

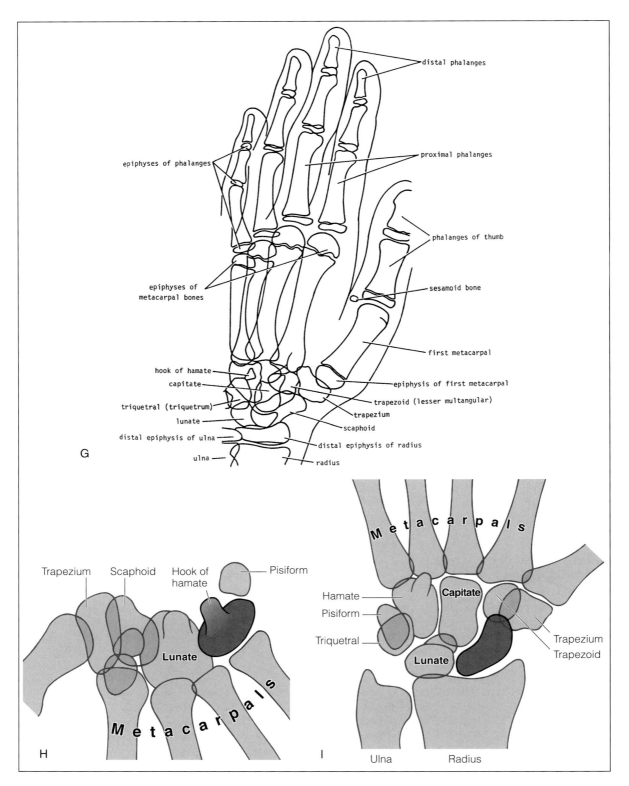

FIGURE 9-3

(*Continued*) (F, G) Oblique views. As in *B*, but the hand is rolled or very slightly pronated to bring the scaphoid into its long axis and bring the metacarpals out of line so that each one can be seen. (H) Hamate view. Oblique views taken with the forearm supinated and the wrist dorsiflexed show the lateral profile of the hook of the hamate and will demonstrate a fracture. (Reproduced by permission from Zemel NP, Stark H. Fractures and dislocations of the carpal bones. Clin Sports Med 1986;5:717.) (I) Scaphoid view. PA views of the wrist in maximum radial and maximum ulnar deviation with the fingers clenched into a fist bring the scaphoid into a horizontal position.

supplemented by oblique (OBLQ) views intended to "open up" the overlapping shadows of the metacarpals and carpals. As it is positioned over the x-ray cassette, the hand usually takes a "prone oblique" posture (1). Special views such as the *carpal tunnel view* take advantage of the natural concavity of the carpus. Figure 9-3 shows a schematic of several of these. Despite the view selected, the bony structure closest to the cassette (film) will be the sharpest image with the least magnification. The lucent line a fracture produces can be confused with an open physis, and vice versa. The fracture line may be broader and lighter (more dense due to impacted fragments) and more jagged than the open physis, which appears darker (lucent), gently undulating, and sclerotic. Almost any disruption in the cortex, from a buckle to a crack, indicates a fracture.

Eponyms of specific pathologies in this region of the body are many and confusing. Some of the more common ones include *Colles', Barton's,* and *Bennett's fractures.* Generally, it is best to use anatomic terminology rather than eponyms. To further complicate the matter, some activities lend themselves to diagnoses. *Boxer's fracture, jersey finger, gamekeeper's thumb,* and *chauffeur's fracture* are a few of these. Again, the anatomic pathology should be described. The x-ray diagnosis and the clinical diagnosis may not always be the same.

Thumb Trauma

Fractures of the thumb phalanges are the second most common of all phalanx fractures. The mechanics are similar to those of the other fractures, with the exception that the soft tissue considerations include disruption of the collateral ligaments and the need to preserve the function of the extensor and flexor mechanisms, which are enhanced by the abductor and adductor functions. Combinations of axial compression, angular deforming forces, torque/twist, and crushing can cause a variety of fracture patterns. The pincer grasp, fine-touch ability, apposition, and extremes of abduction differentiate the thumb as a phalanx. Skeletal integrity must be maintained to perform these functions.

X-Ray Findings

The common fractures include comminuted yet minimally displaced distal phalanx fractures, short oblique fractures of the proximal phalanx, and complex fractures of the thumb metacarpal. The increased mobility of the thumb allows for more accepted deformity in the final result. The size of the thumb, however, lends itself to different types of rigid fixation techniques ranging from plates and screws to external fixators.

Ligamentous Injuries

Some common ligamentous injuries deserve x-ray evaluation because of the commonly associated bony pathology. Disruption of the thumb metacarpophalangeal joint (MPJ) ulnar collateral ligament is commonly termed *gamekeeper's thumb.* This can result acutely from abrupt forced abduction of the thumb MPJ. It also can develop from chronic excessive abduction stressing (valgus stress). *Skier's thumb* is the common name given to this injury, but it is seen in many other activities, particularly volleyball, football, baseball, softball, and rugby. In addition to the ulnar collateral ligament, the volar plate of the thumb may be torn. The athlete presents with the appropriate story and a tender, swollen thumb MPJ. The volar aspect of the proximal phalanx where the ulnar collateral ligament inserts is the point of maximal tenderness. By performing an abduction stress test with the thumb MPJ slightly flexed, the physician can determine whether there is an endpoint, signifying a partial tear, or whether the thumb abducts widely and freely, as with a complete tear of the ulnar collateral ligament.

X-Ray Findings

Although pre-examination x-rays have been recommended to prevent iatrogenic displacement of a nondisplaced fracture, the common management on the playing field includes a gentle stress test. Nonetheless, a few common fracture patterns are seen with this injury. Avulsion fracture at the base of the proximal phalanx is common. This is a true intra-articular fracture into the MPJ. Most of these bony avulsions are small. Another type of fracture involves avulsion of 25% or more of the articular surface of the base of the proximal phalanx (Fig. 9-4). Yet another type of avulsion fracture involves a bony avulsion attached to the volar plate. The initial x-rays obtained are usually true PA and relaxed oblique prone views. When stress views are obtained, if the injured thumb opens up 20% more than the uninjured contralateral joint, the ulnar collateral

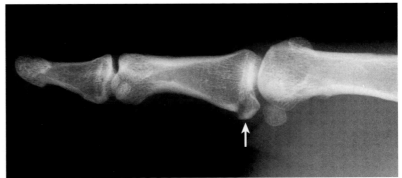

FIGURE **9-4**

Gamekeeper's thumb: the Stener lesion. Avulsion off the proximal end of the proximal phalanx.

ligament is considered torn. The extent of the tear is debatable. Arthrograms have been used in the past, but magnetic resonance imaging (MRI) is used more commonly today. At question is whether fracture fragments or the torn end of the ulnar collateral ligament, or both, or the aponeurosis of the adductor pollicis is a mechanical block in the MPJ or at least interposed between the torn ends of the ulnar collateral ligament. Not only could this occur during the trauma, but it also could happen during the examination. This intra-articular lesion is called the *Stener lesion* (2). Current management is controversial; mandatory MRI and arthrotomy leading to MPJ capsulorrhaphy and adductor reconstruction are practiced in some centers, whereas thumb spica immobilization is still accepted as leading to a reasonable outcome. The ulnar collateral ligament injury with a strong endpoint and negative x-rays may be managed with a thumb spica brace. The ulnar collateral ligament injury causing instability and poor pincer grasp strength with a problematic Stener lesion seen on MRI warrants formal arthrotomy and anatomic repair to obtain a good function result.

Thumb Metacarpal Fractures

Fractures at the base of the thumb are complex and fraught with complications, both short and long term. The reasons for this include that these fractures are intra-articular and the musculotendinous forces across this joint cause inherent disability of the complex joint comprised of the proximal end of the thumb metacarpal and the radial side of the distal carpal row (trapeziotrapezoid joint). Sesamoid bones are commonly found near the head of the thumb metacarpal and should not be mistaken for an avulsion fracture. The Bennett fracture involves an intra-articular fracture of the base of the thumb metacarpal with radial-ward subluxation of the carpometacarpal joint (CMCJ). The Rolando fracture involves an intra-articular fracture of the base of the thumb metacarpal, but it differs from the Bennett type in that the fracture can have a T or Y pattern with dorsal and/or volar intra-articular fracture fragments. The pull of the flexors and extensors pollicis may wedge these fragments around the trapezius. Both the Bennett and the Rolando fractures result from axial loading of the thumb metacarpal against the carpus. The main variables of these two fractures are the size of the fragments and the degree of displacement and disruption (Fig. 9-5). The athlete presents with a grossly swollen hand with tenderness at the base of the thumb. The thumb appears shortened, and motion is limited due to pain.

X-Ray Findings

The PA, lateral, and oblique views demonstrate the fractures; in the Bennett fracture the volar fragment is held to the trapezium while the distal metacarpal dislocates radially, whereas in the Rolando fracture comminution may be greater and the fragments are found dorsally. Both fractures are subsequently typed according to various severities of comminution that portend worse functional outcome.

Closed, conservative treatment of either fracture is associated with post-traumatic arthritis, chronic pain, and decreased function. Closed reduction is difficult to maintain. Articular surfaces need to be anatomically restored. Open reduction and pin fixation are the usual treatment.

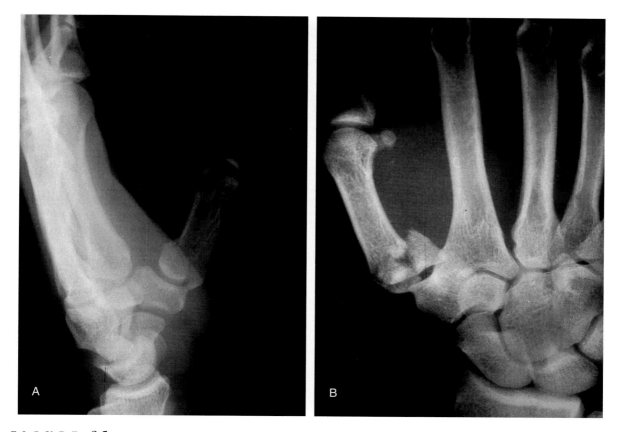

FIGURE 9-5

Bennett's fracture and Rolando's fracture. (A) Bennett's fracture is an intra-articular fracture at the base of the thumb with radialward sub-luxation of the carpometacarpal joint. (B) Rolando's fracture differs from *A* in that the fracture has a T or Y pattern with displaced fracture fragments.

Finger Trauma

Phalanx Trauma

Jersey Finger

Jersey finger refers to an injury commonly sustained by a football player who avulses the profundus tendon of the fourth finger when the fingertip is grasping an opponent's jersey and is forcibly pulled away. This injury is also known as *sweater finger* and *rugby finger*. It is seen in sports where grabbing an opponent is common, as in martial arts. The mechanism of injury includes avulsion of the flexor digitorum profundus tendon due to the forced passive extension of the distal interphalangeal (DIP) joint while the athlete is actively flexing the finger in a grasping motion. Any finger can be involved, but the ring finger is most common (3). This injury is usually sustained during a tackle. Because there is no obvious deformity, this injury is commonly misdiagnosed. The injury is demonstrated by the lack of active flexion of the DIP joint and weakness of the grip. Tenderness may be found in the proximal finger or hand, where the avulsed tendon retracts.

X-Ray Findings The x-ray is frequently normal but is still taken to assess for associated fractures or avulsion of the volar lip of the distal phalanx (Fig. 9-6). The volar plate may remain attached to the fracture fragment, which limits further retraction of the tendon. If avulsion has occurred, oblique views, in addition to PA and lateral views, may help localize the tendon. The proximal hand also must be assessed, because if the tendon has retracted into the palm, the ten-

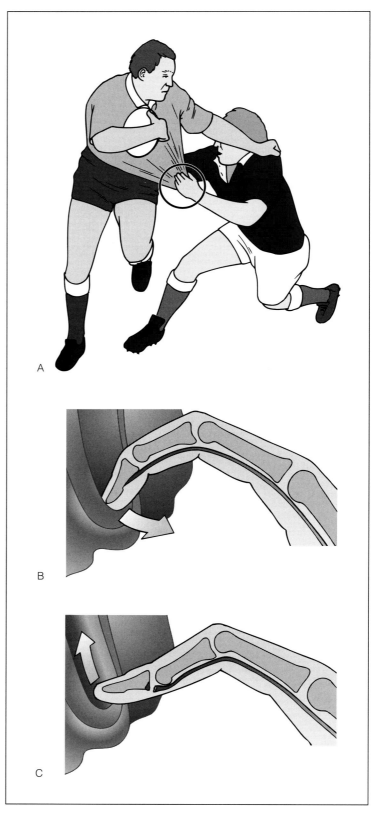

FIGURE 9-6

Jersey finger. (A) Grabbing a jersey. (B) Active flexion of the flexor digitorum profundus. (C) Passive extension avulsing the insertion of the flexor digitorum profundus from the distal phalanx.

don must be repaired within 7 to 10 days. Extensive tendon retraction may lead to secondary tendon rupture due to ischemic necrosis. Failure to diagnose and treat promptly may result in a permanent disruption with a "floppy finger" and a weak grasp.

Mallet Finger

Mallet finger refers to an injury sustained by the extensor digitorum tendon as it inserts on the distal phalanx. This injury is usually incurred in a ball sport. The common name is *baseball finger,* but other labels include *drop finger.* This is the most common fingertip injury, where a ball is thrown against an extended finger. It is seen in baseball, volleyball, basketball, and football. The mechanism of injury includes overloading the extensor digitorum tendon as the DIP joint is forcibly flexed by the ball contacting the fingertip. The ruptured tendon allows the finger to flex at the DIP joint because the flexor digitorum profundus acts unopposed. The athlete presents with the finger flexed and swollen at the DIP joint, while the interphalangeal joint, the middle joint, has an associated hyperextension. The point of maximal tenderness is over the proximal end of the dorsum of the distal phalanx (4).

X-Ray Findings The x-ray may be normal if no bony avulsion has occurred. Nonetheless, the DIP joint is postured in flexion. When a bony avulsion of the tendon insertion has occurred, the important factor is whether the bony fragment represents a significant part of the articular surface of the distal phalanx. Usually only PA and lateral views are needed. When greater than 30% to 50% of the articular surface of the distal phalanx is involved and there is volar subluxation, the best functional result will be attained when an anatomic reduction is pursued (Fig. 9-7). Rigid fixation may be necessary. More commonly, there is just a tiny spicule of avulsed bone that is only minimally displaced, less than 2 mm. These injuries could be treated with immobilization, placing the DIP joint in full extension for 6 weeks. In skeletally immature athletes, epiphyseal injury may take the form of a Salter-Harris type IV fracture, which, if ignored, would lead to a chronic deformity. Regardless of the severity and the appropriateness of treatment, most athletes seem to tolerate this well, with the possible flexion deformity of the terminal digit not causing much impairment if flexion tasks can be performed.

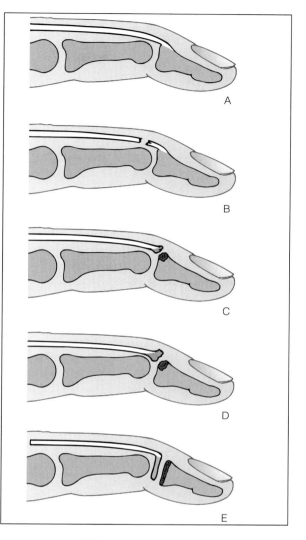

FIGURE 9-7

Mallet finger. There are five distinct patterns to the mallet finger injury complex, but only fracture, avulsion, and slipped epiphysis are seen on x-ray. (Reproduced by permission from McCue FC, Wooten L. Closed tendon injuries of the hand in athletics. Clin Sports Med 1986;5:743.)

Phalanx Fractures

Phalanx fractures are considered from the aspect of different regions: proximal, middle, and distal phalanges.

The *distal phalanx* is prone to being caught in a pinch or crush injury. The typical injury is a fingertip caught between two bowling balls. The pulp of the finger is usually swollen and tense, and a subungual hematoma is common. X-ray findings show a stellate type of fracture with little or no displacement of the many, yet tiny, fragments and no intra-articular extension of the fracture. The PA view is most helpful, but the lateral view is included to assess the articular surface of the phalanx. The volar aspect of the most distal end of the phalanx or "tuft" of the distal phalanx is common in crush-pinch injuries. This is seen as a cortical defect in the tuft. Sometimes these are incomplete fractures. Care is usually directed toward the associated soft tissue injury, management of the edema, and early motion of the DIP joint.

The *middle* and *proximal phalanges* pose a more complicated situation. Since these are "mini-long bones," the mechanics of grasping must be kept in mind. Fractures of these two bones may or may not involve the joint (Fig. 9-8). When the joint is involved, anatomic reduction is preferable. When the joint is not involved, the length and orientation of the phalanx must be considered. Oblique and spiral fractures result from twisting and angular forces. Shortening, rotation, and angular deformity can result. These complications can cause decrements in the functional abilities of the hand. The initial PA and lateral views usually are supplemented with oblique views intended to assess the degree of angulation and rotation and amount of over-riding. This takes on more importance when there are three or more parts to the fracture. In these instances, the periosteal sleeve and dorsal hood cannot stabilize the fracture fragments, and open reduction, pin fixation, and plating may be necessary to allow the best functional outcome. Open fractures and fracture-dislocations involving these two bones are not uncommon. Because of contamination, these fractures are not reduced outside the operating room. Formal wound lavage and debridement are carried out under tourniquet control and adequate lighting so that associated neurovascular and tendon injuries can be found and treated. Fractures involving the open physis at the proximal end of the proximal phalanx are often accompanied by metaphyseal extension of the fracture. Many times these are only minimally displaced and, like closed Salter-Harris type II fractures, can be managed in a closed, conservative fashion.

Dislocations of the proximal interphalangeal (PIP) joint are found commonly in the middle three fingers. Forced hyperextension of the PIP joint can cause dorsal dislocation, in the coronal plane, accompanied by volar plate disruption. Angular deforming forces applied to the distal phalanx can cause PIP joint dislocation, in the frontal plane, accompanied by collateral ligament disruption. Because the proximal ends of the middle phalanges contain the growth plate of the bone, epiphyseal trauma should be suspected in PIP joint dislocations. Volar PIP joint dislocations are much more uncommon, but when they are found, disruption of the central slip must be suspected. Boutonniere deformity will result if this is diagnosed in later stages (5). All these PIP joint dislocations can be open dislocations, and all can be accompanied by marginal fractures of the distal end of the proximal phalanx. Open fracture-dislocations warrant formal open arthrotomy and lavage prior to reduction.

Metacarpal Fractures

The palm of the hand is susceptible to trauma as the hand is used defensively to protect the face, as well as being used as an offensive weapon. The mobility of the thumb and little finger metacarpals allows for retained function despite deformity. The middle three metacarpals are less mobile and require more effort to regain their anatomic reduction. The transverse metacarpal arch should be maintained for hand mechanics and grip strength (6). The following fractures are the more common nonthumb metacarpal fractures.

Boxer's Fracture

Despite this label, most of these fractures are incurred by hitting inanimate objects in a fit of rage. This fracture involves a transverse or short oblique fracture of the neck of the distal metacarpal (Fig. 9-9). Usually the little finger metacarpal is involved. The head of the metacarpal rolls palmarward so that there is dorsal angulation, loss of the little finger knuckle when a fist is made, and a diagnostic bulge in the palm on the ulnar side. Since this deformity is in the plane of flexion of the MPJ, considerable angulation can be accepted, and closed reduction with cast immobilization is the common treatment. To maintain the length of the dorsal extensor soft tissues, the MPJ is casted at 90 degrees of flexion.

Metacarpal Diaphyseal or Shaft Fractures

The diaphysis of a metacarpal is subject to angular deforming forces and axial loading forces. The common fracture patterns include a variety

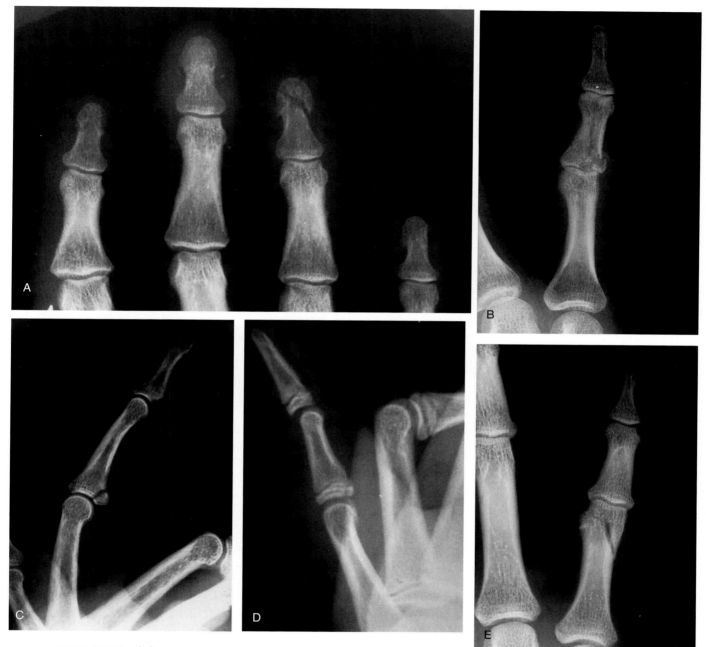

FIGURE   **9-8**

Phalanx fractures. (A) Distal phalanx fracture. A stellate, multipart fracture with minimal displacement. (B) Middle phalanx fracture. An inverted T-shaped fracture with no displacement when the PIP joint is extended. (C) Middle phalanx fracture. A volar plate avulsion fracture with minimal displacement. (D) Interphalangeal dislocation. This postreduction x-ray shows injury to the physis at the proximal end of the middle phalanx. (E) Proximal phalanx fracture. This fracture was sustained from forceful hyperabduction. The peristeal sleeve keeps the widening to a minimum.

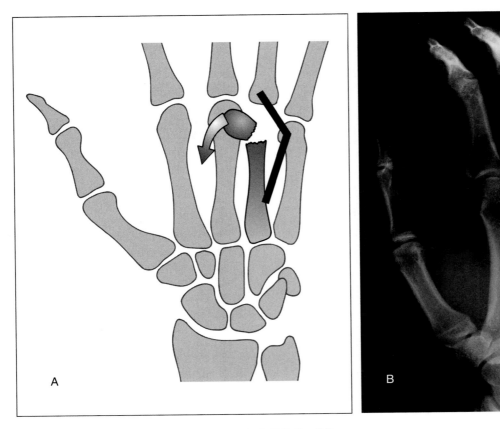

F I G U R E   **9-9**

Boxer's fracture. An illustration (A) and an x-ray (B) of a fracture of the neck of the metacarpal. The fracture allows the metacarpal head to displace palmarward. The ring and little fingers are the usual sites of this fracture.

of oblique fractures and "butterfly fragments" or rhomboid-shaped comminution. The intrinsic hand muscles, the interossei and lumbricales, as well as the extensor hood and the metacarpal periosteal sleeve, help to stabilize the fracture. Like rib fractures, where there are three bones involved, stability with closed techniques tends to be poorer than with isolated solitary metacarpal fractures (Fig. 9-10). Open fractures may look obvious or be suspected from overlying puncture wounds. These hand fractures present with the patient demonstrating a grossly swollen hand offering no motion due to pain.

X-Ray Findings The PA and prone oblique views demonstrate these fractures. The main concern is determining whether there is intra-articular extension of the fracture line. The articular surface must be restored to avoid post-traumatic arthritis and chronic pain. Over-riding of

long, oblique fractures causes shortening of the bone. Torquing causes rotation, and severe angulation causes deformation of the plane of flexion. These changes decrease the effectiveness of hand function. The lucency of the cortex where a nutrient artery lies can be mistaken for a fracture line. The metacarpal epiphyses are all located distally, as opposed to the proximally located phalangeal epiphyses, except for the thumb metacarpal, which has a proximally located epiphysis. These can complicate an assay for fractures. Soft tissue swelling and the soft tissue shadow it creates must be used as a clue.

Management options include closed reduction, immobilization using percutaneous transfixing pins, pin and plaster cast immobilization, miniature plates and screws, intramedullary pinning, and external fixators. In addition to restoring length and decreasing rotation and angulation, reduction with the aforementioned

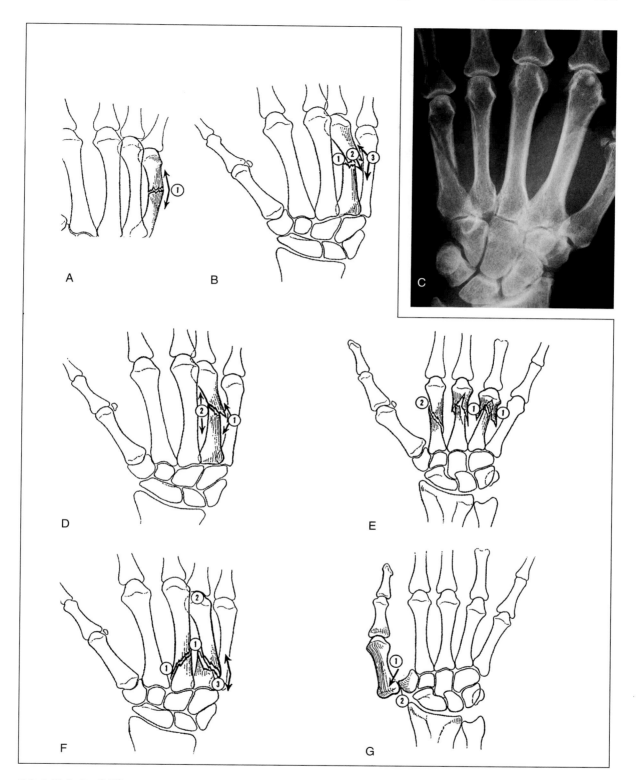

Metacarpal fractures. Metacarpal fractures can be transverse, short oblique, or long oblique. The latter has potential for shortening but is usually stable due to the palmar interossei muscles that adduct the metacarpals.

immobilizing techniques helps minimize the potential for complications such as reflex sympathetic dystrophy because early motion can be attained.

Carpal Trauma

The carpus is comprised of two rows of irregularly shaped, small, interlocking bones that function with the radiocarpal and the carpometacarpal joints to enhance flexion, extension, radial and ulnar deviation, supination, and pronation. The rows of carpal bones are curved in two planes. The carpus protects the neurovascular structures supplying the digits and provides a conduit for the bundles of flexor tendons. With the tightly adherent volar retinaculum/aponeurosis, the carpus forms the *carpal tunnel.* The following conditions are unique in that no carpal bone can sustain any pathology without adversely affecting the other parts of the hand. The common presentation of these problems includes a history of a fall onto the extended wrist with the hand open. There is variable pain and swelling, poor hand grasping function, and variable degrees of reflex dystrophy in older, long-standing injuries. The distal carpal row is made up of the trapezium and trapezoid (greater and lesser multrangulars), capitate, and hamate. The proximal carpal row is made up of the scaphoid (carpal navicular), lunate, triquetrum, and pisiform.

Scaphoid Fractures

The scaphoid is the most commonly fractured bone of the wrist, accounting for 70% of all carpal bone fractures. It is a key stabilizer, bridging the proximal and distal carpal rows. It is uncommon in children but very common in young males. The most common mechanism of injury is falling onto the outstretched hand with near-right-angle dorsiflexion. This trauma causes axial compression along the long axis of the scaphoid. The scaphoid tubercle can fracture when the athlete's hand sustains a blow to the radial side of the hand. Examination reveals tenderness localized to the anatomic snuff box at the wrist just distal to the radial styloid. The *snuff box* is defined by the prominences of the extensor pollicis longus and brevis and the abductor pollicis tendons. (Grated tobacco was

placed into this depression on the back of the wrist. The wrist was brought up to the nose, where the tobacco was snorted into the upper airway.) In addition to decreased range of motion, the athlete has decreased grip strength. An unstable scaphoid can be felt to snap with passive extreme wrist dorsiflexion.

X-Ray Findings

Common views, PA, lateral, and oblique, can show a variety of fracture patterns: horizontal, transverse, and vertical fractures (Fig. 9-11). Among these, there can be variable degrees of displacement. The oblique view is the best for demonstrating this fracture. A special view, the *scaphoid view,* is taken AP with 30 degrees of supination and slight ulnar deviation. Because the blood supply of the scaphoid enters from the distal end, the location of the fracture is important to determine. A nondisplaced fracture of the waist of the scaphoid has the best chance of an uncomplicated outcome even when treated in a short-arm thumb spica plaster cast. A long-arm cast also can be considered because of the micromotion of the scaphoid involved in supination and pronation. Tubercle fractures and proximal pole fractures have increased complications such as malunion, fibrous union, and nonunion. Because of the chronic pain and hand weakness these cause, screw fixation or plating can be considered. Many times this fracture, if nondisplaced, is mistaken for an inconsequential wrist sprain. Degenerative joint disease or avascular necrosis can result. When clinical suspicion runs high, thumb spice immobilization for 10 to 14 days with repeat x-rays can be helpful. Pinhole, triple-phase SPECT scanning can confirm the clinical picture. Chronic instability due to scapholunate dissociation or dorsiflexion of the lunate also may occur if this injury is overlooked.

Scapholunate Dissociation

This is one of the most common and arguably the most significant problem because of the chronic pain and grasp weakness it can cause. It is caused by a fall on the athlete's outstretched and ulnar-deviated hand. Lighter, yet repetitive trauma also can cause this injury. The athlete presents with a tender and swollen wrist with guarded and limited motion. Sudden vigorous gripping produces pain. A provocative test, the

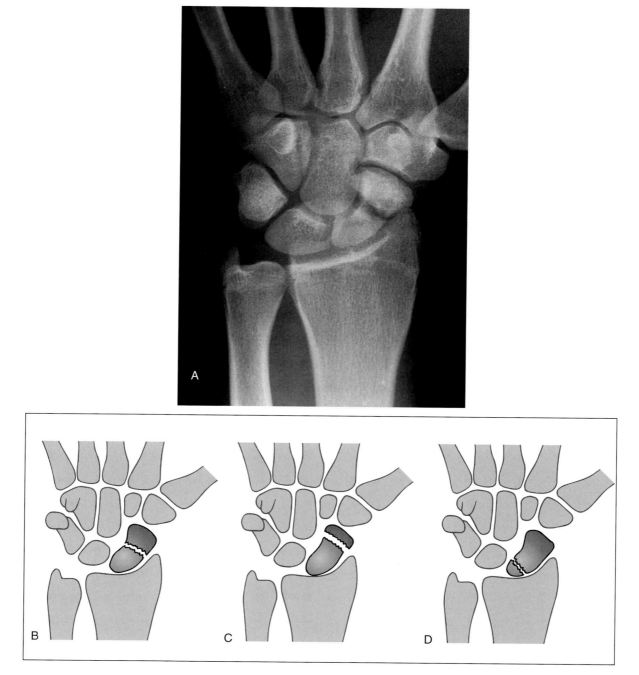

F I G U R E   **9-11**

Scaphoid fractures. (A) Fracture through the waist or middle third. These are the most common. (B and C) Fracture through the tubercle or distal third. These are the least common. (D) Fracture through the body or proximal third. These account for about 20% of all scaphoid fractures. Because of deficient circulation, these take longer to heal and are associated with avascular necrosis.

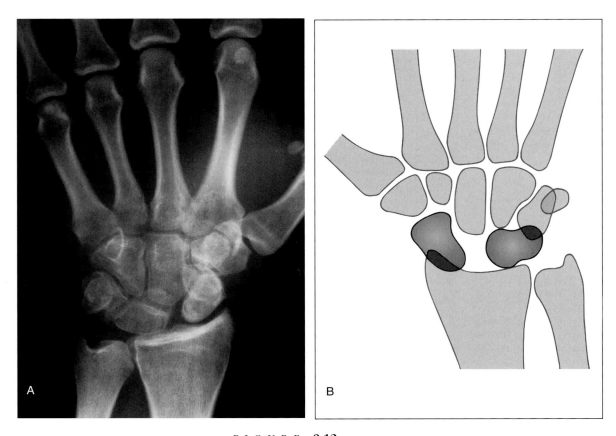

FIGURE 9-12

Scapholunate dissociation. A scapholunate interval greater than 2 mm is indicative of a scapholunate dissociation.

Watson test, is performed by the physician. This involves compressing the scaphoid with the examiner's thumb and moving the athlete's wrist from ulnar to radial deviation.

X-Ray Findings

The *Terry Thomas sign* refers to a space, the scapholunate interval, greater than 2 mm between the scaphoid and lunate on the PA projection (Fig. 9-12). (Terry Thomas is not a famous hand surgeon but rather a British comedian who has a space between his upper central incisors.) The PA view also may show a foreshortened scaphoid. An oblique PA view can show the scaphoid "on end," giving a ringed appearance, or the *ring sign,* sometimes called the *cortical ring sign.* The lateral view shows a dorsiflexed lunate or dorsal intercalated segment instability (DISI) pattern. The scapholunate angle is greater than 65 degrees, and the capitolunate angle is greater than 15 degrees. (An angle between the long axis of the scaphoid and the lunate of greater than 70 degrees is abnormal and indicative of scapholunate dissociation, whereas an angle less than 30 degrees is also abnormal and indicative of ulnar instability (7). Grip stress views force the scaphoid and lunate further apart to help cinch the diagnosis.

When these injuries are not diagnosed, the athlete has chronic instabilities due to the sum of this and frequently associated injuries such as degenerative arthritis, triangular fibrocartilage tear, and additional intercarpal ligament tears such as lunotriquetral and radiotrapezial ligament tears.

Trans-Scaphoid/Perilunate Fracture-Dissociation

Perilunate instabilities are the most common type of carpal instabilities. The mechanism of injury is axial loading of the wrist with severe, forced hyperextension with pronation and radial deviation. This occurs when the athlete falls with the arm behind him or her, as happens in falling on ice skates or in-line skates. The athlete presents with a swollen, tender wrist having palmar angulation of the wrist with lost wrist extension.

X-Ray Findings

Widely separated transverse fracture of the scaphoid, with the distal carpal row dorsal to the lunate, is seen on PA views. The proximal pole of the scaphoid and the distal carpal row are seen to maintain their relationship with the radius on lateral view. As with perilunate dissociation, the lunate takes on a triangular contour and looks like a "spilled teacup" on the lateral view (Fig. 9-13). If the athlete can tolerate it, a traction view can be taken with the fingers in 5 to 10 lb of finger trap traction.

Treatment options revolve around open exploration and re-establishing the normal intercarpal relationships. When left untreated, radial and ulnar neuropathy and hand atrophy develop. Even when presumably adequate treatment is provided, scapholunate dissociation often can remain as a residual problem.

Perilunate Dissociation

This injury is fairly common. It is caused by a fall on an outstretched hand. This injury presents similarly to trans-scaphoid/perilunate fracture-dislocation. Untreated injuries are associated with median neuropathy and chronic carpal instability.

X-Ray Findings

The PA view shows a triangular-appearing lunate instead of its usual trapezoid contour. The lateral view shows the lunate as a "spilled teacup" and the distal carpal row dorsal to the lunate and radius. Special views can enhance this appearance by repeating the PA view in extremes of ulnar and radial deviation and repeating the lateral view in maximal volar and dorsal flexions.

Hamate Fracture

Falling onto the hypothenar eminence or ulnar border of the hand in a forced dorsiflexion position or repetitive vibratory trauma can fracture the base of the hook of the hamate. Bat and rac-

quet sports, cycling and motor cross, gymnastics, volleyball, and open-handed ball handling have been implicated in this injury. Tenderness may be palmar, dorsal, or both.

X-Ray Findings

A supination oblique view shows a transverse fracture through the base of the hamate. The hamate view is obtained with the wrist in midsupination and slight dorsiflexion. The carpal tunnel view shows the hamate and pisiform well (Fig. 9-14). Negative x-rays with ongoing clinical suspicions can be answered with technetium-99m pertechnetate scanning to assess for abnormal uptake or an MRI with STIR imaging. Further evaluation using CT scanning remains an alternative. Undiagnosed fractures can lead to symptoms due to ulnar nerve compression in Guyon's canal, hand paresthesias, weakness of the intrinsic hand muscles (abductor digiti quinti), and pain provoked by palpation over the bony eminence of the hamate or forceful dorsiflexion with ulnar deviation.

Lunate Fracture

The lunate is the second most injured carpal bone (behind the scaphoid). Abrupt, forceful dorsiflexion of the wrist can cause this fracture. Sometimes there is no trauma history, but the athlete complains of a stiff and painful wrist and of hearing or feeling a snap in the wrist with repetitive dorsiflexion. Carpenters, carpet layers, and riveters acquire this injury. Keinbock's disease (avascular necrosis of the lunate) is a complication of this fracture. This may occur due to the same microfracture mechanics with ischemia due to interruption of the vertically oriented (dorsovolar) blood supply. Limited motion and dorsal tenderness are usually found.

X-Ray Findings

Superimposed structures can make it difficult to visualize this injury even with PA, lateral, and oblique views. Early on this condition has normal x-rays. Later stages of avascular necrosis give the lunate a dense, chalky-white, sclerotic appearance (Fig. 9-15). Still later, cystic degeneration, fragmentation, collapse, loss of carpal height, and scaphoid rotation can be seen (8). On bone scanning, the lunate takes up little to no isotope tracer as compared with the opposite hand late in this "disease," whereas early in the

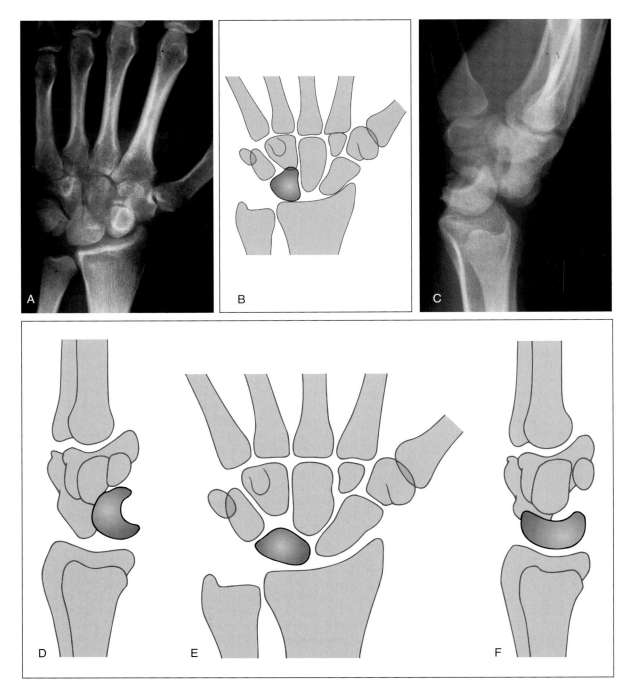

FIGURE 9-13

The PA view shows the lunate having a triangular contour instead of its usual quadrilateral contour. The lunate takes on the "spilled tea-cup" appearance on lateral view.

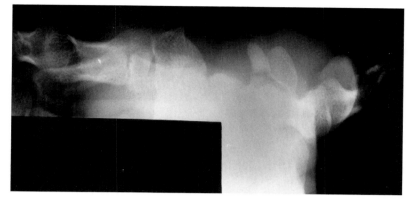

FIGURE   **9-14**

Hamate fracture. The hamate view is an oblique view taken with the forearm supinated and the wrist dorsiflexed to bring the hook of the hamate into profile. The carpal tunnel view seen here is also taken with the wrist maximally dorsiflexed with the x-ray beam angled through the carpus, also imaging the lateral profile of the hook of the hamate. Note the fracture of the hamate in this x-ray.

course of this problem the bone scan may look "hot" due to the reactive synovitis consistently seen in this condition. Treatment can include a short-arm cast in a conservative treatment plan or a variety of surgical interventions that remain controversial.

Distal Radius and Ulna Trauma

Extension and Flexion Fractures

Fractures of the distal radius and ulna are common because we try to use the upper extremities to protect the head and trunk in falls. Falling with the wrist extended (dorsiflexed) produces a different fracture than falling with the wrist flexed (volarflexed). Additionally, the same mechanism of injury in a skeletally immature athlete will produce an epiphyseal injury, whereas in the osteoporotic athlete a comminuted fracture will be sustained, and in others a variety of angulated, malrotated, over-ridden, and displaced one- and two-bone fractures can be seen. Regardless of the type of fracture, a few underlying common threads of importance should be understood.

X-Ray Findings

The normal x-ray anatomy must be remembered so that the extent of the trauma and the adequacy of the reduction can be appreciated. The metaphysis of the radius is characterized by lines of stress. An athlete whose wrist has "poor bone stock" due to osteoporosis cannot be expected to maintain a reduction. The radial styloid is about 1 cm distal to the ulnar styloid in the adult. The articular surface of the radius is inclined ulnarward 23 degrees and palmarward

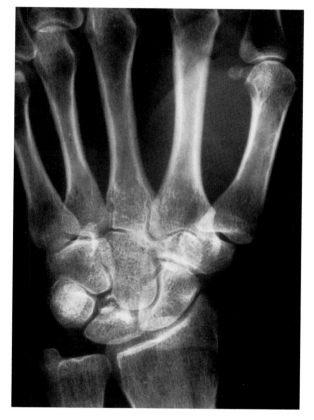

FIGURE   **9-15**

Lunate fracture. Compressive forces on the lunate result when an athlete sustains an axial load from falling in forced hyperextension with pronation and radial deviation, such as when the athlete falls with the arm behind him or her. This can produce a trans-scaphoid/perilunate fracture-dissociation.

11 degrees (Fig. 9-16). Extension fractures are commonly and sometimes erroneously called *Colles' fractures*. (Dr. Colles, a Scotsman, pronounced his name "Cols," whereas in the United States the common pronunciation is "Collies.") A

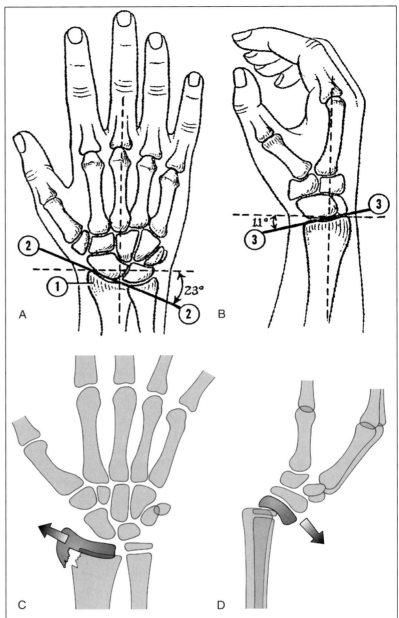

FIGURE **9-16**

Wrist joint angles. The x-ray appearance of the normal wrist shows the styloid process of the radius extending 1 cm beyond the ulnar styloid. The articular surface of the radius is inclined ulnarward 15 to 30 degrees (23 degrees average) and palmarward 1 to 23 degrees (11 degrees average). These anatomic relationships are deranged in wrist fractures.

true Colles' fracture is a transverse fracture of the distal radius about 4 cm proximal to the radiocarpal joint with posterior and dorsal displacement of the distal fragment. The universal classification of dorsal displaced distal radius fractures was described by Gartland and Werley in 1951 (9) and Sarmiento in 1975 (10) (Fig. 9-17). Type I is a nonarticular and undisplaced fracture. Full recovery with no disability should be expected after conservative splinting. Type II is a nonarticular but dorsally displaced fracture that should give a good functional result if the

dorsal displacement and angulation are reduced, usually by closed reduction manipulation, and maintained by a well-molded cast or pin casting. The higher grades of this fracture are intra-articular, with type III being undisplaced and type IV displaced. Type IV is further subtyped according to its inherent stability, with type IVA being reducible and stable, IVB being reducible yet unstable, and IVC being both irreducible and unstable (9,10).

Flexion fractures are not nearly as common and carry the eponym *Smith's fracture*. As

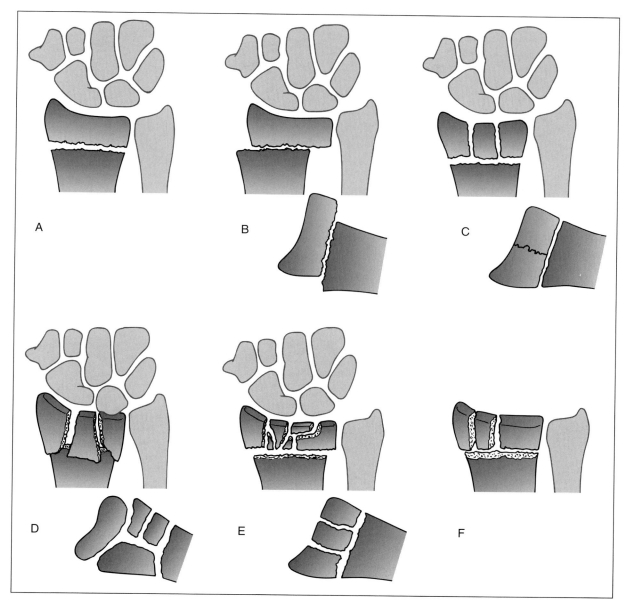

F I G U R E   **9-17**

Classification of wrist fractures. The classification of wrist fracture and dislocations was modified from Gartland and from Sarmentio. This classification differentiates between joint involvement, fragment proximity, and the ability to maintain a closed reduction. (A) Type I: extra-articular and undisplaced. (B) Type II: extra-articular but displaced. (C) Type III: intra-articular and undisplaced. (D) Type IVA: intra-articular and displaced, reducible, and stable. (E) Type IVB: intra-articular and displaced, reducible, and unstable. (F) Type IVC: intra-articular and displaced, irreducible, and unstable.

dramatic as these appear, both clinically and radiologically, attention must be paid to areas distant from the excitement. Commonly associated trauma involves the *proximal* radioulnar joint, the radiocapitellar joint, and the *distal* radioulnar joint. Any of these could undergo subluxation or even dislocation as part of the response to a traumatic energy transfer. What may look like a simple Colles' fracture (no such thing exists) or a Smith's fracture may really be a variant of a complex two-bone fracture, such as Monteggia's and Galliazzi's types. Generally speaking, unless the reduction restores the articular surface of the radius, the length of the radius, and the ulnar and volar inclinations of the radiocarpal joint, chronic pain, hand weakness, and disability should be expected. *Barton's fracture* refers to a posterior marginal fracture, more correctly described as an oblique fracture of the posterior lip of the distal end of the radius directed upward and backward (Fig. 9-18). These fractures are usually minimally displaced and can be managed with the forearm pronated in a cast for 6 to 8 weeks. The anterior analogue of this marginal fracture is a type of Smith's fracture. It, too, is usually minimally displaced and can be managed in a cast but with the forearm

supinated. The *chauffeur's fracture* refers to a triangular distal radius fracture involving a significant metaphyseal fragment (Fig. 9-19). The fracture line is directed upward and outward. The articular surface of the radius is involved, and the carpus is shifted to the radial side of the radial fragment. Because this is basically a metaphyseal fracture, it does well with 4 to 6 weeks of cast immobilization. One of the supposed mechanisms of injury was the whipping of the automobile starter crank against the dorsum of the chauffeur's wrist.

Intra-articular fractures of the distal radius result from the characteristic "die punch" mechanism of injury. The convex aspect of the lunate pounds the articular surface of the radius, producing a consistent fracture pattern comprised of an unstable four-part articular fracture (Fig. 9-20). Melone described the pivotal position of the medial fragments of this fracture because both the radioulnar and the radiocarpal joints become disrupted (11). The four parts of this fracture are the distal shaft of the radius, the radial styloid, the dorsal medial part, and the palmar medial part. This is a grossly unstable fracture needing expert anatomic reduction to restore the articular surface of the distal radius.

F I G U R E   **9-18**

Smith's fracture and Barton's fracture. (A, B) Smith's fracture is a flexion fracture of the distal radius, sometimes called a *reverse Colles' fracture*. (C, D) Barton's fracture is a marginal distal radius fracture. The anterior marginal distal radius fracture can be sustained in a flexion mechanism. The posterior marginal analogue is sustained from an extension mechanism.

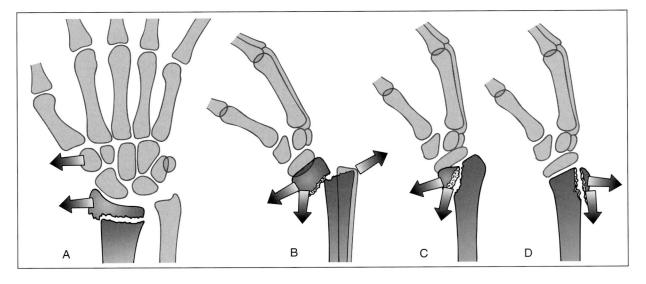

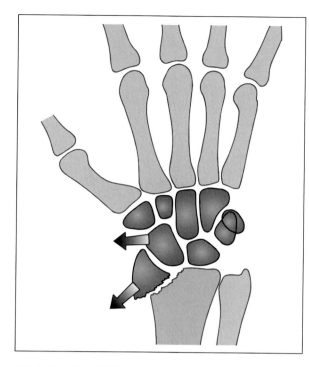

FIGURE **9-19**

The chauffeur's fracture. This fracture involves the articular surface of the radius. Usually there is no or minimal displacement of the fracture fragment. The carpus is shifted slightly radialward with the radial fragment.

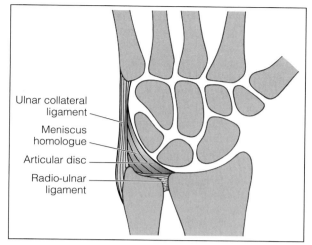

FIGURE **9-21**

The triangular fibrocartilage complex. The triangular fibrocartilage complex is a confluence of structures whose contribution to the distal radioulnar joint stability changes with forearm position.

Triangular Fibrocartilage Tear

The triangular fibrocartilage is a tough fibrocartilaginous structure located on the ulnar side of the wrist providing intrinsic stability to the wrist. (Extrinsic stability is provided to the wrist joint by the pronator quadratus, flexor carpi ulnaris, and extensor carpi ulnaris muscles as well as the interosseous membrane.) The triangular fibro-

cartilage complex is a confluence of structures contributing to the stability of the distal radioulnar joint. It is composed of meniscus homologue, prestyloid recess, articular disk, ulnar collateral ligament, and radioulnar ligament (12) (Fig. 9-21). The triangular fibrocartilage complex can tear and causes ulnar-sided wrist pain worsened by extremes of forearm rotation, radioulnar compression, and dorsal-volar translation of the distal ulna. Treatment can range from cast immobilization for 6 weeks to surgical excision, which has shown inconsistent results, particularly in patients over 40 years of age. Arthroscopic debridement resulted in a favorable outcome in 80% of Bitter and Dell's study group. Patients who have concomitant lunotriquetral

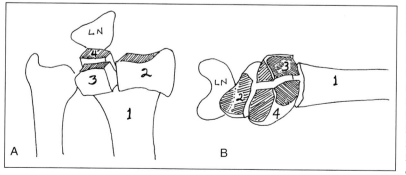

FIGURE **9-20**

Melone's intra-articular fracture classification. The "die punch" mechanism of distal radius fractures caused by the lunate forcing apart the articular surface of the radius produces a consistent fracture pattern. The medial complex is comprised of the medial fragments of the radius. These fragments include the radiocarpal and distal radioulnar joints.

tears need those lesions repaired. Patients who continue to have radioulnar joint instability after virtual healing of their radial fracture should be suspected of having a triangular fibrocartilage complex disruption. An ulnar styloid fracture, with or without nonunion, can contribute to chronic instability.

REFERENCES

1. Snell RS, Wyman AC. An atlas of normal radiographic anatomy. Boston: Brown, Little, 1976:64–85.

2. Stener B. Displacement of the ruptured ulnar collateral ligament of the metacarpophalangeal joint of the thumb. J Bone Joint Surg 1962;44B:869.

3. Blazina M, Lane C. Rupture of the insertion of the flexor digitorum profundus tendon in student athletes. J Am Coll Health Assoc 1966;14:248.

4. McCue FC, Wooten L. Closed tendon injuries of the hand in athletics. Clin Sports Med 1986;5:743.

5. Brunet M, Haddad R. Fractures and dislocations of the metacarpals and phalanges. Clin Sports Med 1986;5:773–781.

6. Gieck J. Protective splinting for the hand and wrist. Clin Sports Med 1986;5:795–807.

7. Culver JE. Instabilities of the wrist in injuries to the elbow, forearm, and hand. Clin Sports Med 1986;5:725–740.

8. Lichtman DM, Gelberman RH, Bauman TD, et al. Kienbock's disease: update on silicone replacement arthroplasty. J Hand Surg 1982;7:343.

9. Gartland J, Werley CW. Evaluation of healed Colles' fractures. J Bone Joint Surg 1951;33A:895–907.

10. Sarmentio A. Colles' fractures: functional bracing in supination. J Bone Joint Surg 1975;57A:311–317.

11. Melone CP. Unstable fractures of the distal radius. In: Lichman DM, ed. The wrist and its disorders. Philadelphia: WB Saunders, 1987.

12. Palmer AK, Werner FW. The triangular fibrocartilage complex. J Hand Surg 1981;6:153–162.

CHAPTER 10

Abdominal Injuries and Their Radiographic Assessment

PAUL R. STRICKER
JAMES C. PUFFER
BARBARA KADELL

*A*bdominal injury is perhaps one of the most challenging diagnostic and management problems that the clinician encounters, and this is particularly so when it occurs to a competitive athlete. The unprotected abdomen is obviously vulnerable in collision or contact sports, and what may seem to be a relatively minor trauma with minimal physical findings may quickly turn into a potentially catastrophic injury. The advent of modern diagnostic imaging, heralded by the development of computed tomography (CT), has been instrumental in facilitating a rapid and precise diagnosis in such injuries, and this chapter will explore the use of radiography and advanced imaging in the diagnosis and management of acute abdominal injury. However, as a preface, we will first explore the incidence of abdominal injury in athletes, the mechanisms by which injury occurs, the role of physical examination in initially assessing the injured athlete, and initial management strategies.

Incidence

Injuries to the abdomen have been found to account for as many as 7% of sporting injuries in the United States (1). Abdominal injuries account for 10% of all athletic injuries in Sweden (2,3), and they make up 7% of the sports injuries in children less than 14 years of age (4). In children 11 to 14 years of age, abdominal injuries most frequently result from sporting activities and accidents. While abdominal injury occurs infrequently, a wide variety of intra-abdominal injuries can be encountered, including injury to both hollow and solid organs as well as vascular structures. Of the abdominal viscera, the spleen, liver, and kidney are the most commonly injured organs (3,5–9). Reported incidences of renal injury range from 10% to 50%, splenic injury from 11% to 16%, hepatic injury from 4.4% to 4.9%, bowel injury from 2.2% to 4%, and pancreatic injury from 0.7% to 1% (2,4,7,10–13).

Mechanisms of Injury

The abdomen is unprotected and vulnerable to injury during sports participation. Although the abdominal contents are not usually protected by external equipment in athletes, they are somewhat protected by musculoaponeurotic tissue and the bony ribs. The spleen and liver have partial protection from the diaphragm and ribs, whereas the kidneys and pancreas are surrounded in part by the lower ribs, spine, and paraspinal musculature. The intestines may not have much protection other than the abdominal musculature, but they have the advantage of being soft, pliable, and mobile. Solid organs are more vulnerable to trauma because they are fragile and relatively fixed. The hollow organs are susceptible to rupture from rapid increases in intra-abdominal pressure from forceful compression of the abdomen. Compression of a small abdominal area easily can result in intra-abdominal injury, even if caused by a low-energy event (2).

Mechanisms of injury can vary, and the location of pain is not necessarily the location of the actual injury. For the most part, however, obtaining a history of the mechanism may help the physician begin to specifically locate the site of injury. Early recognition of potential abdominal injury is critical due to the deceiving nature of these injuries. Abdominal injuries arise from either an object striking the athlete or the individual striking another object or individual. Direct blows account for many of the injuries, but deceleration forces also create shearing and vascular injuries. Generally, blows to the left side of the abdomen or ribcage cause splenic injury, and trauma to the right side can injure the liver, although contracoup injuries have been reported (14). Renal injury usually results from trauma to the flank, pancreatic problems arise from forces to the upper midabdomen, and hollow viscus injuries can occur from direct blows or deceleration injuries. Rib fractures additionally can produce injuries to many of these organs.

Physical Examination

Since hemorrhage is the most common cause of death from abdominal injury, awareness of the potential for catastrophic injury following abdominal trauma is crucial. Fortunately, significant internal injuries are uncommon, but the subtlety of these injuries may result in a low index of suspicion that can affect outcome adversely. Although physicians routinely rely on the initial physical examination of other injuries to guide treatment decisions, the physical examination in abdominal injury is an unreliable indicator of the severity of injury. It has been demonstrated that in patients with negative initial examinations, a 43% incidence of significant abdominal injury existed (6,15), and as many as 20% of patients with acute hemoperitoneum had a benign abdominal examination when first examined (16). Abdominal injuries can progress

quickly to shock or result in insidious bleeding that can lead to vascular collapse at a later time. If any suspicion of serious abdominal injury exists, vital signs and volume status should be assessed and monitored carefully, intravenous access should be established quickly, and the injured athlete should be placed in the Trendelenburg position until transport can be carried out.

Management of Abdominal Trauma

Prompt surgical exploration is required if gross hemorrhage and hemodynamic instability, abdominal distension, obvious peritonitis, abdominal wall disruption, or other entities that require emergency treatment are present. However, many abdominal injuries may not present with the obvious, and certain diagnostic procedures necessarily will be performed to determine the seriousness of the injury. If the patient is stable, time may permit these tests to be carried out. Constant observation, vital sign determination, and assessment of hemodynamic status are crucial. Nonoperative management should be abandoned if there is any indication of deteriorating hemodynamic status, unstable vital signs, falling hematocrit, hematocrit not responding to transfusion, or abdominal distension.

Laboratory tests to be obtained are few. Hematocrit, urinalysis, and stool for occult blood should be performed. Serum amylase and liver transaminase levels are additional tests that may help in the diagnosis of occult pancreatic or liver injury.

The remainder of the diagnostic process may consist of diagnostic peritoneal lavage (DPL) and diagnostic imaging. Nonoperative diagnostic sensitivity has improved dramatically due to the technological advances that have occurred in diagnostic imaging, increasing the potential for detecting injuries in single and multiple organ systems.

Diagnostic Imaging

Plain Films

Historically, plain radiographs of the chest (anteroposterior and lateral views) and abdomen (supine and upright views) were used routinely as the first diagnostic step in abdominal injuries. They are still frequently used in this capacity, but initial imaging procedures now are usually tailored to the nature of the presenting problem. Nevertheless, plain radiographs are readily available, easy to obtain, and relatively inexpensive. They may be helpful in detecting pneumothorax, rib fracture, spine or transverse process fracture, abnormal gas patterns or free air, masses, abnormal diaphragm contour, and loss of psoas shadows or enlargement of splenic or renal contour. Any of these findings may aid in determining injury or in deciding the next diagnostic test to perform. Fractures of the ribs or transverse processes should raise the suspicion of possible hepatic, splenic, or renal injury. Loss of normal organ, fat, or muscular shadows may be indicative of blood, mass, or enlarged organ, such as occurs with a capsular hematoma (Fig. 10-1). Loss of the normal diaphragmatic contour can be obvious but more often is subtle and missed on initial readings, usually due to the lack of a high

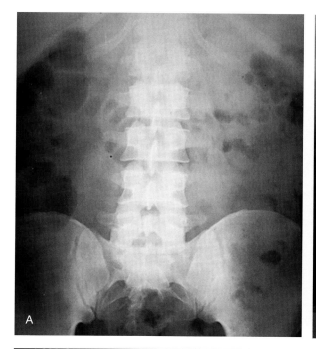

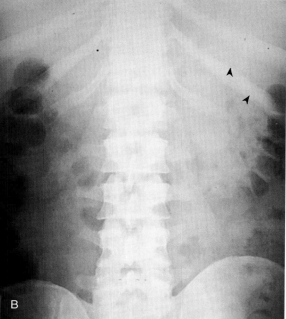

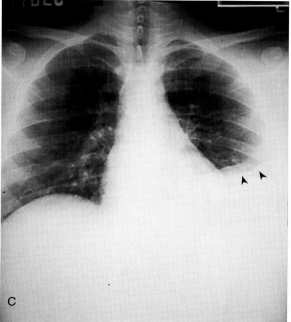

FIGURE **10-1**

Splenic laceration, plain radiographs. (A) Initial abdominal radiograph taken shortly after trauma shows no evidence of splenic enlargement. (B) Six hours later. A left upper quadrant mass is due to a splenic laceration and delayed hematoma. (C) The left hemidiaphragm is elevated, and a left pleural effusion is present.

index of suspicion. A raised hemidiaphragm, unusual position of bowel gas, mediastinal shift, or pleural effusion after abdominal trauma requires closer attention to the integrity of the diaphragm.

Abnormal gas patterns or air-fluid levels necessitate further investigation. Upper gastrointestinal (GI) contrast studies (as well as CT) can provide more definitive information for duodenal or proximal jejunal hematomas. Free air from a bowel perforation often appears on plain radiographs, but small amounts may be missed. Free air appears on plain radiographs about 80% to 90% of the time (17). Gut perforation may be seen with air outside the lumen of the bowel or as air under the diaphragm on upright chest radiograph. Probably more sensitive is the left lateral decubitus film, performed after the patient has been in position for at least 5 to 10 minutes if possible (18). Larger amounts of free air can present as a double-wall sign, since both the mucosal and serosal surfaces are outlined by air. If perforation is retroperitoneal, then air will be present in the various retroperitoneal compartments, often outlining the psoas muscle or kidney. Retroperitoneal air is relatively fixed with respect to position, unlike intraperitoneal air, and if it is beneath the diaphragm, it appears more lateral and crescent-shaped than under the dome of the diaphragm with a straight inferior border. Water-soluble contrast studies are advantageous in locating the exact site of perforation.

Another contrast study that may be helpful after abdominal trauma and suspected renal injury would be the intravenous pyelogram (IVP). This study helps to ensure at least one functioning kidney. Abnormal findings can present as decreased contrast density and/or excretion, displacement of, or extravasation from the injured kidney. In the patient with localized flank trauma and a high clinical suspicion of an isolated renal injury, an IVP is a viable and cost-effective diagnostic option. However, because an IVP provides limited information in the trauma patient, CT is often preferred. CT is quicker, noninvasive, and has greater diagnostic accuracy (7,11,15). Hematomas of the kidney and retroperitoneum may be apparent on CT as well as perfusion abnormalities or contrast and urine extravasation (Fig. 10-2). CT also can reliably detect renal arterial occlusion.

Nuclear Scintigraphy

Nuclear medicine procedures, such as liver-spleen scintigraphy, are very organ specific and

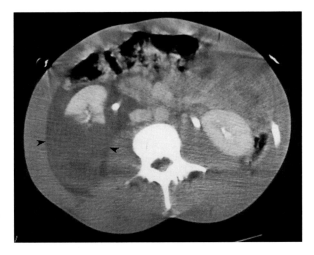

F I G U R E   **10-2**

Right renal trauma. This is a shattered right kidney following blunt trauma to the abdomen. The anterior portion of the kidney has maintained its vascular supply. The posterior portion has lost its arterial blood supply and did not develop a nephrogram (*arrows*). **There is also a large perinephric hematoma.** (Courtesy of Sachiko T. Cochran, MD, UCLA School of Medicine.)

may have a follow-up role for functional assessment after an abdominal organ injury. This imaging modality also has been used in the past to assess spleen size in the athlete recovering from infectious mononucleosis (although this has now been replaced by ultrasound, which is quicker and more accurate). However, because of its infrequent use in the acute trauma patient, scintigraphy will not be discussed in this chapter.

Diagnostic Peritoneal Lavage Versus Imaging

Diagnostic peritoneal lavage (DPL) can be performed to look for hemoperitoneum after abdominal injury and is often used in the evaluation of blunt abdominal injury (15,19). Since its introduction by Root in 1965 (20), it has remained consistently accurate. It is a time-honored procedure that is reliable, fairly quick, and easily available. A distinct advantage of the procedure is the ability to distinguish the type of free intra-abdominal fluid, such as blood, ascites, or bowel contents. The procedure has evolved over time from the original closed procedure to the more open procedure that is widely accepted today. This has helped to decrease the complication rate, yet there is always increased risk because it is an invasive procedure. Its high sensitivity of 98.5% has been criticized for increasing the number of nontherapeutic operations or laparotomies when compared with evaluation by CT scan, and evidence exists to suggest that CT scan localizes specific abdominal injury that would otherwise be questioned by indeterminate DPL findings, thus allowing earlier diagnosis with a less invasive procedure (19). Additional limitations of DPL include uncertainty of the source of bleeding, poor ability to detect retroperitoneal bleeding or diaphragmatic injury, and the questionable significance of analysis of the fluid (21,22). Chemical and microscopic analyses for white blood cells and enzymes have not increased the diagnostic precision of DPL (10). Furthermore, controversy exists over the management of a patient with an indeterminate DPL result (20,000–99,999 RBC/mm^3). Despite the development of other noninvasive techniques, DPL has a proven track record of performance for its primary objective—to determine the presence or absence of hemoperitoneum. It still plays an important role in the early management of abdominal injuries in many centers.

Ultrasound

Ultrasonography (US) threatens to replace DPL in Europe but is rarely used in the United States (23,24). It should be noted, however, that in Europe, virtually all ultrasound procedures are performed by surgeons or emergency physicians rather than by radiologists or ultrasound technicians, as is done in the United States. This makes the results of their research difficult to generalize to centers in our country. Diagnostic US is used as an initial approach to the abdominally injured patient in a manner similar to DPL; that is, the major objective is to determine the presence of intra-abdominal fluid. Fluid accumulates in areas that are considered "acoustic windows" well suited for US such as the subphrenic, subhepatic, perirenal, and pelvic areas. European studies have found sensitivities for US to determine intra-abdominal fluid to range from 81% to 100% (23,24). One study showed that US had a sensitivity of 89% for detecting lesions requiring surgical repair (with a 5% rate of false-positive results leading to unnecessary laparotomy), whereas others have found it poorly sensitive for determination of actual organ injury (24).

Disadvantages of this imaging modality include the high level of experience required to perform the procedure and the operator-dependent nature of the results. It is virtually impossible to perform ultrasonography with obese patients or those with subcutaneous emphysema. It is not helpful in assessing diaphragmatic injuries, and assessment of pancreas injuries may be exceptionally difficult secondary to overlying bowel gas. It cannot assess the type of intra-abdominal fluid present. Given these limitations, it cannot substitute for CT in the assessment of the patient with abdominal trauma.

Computed Tomography

Due to its high sensitivity (95%–96%) and accuracy (97%) in diagnosing injuries to the abdomen, CT has been supported as one of the most important imaging methods for the evaluation of patients with abdominal trauma (17,25). Organ subcapsular hematomas and lacerations are well seen by CT in spleen, liver, kidneys, and even pancreas, which is a difficult organ to image by other means. The size of the hematoma can be measured by CT, and the extent of lacerations can be seen as small linear lacerations to large branching areas of decreased attenuation in the organ parenchyma.

CT is notably less accurate for detecting diaphragmatic injury and for intestinal trauma (26). Most of the pitfalls of imaging GI lesions with CT are related to early scanning before significant abnormalities are detectable. In addition to the limited ability to detect hollow viscus injuries, other major disadvantages of CT include the need for transport to the scanner, limited availability in some areas, the length of time required to perform the procedure on older equipment, and its nonfeasibility for unstable patients.

Despite these shortcomings, CT is extremely effective for noninvasive detection of intra-abdominal injury. It has the great capacity to image the entire peritoneal and thoracic cavities, pelvis, and retroperitoneum. Being able to quantify hemoperitoneum and determine the extent of lacerations has been increasingly beneficial, especially for selected organ injury. For example, with the capability to quantify blood loss, work has shown that the need for surgery can be correlated more with the extent of hemoperitoneum than with the actual size of a hepatic laceration (21). CT seems to provide the best features of all available diagnostic techniques in evaluating abdominal injury patients noninvasively. The correlation of CT images with clinical findings can provide the basis for individualized treatment, thereby decreasing the number of nontherapeutic laparotomies.

While CT has gained increasing favor as a primary diagnostic tool, it also can complement other diagnostic imaging procedures. It can add to plain film findings of a mass effect or loss of anatomic shadows by defining actual pathology. CT "lung window" images are best for detecting small pneumothoraces or a small pneumoperitoneum (17), although CT is notably less than optimal for evaluation of hollow viscus injuries. Air usually can be found along the anterior liver surface or falciform ligament, in the porta hepatis, or among folds of mesentery.

If DPL is positive for blood and the patient is stable, CT can aid in further diagnosis of organ injury without the need of a diagnostic laparotomy.

Angiography

Diagnostic angiography is rarely performed immediately after abdominal trauma but may be valuable after CT has suggested the source of a patient's bleeding. The interventional angiographer may embolize bleeding sites in the liver, spleen, and kidneys as well as occlude pseudoaneurysms formed as a result of trauma. Retroperitoneal hematomas and trauma-induced arteriovenous fistulas may be treated in this manner and thereby circumvent the need for surgery (27). Coils, balloons, and hemostatic agents are introduced via angiographic catheter to stop bleeding after angiography has demonstrated the precise bleeding site.

Magnetic Resonance Imaging

While the use of CT has exceptional utility in imaging abdominal injury, newer technologies are being explored. MRI is a well-known, highly used procedure with demonstrated application for imaging the musculoskeletal, cardiovascular, and central nervous systems, and it is now being investigated with respect to assessing abdominal injury. However, trying to apply this technique to the abdomen has not been as successful and to date has been of limited usefulness (28). Growth of the use of MRI for the abdomen will be dependent in part on the ability of newly developing applications to increase diagnostic accuracy. Multiple problems exist with imaging the abdomen, the most common being motion artifact image degradation from physiologic cardiorespiratory movements and bowel peristalsis, although these pose slightly less detriment to retroperitoneal or pelvic imaging. Refinement in technique and computer software may help somewhat but poses the problem of greatly increasing the scan time (29).

Despite its high technology, nonionizing radiation, multiplanar imaging capabilities, and superior soft tissue contrast, MRI still remains of limited usefulness in the evaluation of abdominal trauma and has inherent drawbacks. Patient transport to the scanner is required, examination time is long, motion artifact interferes with quality images, and cost is prohibitive (29). In 1990, the mean cost of an MRI examination was approximately $950 (with a range of $540 to $1308), whereas typical CT charges ranged from $350 to $600 and ultrasonography from $150 to $300 (28). As imaging time decreases, the cost eventually may decrease. With decrease in imaging time and improvement in artifact control, the technical limitations of abdominal imaging may improve. It is expected that the role of MRI will increase somewhat over time in this area, but mainly for very select patients.

Specific Injuries

Abdominal Wall

Contusion of the muscular abdominal wall often coexists with intra-abdominal injury after blunt trauma, but the pain from superficial muscular contusion or muscular hematoma usually occurs only over the area of impact or with contraction of the abdominal muscles. Signs of rigidity, referred pain, or loss of bowel sounds is not present. This diagnosis usually can be made clinically, although the injury can be visualized easily on CT scan in instances in which the diagnosis is in doubt. A complication of trauma to the rectus abdominis muscles is laceration of the inferior epigastric artery, which can produce a rapidly expanding hematoma that requires surgical ligation.

Spleen

The spleen is one of the most commonly injured organs after blunt athletic trauma (6) and is more susceptible to injury and rupture during infectious mononucleosis. Fractures at the seventh to eleventh ribs on the left can lead to splenic laceration (Fig. 10-3). One must remain alert for

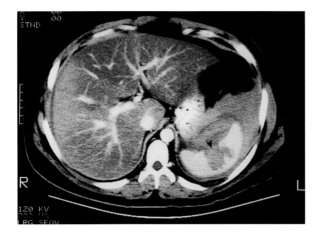

F I G U R E   **10-3**

Splenic laceration. Arrow indicates splenic laceration extending to the splenic hilum. The spleen is surrounded by hemorrhage.

concomitant injury to the left kidney with this mechanism of injury (Fig. 10-4). The spectrum of splenic trauma includes contusion, subcapsular hematoma, and frank rupture. A subcapsular hematoma results from the slow accumulation of blood beneath the capsule after splenic laceration (Fig. 10-5). This serious injury can be asymptomatic initially, but rupture of the accumulated hematoma can occur even several weeks after the initial injury. If frankly ruptured, the spleen bleeds quickly in approximately 85% of cases,

leading to hypovolemia, peritoneal irritation, and possible referred pain to the left shoulder, which is present in approximately 50% of patients (6,7). Observation and/or surgical repair of splenic lacerations has become standard, leaving splenectomy for only unsalvageable cases.

Liver

In contrast to splenic injuries, laceration of the liver rarely results in immediate serious bleeding (6), and ribs may or may not be fractured (3,30). Liver injury does not require concomitant rib fracture, since the liver is larger and more exposed than the spleen. Approximately 50% of liver injuries involve only the capsule or superficial parenchyma, so bleeding is often self-limited (15). The attachment of the liver by the falciform ligament along its left one-third, the larger volume of the right lobe, and the proximity of the right lobe to the lower ribs most likely explain why almost 80% of injuries to the liver involve the right lobe following blunt abdominal trauma (20,31). Hepatic contusions usually produce mild symptoms of right upper quadrant pain and occasional nausea and vomiting. This type of injury and most hepatic injury that does not result in continued bleeding, progressive liver enlargement, or shock can be treated by bed rest, observation, and exclusion from athletic activity for at least 2 to 3 weeks (30). Actual lacerations of

F I G U R E   **10-4**

Splenic and left renal injury in the same patient. (A) Splenic fracture. Arrow indicates a deep laceration extending to splenic hilum. Blood surrounds the spleen. (B) Subcapsular renal hematoma of left kidney (same patient). Arrow indicates hematoma within the left renal capsule. Left subcutaneous emphysema is also present due to accompanying rib fractures.

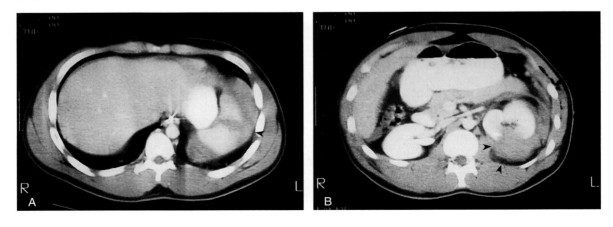

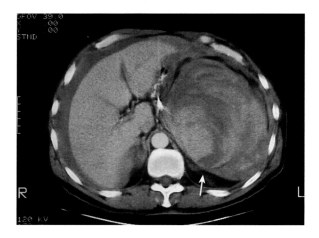

F I G U R E   **10-5**

Splenic hematoma. "Onion skin" appearance is due to repeated episodes of delayed bleeding on this CT scan performed 1 week after injury.

the liver can range from small tears with little bleeding to deeper, more severe lacerations that cause significant bleeding, peritoneal signs, and shock and result in surgical intervention.

Nonoperative therapy is now commonplace in the management of splenic trauma, and several reports in the literature have advocated nonoperative management in selected blunt liver injuries (32) (Fig. 10-6). The usual criteria for nonoperative management are hemodynamic stability, the absence of symptoms of he-

moperitoneum, and the lack of significant extrahepatic injury (20,33). In patients who are hemodynamically stable with no other injuries, nonoperative management can be supported further by the facts that most liver trauma leads to subcapsular or small intraparenchymal hematoma with minimal hemoperitoneum and up to 70% of liver lacerations will have stopped bleeding spontaneously by the time of laparotomy (32,33). Associated injuries involving the right kidney or the right adrenal gland may be present (Fig. 10-7).

Kidney

Various types of renal injuries can result from blunt trauma and include contusion, hematoma (perinephric, subcapsular, or intrarenal), laceration (cortical or caliceal), complete fracture, or vascular pedicle injury (7,11,34). Although kidney injuries are fairly common in sports, most are minor and are contusions. Whereas gross hematuria requires hospital evaluation, microscopic hematuria does not necessarily indicate significant injury and often has been reported with such sports as football, rugby, boxing, basketball, and long-distance running (3,7,35). It has been shown that pre-existing renal anomalies increase the risk of renal injury (7). Most renal injuries short of complete fractures and pedicle injuries (Fig. 10-8) can be managed conservatively, allowing the hematuria to clear and

F I G U R E   **10-6**

Liver laceration and contusion treated conservatively. (A) Liver laceration (arrows indicate linear defects) and large hematoma in the posterior segment of the right hepatic lobe. (B) Five weeks later. Only a small hypodense defect remains (likely a biloma or residual hematoma).

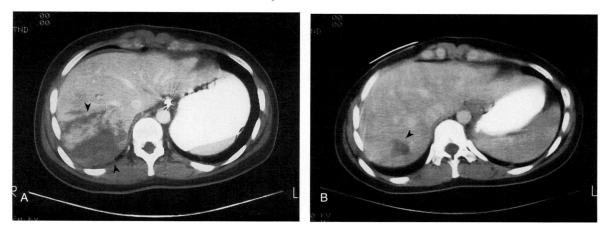

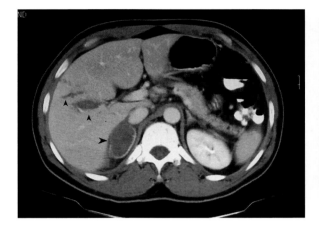

Liver lacerations and adrenal hematoma. Arrows indicate hypodense linear defects indicating traumatic lacerations. Larger arrow points to an enlarged right adrenal as a result of trauma-induced adrenal hemorrhage.

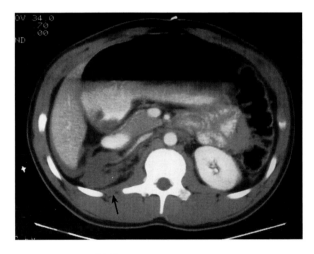

F I G U R E   **10-8**

Renal pedicle injury. The CT scan shows an infarcted right kidney (*arrow*). Notice the lack of arterial perfusion to the right kidney resulting in no nephrogram. Notice the reflux of contrast material into the right renal vein from the IVC. (Courtesy of Sachiko T. Cochran, MD, UCLA School of Medicine.)

healing to occur before return to sports participation at around 4 weeks.

Bowel

Although the liver, spleen, and kidney are the most common abdominal organs injured in blunt abdominal trauma, bowel and mesenteric injuries are found in 5% of trauma patients un-

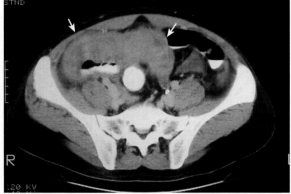

F I G U R E   **10-9**

Mesenteric hematoma. Arrows indicate large high-density hematoma surrounding the bowel. There was no evidence of bowel perforation.

dergoing laparotomy. Bleeding in the mesentery is more common than bowel lacerations and often may be treated conservatively in stable patients (Fig. 10-9). Lacerations of the bowel, however, may be life threatening and, unfortunately, are often difficult to detect early using even our most sensitive imaging methods because of minimal radiographic findings.

CT is the preferred imaging method, and it is important that oral and intravenous contrast agents are used for the examination (36). Small amounts of free air, contrast material extravasation, and intra-abdominal or bowel wall hematoma may be subtle findings (Fig. 10-10). If initial scanning is inconclusive but fever or peritoneal findings increase, a follow-up CT scan may show more conclusive findings such as blood, bowel wall thickening or extraluminal gas, bowel contents, or gas.

Deceleration Injury

Any deceleration injury warrants consideration of the potential for shearing or vascular disruption. While not common, contusion, hematoma, laceration, and even rupture can result from the shearing forces placed on the abdominal organs. The duodenum and pancreas are especially vulnerable where they traverse the spine. Duodenal hematoma and jejunal perforation have been reported following abdominal injury in football players (37,38). Even less common is injury to the stomach and its attachments (Fig. 10-11); however, the stomach is more vulnerable to injury when dilated, such as following a large

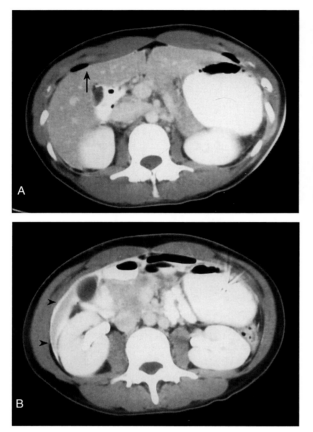

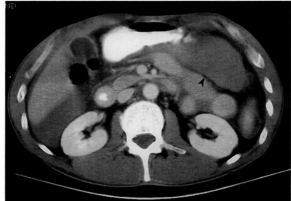

FIGURE 10-11

Gastrocolic ligament hematoma. Arrows indicate large hematoma in the gastrocolic ligament sustained as a result of a football injury. A large amount of blood is also present around the liver.

FIGURE 10-10

Bowel perforation as a result of blunt trauma. (A) Arrow indicates pneumoperitoneum. (B) Extravasated contrast material in the perihepatic region (*arrows*) is due to a postbulbar duodenal laceration.

meal (39). Deceleration injury also should lead to the consideration of diaphragmatic rupture (Fig. 10-12), especially if there are other associated injuries such as liver or spleen lacerations or rib fractures. This is the most common injury to the diaphragm following blunt athletic trauma (30), with rupture located on the left side in 70% to 90% of cases due to the protective effect of the liver on the right side (40).

Summary

Abdominal injuries must be evaluated with a high index of suspicion. Appropriate and expe-

FIGURE 10-12

Rupture of the left diaphragm. (A) Left pneumothorax, subcutaneous emphysema, left pleural effusion, and unusually elevated position of the gastric body (*arrows*) suggest diaphragmatic laceration. (B) Arrow indicates point of gastric torsion as a portion of the stomach passes through the site of laceration.

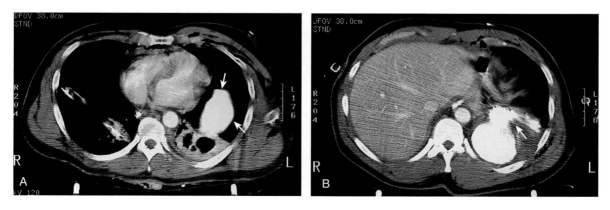

dient treatment is crucial in the prevention of a potential catastrophic event. The choice of the optimal diagnostic procedure and/or imaging modality should be based on the specific clinical situation and the stability of the patient. Computed tomography is the imaging procedure of choice in the evaluation of abdominal injury in the stable patient because it provides the greatest diagnostic accuracy.

REFERENCES

1. Davis JM, Kuppermann N, Fleisher G. Serious sports injuries requiring hospitalization seen in a pediatric emergency department. Am J Dis Child 1993;147:1001–1004.

2. Bergqvist D, Hedelin H, Karlsson G, et al. Abdominal injury from sporting activities. Br J Sports Med 1982;16:76–79.

3. Diamond DL. Sports-related abdominal trauma. Clin Sports Med 1989;8:91–99.

4. Bergqvist D, Hedelin H, Lindblad B, et al. Abdominal injuries in children: an analysis of 348 cases. Injury 1985;16:217–220.

5. Bergqvist D, Hedelin H, Karlsson G, et al. Abdominal trauma during thirty years: analysis of a large case series. Injury 1981;13:93–99.

6. Green GA. Gastrointestinal disorders in the athlete. Clin Sports Med 1992;11:464–470.

7. Kenney P. Abdominal pain in athletes. Clin Sports Med 6:885–904.

8. Wilson DH. Incidence, aetiology, diagnosis and prognosis of closed abdominal injuries. Br J Surg 1963;50:381.

9. DeHaven KE. Athletic injuries in adolescents. Pediatr Annu 1978;7:704–714.

10. Schimpl G, Schmidt B, Sauer H. Isolated bowel injury in blunt abdominal trauma in childhood. Eur J Pediatr Surg 1991;2:341–344.

11. Cianflocco AJ. Renal complications of exercise. Clin Sports Med 1992;11:437–452.

12. Kuzmarov IW, Morehouse DD, Gibson S. Blunt renal trauma in the pediatric population—a retrospective study. J Urol 1981;126:648–649.

13. Mandour WA, Lai MK, Linke CA, et al. Blunt renal trauma in the pediatric patient. J Pediatr Surg 1981;16:669–676.

14. Stricker PR, Hardin BH, Puffer JC. Unusual presentation of liver laceration in a thirteen-year-old football player. Med Sci Sports Exerc 1993;25: 667–672.

15. Olsen WR. Abdominal trauma in the athlete. In: Schneider RC, Kennedy JC, Plant ML, eds. Sports injuries—mechanisms, prevention, and treatment. Baltimore: Williams & Wilkins, 1985:809–817.

16. Abdominal trauma. In: Advanced trauma life support student manual. Chicago: American College of Surgeons, 1989:113–123.

17. Balthazar EJ, Chako AC. Computerized tomography in acute gastrointestinal disorders. Am J Gastroenterol 1990;85:1445–1452.

18. Shaffer HA Jr. Perforation and obstruction of the gastrointestinal tract. Radiol Clin North Am 1992;30:405–426.

19. Demaria EJ. Management of patients with indeterminate diagnostic peritoneal lavage results following blunt trauma. J Trauma 1991;31:1627–1631.

20. Root HD, Keizer PH, Perry JF Jr. The clinical and experimental aspects of peritoneal response to injury. Arch Surg 1967;95:531–537.

21. Moon KL, Federle MP. CT in hepatic trauma. AJR 1983;141:309–314.

22. Smithers BM, O'Loughlin B, Strong RW. Diagnosis of ruptured diaphragm following blunt trauma: results from 85 cases. Aust NZ J Surg 1991;61:737–741.

23. Hoffman R, Nerlich M, Muggia-Sullam M, et al. Blunt abdominal trauma in cases of multiple trauma evaluated by ultrasonography: a prospective analysis of 291 patients. J Trauma 1992;32: 452–458.

24. Rothlin MA, Naf R, Amgwerd M, et al. Ultrasound in blunt abdominal and thoracic trauma. J Trauma 1993;34:488–495.

25. Dang C, Schlater T, Bui H, Oshita T. Delayed rupture of the spleen. Ann Emerg Med 1990;19: 399–403.

26. Balthazar EJ. CT of the gastrointestinal tract: principles and interpretation. AJR 1991;156:23–32.

27. Selby JB Jr. Interventional radiology of trauma. Radiol Clin North Am 1992;30:427–439.

28. Edelman RR, Warach S. Magnetic resonance imaging. N Engl J Med 1993;328:785–791.

29. Caron KH. Magnetic resonance imaging of the pediatric abdomen. Semin Ultrasound CT MRI 1991;12:448–474.

30. Mustalich AC, Quash ET. Sports injuries to the chest and abdomen. In: Scott WN, Nisonson B, Nicholas JA, eds. Principles of sports medicine. Baltimore: Williams & Wilkins, 1984:236–240.

31. Coant PN, Kornberg AE, Brody AS, et al. Markers for occult liver injury in cases of physical abuse in children. Pediatrics 1992;89:274–278.

32. Cywes S, Rode H. Blunt liver trauma in children—nonoperative management. J Pediatr Surg 1985;20:14–18.

33. Hiatt JR, Harrier D, Koenig BV, et al. Nonoperative management of major blunt liver injury with hemoperitoneum. Arch Surg 1990;125:101–103.

34. York JP. Sports and the male genitourinary system. Phys Sportsmed 1990;18:116–129.

35. O'Donoghue DH. Treatment of injuries to athletes. Philadelphia: WB Saunders, 1984:341–344.

36. Nghiem HV, Jeffrey RB Jr, Mindelzun RE. CT of blunt trauma to the bowel and mesentery. AJR 1993;160:53–58.

37. Henderson JM, Puffer JC. Abdominal pain in a football player. Phys Sportsmed 1989;17:47–52.

38. Chambers TJ, Fine K, Trad K. Jejunal perforation in a football player. Unpublished case report.

39. Grosfeld JL, Rescorla FJ, West KW, et al. Gastrointestinal injuries in childhood: analysis of 53 patients. J Pediatr Surg 1989;24:580–583.

40. Disler DG, DeLuca SA. Traumatic rupture of the diaphragm and herniation of the liver. Am Fam Phys 1992;46:453–456.

CHAPTER 11

Pelvic Injuries

DAVID O. HOUGH
RANDOLPH PEARSON
EUGENE TRYCIECKY

*A*s the athlete and physician are both well aware, functions of the low back, pelvis, and hip play a very important role in nearly all sports. The pelvis serves as a midpoint for forces that originate in the lower extremities and are transmitted upward through the body. In addition, rotatory movements so important for fluid performance of many athletic endeavors rely on flexible motion of the low back–pelvis-hip unit. Finally, many organs reside at least part time in the pelvis, as well as many muscles and other soft tissue structures that can be injured, resulting in the physician being called on to evaluate and treat athletes with pain in these areas.

Because these areas contain large amounts of soft tissue as well as large areas of bone, physical examination of the low back, pelvis, and hips can be difficult. Radiologic imaging studies can be invaluable in aiding the physician while evaluating low back, pelvic, and hip conditions. This chapter deals with many of the more common injuries and syndromes occurring in these body regions in athletes, outlining radiologic studies of choice and their findings. Charges for imaging techniques are presented in Table 11-1. The actual dollar charge varies from hospital to hospital, city to city, and state to state, but the table gives the reader an approximate cost for pelvic imaging techniques.

Anatomic Considerations

Because the muscles about the pelvis play such an important role in the coordinated movement necessary for participation in sports, a variety of soft tissue injuries and overuse syndromes can present themselves to the physician. At times, radiographic evaluation of these injuries is useful in order to exclude more serious injuries. In addition, some pelvic injuries are due to biomechanical imbalances that can be seen with radiographic evaluation.

In order to understand the relationship between abnormal biomechanics and pelvic injury, a brief discussion of normal anatomy of the pelvis is necessary. The bony pelvis consists of paired innominate bones, each of which is comprised of the ilium, ischium, and pubis, components that are indistinguishable except by shape and location (1). Posteriorly, the innominate bones meet with the sacrum at a cartilaginous joint called the *sacroiliac joint* or *junction*. Anteriorly, the innominate bones articulate across a fibrocartilaginous disk at the pubic symphysis. While the anterior and posterior articulations technically are cartilaginous joints, movement at these sites is restricted by strong ligaments that allow only small amounts of movement. Osteitis pubis is an example of repetitive movement overload at the symphysis pubis that results in

T A B L E   **11-1**

Average Imaging Charges: Pelvic Injuries

X-ray

72170	Pelvis, AP	$40
72190	Pelvis, two views	$78
72202	Sacroiliac joints	$90
73510	Hip, unilateral	$104
73520	Hip, bilateral	$133
73540	Hip, bilateral, 12 years	$104
74480	Urethrogram	$195
50393	Injection of contrast media	$104
74420	Retrograde urethrogram	$187
74455	Voiding cystourethrogram	
51600	Injection of contrast media	$65
74456	Cystogram	$252
51605	Injection of contrast media	$65

MRI

72196	Pelvis	$600
73721	Hips	$685

Ultrasound

76856	Pelvis other than Ob	$300
76870	Scrotal with doppler	$148

CT

72193	Pelvis, with	$446
72194	Pelvis, with, w/o	
73701	CT lower extremity, with	$495
73702	CT lower extremity, with, w/o	
74160	Abdomen, with	$488
74170	Abdomen, with, w/o	

Nuclear Medicine

78300	Bone scan, limited area	$190
78306	Bone scan, whole body	$245
78760	Testicular scan	$200

Note: These imaging charges represent relative costs for each procedure. All numbers represent the total (professional and technical) charge and reflect costs in the authors' locale at a multispeciality health center's radiology department. Costs are those established in February 1996.

inflammation and tenderness of this site (2). Similarly, laxity at the sacroiliac joint may lead to sacroiliitis or sacroiliac joint dysfunction.

The normal radiographic appearance of the sacroiliac joint is that of a small but clearly appearing joint space demarcated by the well-defined cortical lines of the sacrum and ilium. In-dividuals with acute injury to the sacroiliac joint often will have normal-appearing plain radiographs of the joint. Individuals with recurrent pain referrable to the sacroiliac joint, however, may have a hazy or ratty appearance to the joint line on the radiograph. Chronic injury to the joint may lead to irregular calcification and loss of portions of the joint space. Because the ligaments allow very limited motion, subtle subluxation of the sacroiliac that can produce significant pain is indistinguishable on plain radiographs. More advanced studies such as computed tomography (CT) or magnetic resonance imaging (MRI) likewise will show no abnormality but may be useful in distinguishing arthritis or infectious causes of pain. However, sacroiliac joint disease may be indistinguishable from other causes of lumbar spine pain. Generally, imaging of the sacroiliac joint with MRI or CT will evaluate this joint precisely.

Soft Tissue Injuries about the Pelvis

A number of important muscles with recognized injury or overuse syndromes have the bony pelvis as their point of origin. Acutely, patients with these syndromes will have normal radiographs; however, as the syndrome progresses over time, evidence of calcifications may indicate areas of recurrent inflammation (2). Examples of such syndromes include gracilis syndrome, gluteus medius syndrome, and adductor syndrome. Table 11-2 summarizes sites of possible radiographic findings of these pelvic muscle syndromes (3).

T A B L E   **11-2**

Attachments of Muscles within the Pelvis and Locations Where Radiographic Findings May Confirm a Pelvic Muscle Syndrome

Muscle	Attachment
External oblique	Iliac crest
Sartorius	Anterosuperior iliac spine
Rectus femoris	Anteroinferior iliac spine
Hamstrings	Ischial tuberosity
Gracilis	Inferior pubic ramus
Glutus medius and minimus	Greater trochanter
Iliopsoas	Lesser trochanter

Occasionally, an athlete will present with intermittent pain in the inguinal canal or femoral triangle suspicious of inguinal or femoral hernia. Although the physical examination is the diagnostic method of choice for inguinal and femoral hernias, occult hernias may be present and diagnosis may be difficult due to the habitus of the patient. In such cases, ultrasound evaluation of the scrotum or femoral triangle can be of aid. Hernias will appear as complex masses originating in the inguinal canal or femoral triangle, respectively.

Snapping Hip Syndrome

Snapping hip syndrome usually manifests as an annoying but otherwise asymptomatic "snap" that occurs during walking or running. While snapping hip syndrome can be due to a variety of causes, the most common etiology is from a tight iliotibial band stretching and snapping across the greater trochanter of the femur during flexion and extension of the leg on the hip (1). Occasionally, patients with snapping hip syndrome will develop pain overlying the greater trochanter due to repeated mechanical injury to the iliotibial band as it rubs over the underlying bony structures. Painful snapping hip syndromes usually respond to rest and careful stretching of the offending muscle groups over a period of 2 to 6 months.

At times it is useful to obtain plain radiographs of the affected hip, since occasionally abnormal bony protuberances can be seen as the etiology for the syndrome. The snapping hip syndrome also can be caused by subluxation of the iliopsoas tendon over the iliopectineal eminence. Snapping hip generally responds to treatment with nonsteroidal anti-inflammatory drugs (NSAIDs), stretching of the hip flexors, and time. Most cases present no concern for future sports participation, and symptoms should not preclude participation.

Trochanteric Bursitis

Like snapping hip syndrome, trochanteric bursitis occurs as a result of repeated irritation of the trochanteric bursa as it is compressed between the greater trochanter and the iliotibial band. This results in localized pain over the greater trochanter that worsens with passive external rotation and adduction of the hip. Plain radio-

graphs are useful in evaluating the patient for bony causes of irritation to the bursa and should be obtained in chronic cases. In addition, patients with chronic trochanteric bursitis occasionally will show soft tissue calcification within the tendon or bursa itself (Fig. 11-1). MRI may be useful but not necessary in diagnosing this condition by showing a distended fluid-filled bursa and may direct the physician to consider surgical excision of the bursa. The diagnosis is commonly made by a thorough physical examination. NSAIDs and icing should be tried but frequently fail to control symptoms.

Chronic or recalcitrant trochanteric bursitis should be treated by injection of a combination of 1 cc 1% lidocaine and 1 cc betamethasone into the area of maximum tenderness, followed by regular icing. The patient should be re-evaluated in 3 weeks to observe progress. Other

FIGURE 11-1

Tendonitis and trochanteric bursitis. Magnified image from an AP radiograph of the right hip. There are two calcifications (*black arrows*) in the region of the gluteus medius tendon and adjacent trochanteric bursa.

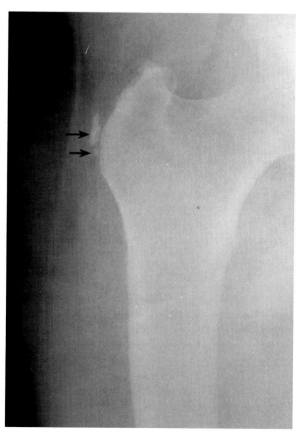

common causes of bursitis around the pelvis include iliopsoas bursitis and ischial bursitis.

Iliopsoas bursitis is characterized by tenderness over the lesser trochanter, medial groin pain, and pain with active flexion, abduction, and external rotation. Ischial bursitis is aggravated by sitting and hamstring contraction. These causes of bursitis are best treated by stretching, ice application, NSAIDs, and physical therapy over 6 to 8 weeks. MRI may show a distended bursa filled with fluid (Fig. 11-2). Bone scan or MRI is indicated to rule out femoral neck

and ischial stress fractures that can mimic bursitis symptoms, unless the diagnosis is clear. Radiographic studies also should look for tumors as a cause of symptoms and bony pathology (2).

Osteitis Pubis

Osteitis pubis is an inflammation of the pubic symphysis that develops as a result of microtrauma to the area occurring from shear forces exerted during running and jumping activities

FIGURE **11-2**

Iliopsoas bursitis. (A) Axial proton density–weighted (TR/TE 2000/30) and (B) axial T2-weighted (TR/TE 2000/90) magnetic resonance images show a curvilinear signal abnormality (*long arrows*) posterior to the right iliopsoas muscle (*arrowhead*) and lateral to the iliopsoas tendon (*short arrows*). It has signal characteristics of fluid and represents a distended iliopsoas bursa. It lies anterior to the femoral neck.

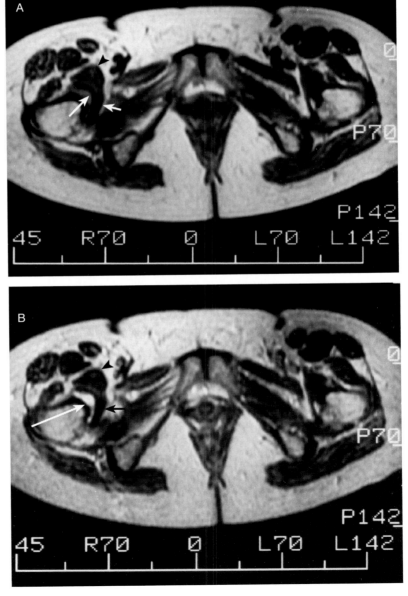

(4). Because of this mechanism of injury, osteitis pubis occurs most often in athletes participating in running and jumping sports such as basketball, baseball, track, and soccer. In addition, because of increased stress on the area by the gravid uterus as well as instability of the pubic joint after childbirth, osteitis pubis can be seen in exercising pregnant women and women who are immediately postpartum.

Osteitis pubis presents as pain in the area of the pubic symphysis, initially during running and jumping activities but later as a more constant pain. Physical examination is often unremarkable, but patients may exhibit tenderness to palpation over the pubic symphysis as well as pain elicited in the area during passive flexion, adduction, and external rotation of the hip (Patrick test).

Radiologic evaluation for osteitis pubis begins with plain anteroposterior (AP) pelvis radiographs. Findings may include irregularity of the edges of the pubic symphysis with adjacent bone resorption or sclerosis (Fig. 11-3). Later in the disease process, a bone scan should be obtained if the diagnosis is in doubt, since some pelvic stress fractures may present with a similar, insidious history. Findings on bone scan include increased uptake along the borders of the pubic symphysis. Bone scan evaluation for osteitis pubis may be technically difficult, however, because the radioactive isotopes are excreted by the kidney and concentrate in the bladder, which may mask a subtle increased uptake at the pubic symphysis. CT may show a healing stress fracture, which

can mimic osteitis pubis, whereas MRI may be helpful in detecting evidence of pubic microtrauma. MRI has advantages over bone scans by providing better anatomic localization of the abnormality and eliminating the problem of the bladder masking the abnormality.

Treatment for osteitis pubis consists mainly of rest and NSAIDs. Many athletes will respond to this regimen after a few weeks. Some injuries, however, are more recalcitrant to treatment, requiring months of inactivity and, occasionally, local injection of corticosteroids.

Iliac Crest Contusion (Hip Pointer)

The iliac crest contusion, or hip pointer, is caused by a direct blow to the iliac crest, either as a result of a collision between two athletes or from falling on the ground. Hip pointers are seen most often in collision sports such as football, hockey, and lacrosse. Athletes present with pain at the iliac crest. Physical examination often reveals a point-tender area at the site of contusion. Radiographic evaluation in the athlete presenting with an iliac crest contusion includes plain radiographs of the affected side of the pelvis in AP and bilateral oblique projections. These films are obtained to rule out the presence of an iliac crest fracture, which may be caused by the strong abdominal muscles that attach to the iliac crest. Because the iliac wing is flared and not completely depicted on the AP view, oblique films are obtained. Film cost is ap-

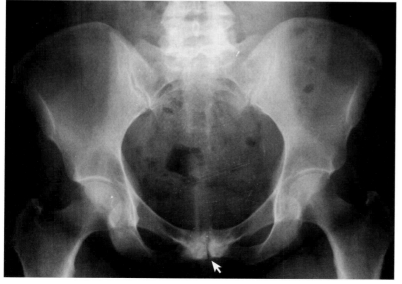

FIGURE **11-3**

Osteitis pubis. AP radiograph of the pelvis showing sclerotic and lytic areas in pubic bones.

proximately $100 using the scale of radiographic procedures provided in Table 11-1.

Iliac crest contusions are notoriously slow to heal, sometimes taking several weeks to become asymptomatic. Follow-up plain radiographs should be considered in the athlete with little or no improvement over a 2- to 3-week period to exclude the presence of an occult iliac crest fracture. Radionuclide bone scanning with a technetium-99m pertechnetate analogue also may be indicated and costs approximately $250. Generally, hip pointers are best treated with icing, protective padding, and NSAIDs. However, an injection of 1% lidocaine and 0.25% marcaine followed by injection of 1 cc betamethasone into the site of maximum tenderness will reduce the period of disability significantly. Gradual return to stretching and progressive activity is indicated over 7 to 14 days following injury. Indications for injection include localized tenderness over the crest that is best appreciated immediately after the injury occurs.

Iliac crest contusions typically take 3 to 4 weeks to heal and allow full participation. If the area of tenderness is relatively small and no tear of the muscles that reflect over the crest is detected, the iliac crest can be injected safely as described. This management technique will reduce the time away from participation dramatically in our opinion. Return to play is allowed when the athlete can perform all functional activities with appropriate strength and flexibility. Padding of the iliac crest with orthoplast (plastic) or foam pads will protect the area from reinjury.

Iliac Crest Avulsion

Iliac crest avulsion occurs most often as a result of traction overload to the crest. This process is seen in adolescent athletes before the closure of the iliac crest ossification centers. While seen most commonly in runners as they increase their mileage, it also can be seen in baseball and softball players and track runners. This condition is a tension apophysitis that manifests with pain and local tenderness at the iliac crest ossification centers.

Radiographic findings of iliac crest avulsion include widening of the physeal plate along the iliac crest. Such widening may be very subtle, and the diagnosis of avulsion may rest in large part with radiographic correlation of the opposite iliac crest. Avulsion of the iliac crest responds well to rest and stopping all activity that causes pain, such as jumping, running, and weight training. A bone scan of the pelvis in iliac crest avulsion reveals increased radioisotope uptake across the iliac crest apophysis. However, this must be distinguished from normal increased uptake in the growth centers; bone scanning is therefore of limited value in this condition.

Follow-up radiographs are indicated at 2- to 3-month intervals because this injury may take up to 6 to 12 months to heal. It is best to follow the patient clinically and not allow running or jumping activities until the crest is totally nontender. Return to activity should follow a gradual but progressive addition of activities over 4 to 6 weeks that produce no pain over the iliac crests. All activity should be followed by regular icing and combined with strength and flexibility training appropriate for the athlete's sport.

Avulsion Fractures

As noted earlier, a number of muscles and muscle groups have their origin and/or insertion within the pelvis. Avulsion fractures at the site of origin or insertion of these muscles can occur (as well as avulsion of ligamentous insertion within the pelvis) as a result of either acute trauma to the area or overuse. The presenting complaint of athletes with such fractures is pain. However, since many muscle attachments are deep within the pelvis, the presenting pain may be relatively nondescript or vague. Initial evaluation of the athlete with deep avulsion fracture may raise suspicion that such a condition exists when stretching of the affected muscle elicits pain.

The radiologic procedure of choice in evaluating athletes with suspected avulsion is the plain radiograph. An avulsion fracture appears as a small bony fragment or separation at the site of muscular or ligamentous attachment (Fig. 11-4). In the young athlete, avulsion fractures may take the appearance of a widened physeal plate, so care should be taken in these age groups to compare films between the affected and unaffected sides. Hypertrophy of an epiphysis or apophysis can be found on radiographs of patients with chronic insertional injury. Table 11-2 summarizes sites of muscular attachment within the pelvis where avulsion fractures may occur. If avulsion fractures are suspected but not apparent on plain films, radionuclide bone scanning can be of aid, with the site of avulsion fracture appearing as a "hot" spot on the scan.

Treatment of avulsion fractures about the

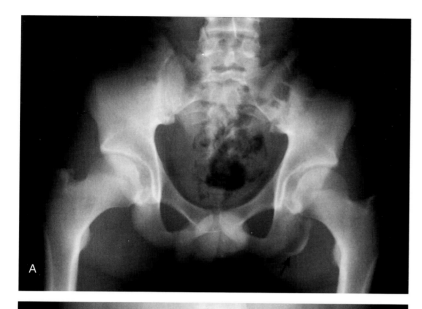

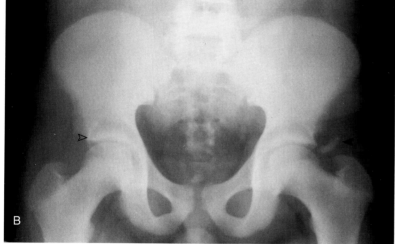

FIGURE 11-4

(A) Avulsion fracture of apophysis of left ischial tuberosity. AP radiograph of pelvis shows a curvilinear bone fragment avulsed from the ischial tuberosity (*arrow*). This is the insertion of the hamstring muscles. (B) Avulsion fracture of the apophysis of the left anteroinferior iliac spine. A crescent-shaped bone fragment (*solid arrow*) is avulsed from the left anteroinferior iliac spine. The rectus femoris muscle inserts here. Note normal right anterior inferior iliac spine apophysis (*open arrow*).

pelvis usually involve the use of rest, occasionally non-weight-bearing activities, NSAIDs, and gradual strengthening and flexibility programs. Fracture care should be individualized to the patient's age, sport, and level of training. Surgical intervention is sometimes indicated for fragments that are displaced more than 1 cm. Other causes of pain such as infection and tumor should be considered.

Pelvic Fractures

Pelvic fractures in athletes can range from simple bone disruptions and avulsions to significant injuries requiring operative intervention. Minor pelvic fractures include avulsion fractures (see preceding discussion), undisplaced sacral frac-

tures, fractures of a single pubic ramus, single ischial fractures, fractures of the coccyx, and ilial wing fractures. Most minor fractures are suggested by the history of injury and location of pain on physical examination. The initial diagnostic method of choice is the standard AP radiograph of the pelvis (5) (Fig. 11-5). The evaluation of the bony pelvis is enhanced by the inlet and outlet views, which are AP projections with caudad and cephalad angulation of the x-ray tube. If a minor pelvic fracture is suspected but not seen on initial radiographs, the films can be repeated in 1 week because fracture lines will become more apparent due to adjacent bone resorption. Alternatively, radionuclide bone scanning can be employed to aid in the diagnosis.

Fortunately, major pelvic fractures are relatively rare in athletes. However, some sports,

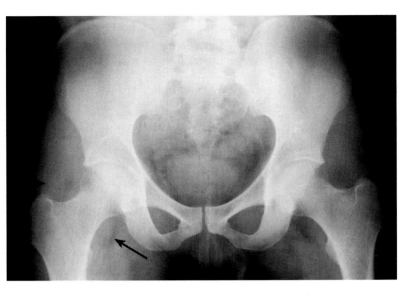

FIGURE 11-5

Normal AP pelvis radiograph. Standard x-ray examination of the pelvis consists of one AP radiograph done with the patient supine. In addition to evaluating the osseous structures, the soft tissues such as the fat planes of the gluteus minimus (*short arrowhead*) and iliopsoas (*arrow*) should be evaluated. These lie on the capsule of the hip joint and may be displaced with joint effusions. The posterior bony margin of the acetabulum projects on the left femoral head.

such as skiing, cycling, and equestrian sports, place the athlete at some risk for suffering a serious pelvic fracture. Major pelvic fractures are those involving more than one area of the pelvic ring or bony portion of the pelvis (Fig. 11-6). By nature, these fractures result in pelvic instability. In addition, certain major pelvic fractures can be associated with bladder and urethral injury. Displaced sacral fractures can have associated neurologic injury.

Initial diagnostic imaging for major pelvic fractures involves a plain AP radiograph. The inlet and outlet views are helpful in detecting and evaluating fractures and joint diastasis. Since these fractures are unstable, care should be exhibited while performing the studies to en-

sure as little movement as possible in the pelvis during transport and the procedure. If a displaced sacral fracture or acetabular fracture is suspected, CT scanning is useful in assessing the degree of displacement and need for further intervention. If urethral or bladder injury is suspected, judicious retrograde contrast imaging can be used to localize any area of disruption of the urethra or bladder.

Leg-Length Discrepancy

Leg-length discrepancy is a relatively common finding in the athlete who presents with chronic knee, hip, sacroiliac, or back pain. An individual

FIGURE 11-6

Malgaigne fracture. There are vertical fractures of the right superior (*black arrow*) and right inferior (*white arrowhead*) pubic rami. The right sacroiliac joint is widely separated, and there is a fracture (*black arrowhead*) through the right sacral ala.

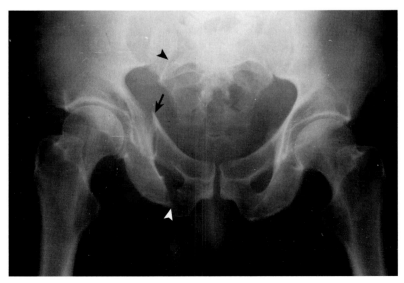

with leg-length discrepancy may have scoliosis but more often has rotation of the sacrum and compensatory changes in leg length (6). Leg-length differences are best examined with the patient lying in the supine and prone position. True leg-length discrepancy is best evaluated radiographically. Many mechanical problems about the pelvic girdle and sacroiliac joint can be diagnosed through careful physical examination of the low back and palpable landmarks of the bony pelvis (6). Radiographs serve a role in the diagnosis of subtle abnormalities of the bony pelvis that lead to pain. The physician must, however, consider all causes of pelvic pain discussed in this chapter and rule out diskogenic disease in particular. The diagnosis can be aided through the use of a standing AP pelvis x-ray. Findings associated with leg-length discrepancy include lateral pelvic tilt with the longer side appearing higher on the radiograph. In addition, films may show an asymmetric appearance of the wings of the ilium if there is compensatory rotation of the longer side.

A more exact measurement of leg-length discrepancy, as described by Greenman (6), involves location of the sacral base plane on the AP standing radiograph. This can be done by location of equal points on the sacrum of one of three areas: 1) most posterior aspect of the superior articular surface of the sacrum, 2) sacral alar sulcus, or 3) medial corner of the sacral articular facet pillars. A horizontal line is drawn on the film connecting the two identified points. Vertical lines are then drawn from the bottom of the film at the femoral shafts, through the femoral heads, and intersecting the sacral baseline. Comparison of the length of these vertical lines determines the amount of leg-length discrepancy (Fig. 11-7). Specific lift therapy can be prescribed based on these findings. The optimal measurement to perform when evaluating patients with suspected leg-length abnormalities is direct measurement of the extremities. X-rays to assess leg length can now be performed with low-dose radiation techniques. While pelvic measurements may indicate the potential presence of a leg-length discrepancy, they do not provide direct evidence. Patient positioning also may create an apparent pelvic tilt.

Genitourinary Injuries Perspective

The genitourinary system is comprised of the internal and external organs that make up the urinary system (kidney, ureter, urinary bladder, and urethra) and the genital organs. These two systems are located in the lower abdomen and pelvic area. Injuries to the kidney, ureter, and bladder are the most frequent abdominal injuries in athletics. Hematuria is the most common symptom that occurs after traumatic injury to the genitourinary systems. Kidney injuries are discussed in Chapter 10, Abdominal Injuries and Their Radiographic Assessment.

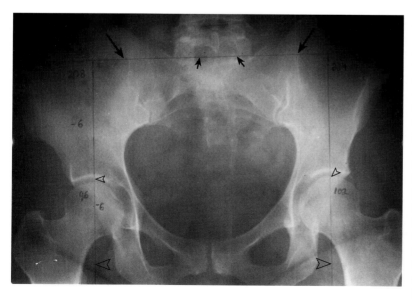

F I G U R E   **11-7**

Standing AP pelvis x-ray. A horizontal line is drawn (*large arrows*) connecting the sacral alar sulci (*small arrows*). Vertical lines (*large arrowheads*) are drawn from the bottom of the film through the highest point of the femoral heads (*small arrowheads*) to the sacral base line. In this case, the distance from the highest point of the femoral heads to the bottom of the film is also 6 mm less on the right. The distance from the sacral base to the bottom of the film is 6 mm less on the right. The right lower extremity is 6 mm less than the left, and the sacral base declines 6 mm to the right.

Anatomy

The organs of the genitourinary systems are well protected, with the kidneys located in the retroperitoneal upper lumbar area of the abdomen. The kidneys are well protected by the twelfth rib as well as the abdominal musculature, large intestine, and other internal organs. Posteriorly, the kidney is protected by the psoas, paravertebral, and latissimus dorsi muscles and rests in a bed of pericapsular fat. In general, the position of the kidney and other organs in the posterior abdominal wall makes these organs particularly prone to blunt trauma in many sports.

The ureters travel along the posterior peritoneal wall and are protected by the lower vertebrae and muscles of the posterior abdominal wall. In general, the ureters are vulnerable when they course over the pelvic rim and into the bladder. The bladder is susceptible to injury only when it is full and then rises above the pelvic rim. Otherwise, the bladder lies well within the pelvis and is relatively free of injury. The entire female reproductive system is located within the pelvis, as are the prostate and internal portion of the male urethra. In the male, the most external organs vulnerable to injury are the penis, scrotum, and testes. These organs are generally protected during sporting activities when held close to the body by an athletic supporter.

Ureteral Trauma

The ureter is the least injured portion of the urinary tract. These uncommon injuries usually are associated with severe abdominal blows with hyperextension of the back. Fractures of the pelvis and lower lumbar vertebrae should be considered when assessing this type of injury. These injuries are rare in sports, and most are due to penetrating trauma. The patient often has other associated injuries and is evaluated in the emergency department with a comprehensive radiographic approach when indicated.

Bladder Trauma

The incidence of bladder injuries in athletics is very low. It is usually associated with a full bladder that is ruptured by a direct blow or in association with a significant pelvic fracture. Traumatic bladder injuries can occur in the martial arts. Typically, the patient will present with symptoms of pain and tenderness in the lower abdomen with muscle guarding, inability to void, hematuria, and ecchymosis of the pubic area. The most common type of bladder injury is a contusion; however, complete ruptures of the bladder can occur but are relatively rare. Bladder trauma can present in 10% to 15% of patients with a fractured pelvis. Repetitive bouncing of the bladder in long-distance running can result in recurrent bladder trauma and contusions.

A urinalysis (use a Foley catheter if necessary), a voiding cystogram, and an intravenous pyelogram should be obtained in this order to establish the diagnosis of a bladder contusion. Urinalysis confirms the hematuria. The voiding cystogram is normal in a bladder contusion and is only performed to rule out other conditions (i.e., tumor) that can cause hematuria. Intravenous pyelogram is performed only to exclude upper urinary tract abnormalities. Athletes with bladder trauma may pass small blood clots and complain of recurrent dysuria.

Treatment of contusions involves bed rest and observation. Severe contusions usually will require the use of an indwelling catheter for upwards of 7 to 10 days and prophylactic antibiotic treatment. A more severe injury involves a bladder rupture that can be intra- or extraperitoneal or a combination of both. These injuries are associated with pelvic fractures and require immediate surgery. A retrograde urethrogram should be performed first to exclude urethral injury. If the urethra is intact, a retrograde cytogram is performed. Contrast material surrounding loops of bowel is diagnostic of an intraperitoneal bladder rupture, whereas contrast material in the perivesical space indicates extraperitoneal rupture.

Treatment of more severe injuries to the bladder should be dictated by the urologist. Follow-up of all injuries with repeat urinalysis examinations will be necessary. The athlete is usually allowed to return to competition after hematuria has cleared and the patient is symptom-free. Prevention of most bladder injuries is accomplished by completely emptying the bladder prior to competition.

Bikers' Bladder

One complication of long distance bicycling is the development of bikers' bladder. Typically, an athlete will have an acute onset of urinary frequency, diminished urinary stream, nocturia, and terminal dribbling. This symptom complex may be confused with prostatitis and is seen in avid bicyclists (5). There are generally no radiographic findings for this problem. This problem may be avoided by frequent emptying of the bladder during long bicycle rides and the use of a cushioned bicycle seat.

Hematuria

Hematuria may occur from cystitis, renal contusion, urogenital laceration, or tumor or be induced by exercise. The major causes of exercise-induced hematuria are listed in Table 11-3. Hematuria is the most common urinary symptom found after vigorous athletic activity (7). Distance swimmers and runners usually have the greatest incidence of exercise-induced hematuria. Hematuria following vigorous exercise usually clears within 48 hours after exercise has been discontinued. The difficulty for the team physician is to distinguish significant organic disease from transient, benign conditions that cause hematuria. Consultation with your urologist, nephrologist, and radiologist is helpful in making this distinction.

The lower urinary tract is regarded as the most common source of hematuria after prolonged and exhaustive exertion. The existence of renal stones, urinary tract infection, or exercise-induced irritation of the urethral meatus from contusion or cold exposure should be eliminated in the differential diagnosis of hematuria (8). The most commonly accepted upper limit of normal is 3 red blood cells per high-powerfield or 1000 red blood cells per milliliter of urine (9). False-positive results can occur from contamination of the urine by menses in the female or by masturbation in the male. Black

T A B L E **11-3**

Causes of Exercise-Induced Hematuria

Kidney	**Bladder**	**Ureter**	**Urethra**
Ischemia	Contusion	Stone	Contusion
Acute renal failure	Stone		Stone
Vascular	Infection		Infection
Fragmentation	Trauma		Trauma
Trauma			Cold
Nephroptosis			
Stone			

athletes with hematuria should be checked for sickle cell disease/trait. A history of drug and medication use should be obtained. The evaluation of the patient with hematuria is presented in Figure 11-8. Appropriate timing of imaging techniques within the first 24 hours is critical in making the proper diagnosis.

Physicians caring for athletes with exercise-induced hematuria from any source should perform repeated urinalyses to ensure that the hematuria has cleared. A clean-catch urine should be cultured if cystitis or infection is suspected. No further testing is indicated if repeated urinalyses are negative. If the hematuria persists or is associated with symptoms such as pain, dysuria, or fever, further investigation is indicated, as seen in Figure 11-8 (9,10). Athletes with persistent hematuria should undergo additional investigation for causes of intrinsic renal disease, as covered in Chapter 10.

Urethral Injuries

Injuries to the female urethra are very rare in sports and are mainly limited to lacerations. The retrograde urethrogram is diagnostic. Most of these injuries should be left to the care of a urologist or gynecologist. Injuries to the male urethra involve two segments of the urethra. The mechanism of injury to the anterior urethra in males involves straddle injuries to the perineum. The patient usually has a history of some form of straddle trauma and pain over the perineum with blood in the meatus. Treatment commonly involves catheterization of the urethra and open resection and realignment of the urethra.

The posterior urethra is injured after severe trauma, which commonly involves a pelvic fracture. The patient presents with gross hematuria and inability to void with a distended bladder or a floating prostate. A retrograde urethrogram is diagnostic of this injury prior to referral to a urologist. Surgical repair with immediate realignment or late urethral reconstruction is required for these relatively rare injuries.

Injury to the Testicles

The testicles are generally well protected in the male athlete. The testes are prone to the development of contusions, epididymitis, or torsion. Direct trauma to the scrotum may cause testicular contusion despite the use of protective de-

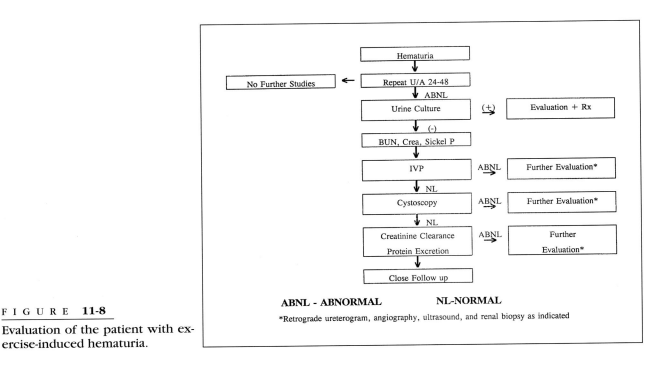

FIGURE 11-8

Evaluation of the patient with exercise-induced hematuria.

vices. Severe pain, nausea, pallor, and anxiety along with scrotal swelling and peroneal ecchymosis are common. The athlete should be placed on his back with the thighs flexed to his chest to release cremasteric muscle spasms. Ice to the scrotum to control bleeding and swelling and elevation of the limbs for 12 to 24 hours are helpful.

If pain and nausea persist, tears of the testicle must be ruled out, and the athlete should be referred to a urologist. Significant testicular injury should be evaluated by the team physician as soon as possible. All expanding masses should be transilluminated. If the mass is not transilluminated or if the epididymis cannot be separated from the testicle, diagnosis of fracture of the testicle or epididymis should be considered.

Fractures of the testes usually result from a rupture of the tunica albuginea. Typically, the athlete will present with pain that seems to be out of proportion to the injury. Scrotal ultrasound may show zones of infarction or hemorrhage in the testis, a hematocele, or in a small percentage of cases, a discrete fracture. Color Doppler ultrasound can detect vascular compromise. A radionuclide testicular scan is not very helpful except in delayed evaluation when the viability of the testicle is being considered (11). Testicular ultrasound should be done quickly to decide whether surgery is indicated. Surgical repairs should be performed rapidly

with a generous scrotal incision, and orchiectomy is performed in most cases (12).

Torsion of the Spermatic Cord

Torsion of the spermatic cord probably represents a genetic predisposition to this type of injury. It is often associated with trauma and should be suspected if pain and swelling in a single testicle occurs after minor trauma. The pain increases with lifting of the testicle above the symphysis, whereas pain from epididymitis is usually decreased by this maneuver. A single ligament normally prevents mobility of the testis by attaching the lower end of the spermatic cord and epididymis to the scrotum. If the tunica vaginalis is loosely attached to the scrotal lining, torsion may occur as the spermatic cord rotates above the testis. Contraction of the athlete's cremasteric muscle draws the testis up over the pubis, and a twist of the cord occurs. Torsion of the spermatic cord is less likely to occur if the athlete wears an athletic supporter.

Localized tenderness, edema, and hyperemia of the scrotal skin with the scrotal contents adherent to the skin are common findings of torsion. The vas deferens is usually inseparable from the swollen, twisted cord. The main differential diagnosis for this condition is epididymitis. Radionuclide scanning using technetium-

99m pertechnetate is 85% to 100% accurate in diagnosing torsion (11) (Fig. 11-9). Color Doppler ultrasound can diagnose testicular torsion with a sensitivity and specificity comparable with that of the testicular radionuclide scan (11). Color Doppler ultrasound is less expensive than a radionuclide scan but is dependent on the operator and the equipment. Accuracy can vary between imaging departments (12).

If the patient presents within 4 to 6 hours after torsion occurs, cooling of the scrotal skin, lidocaine cord block, and manual derotation may be accomplished but should not delay surgical exploration and repair. Surgical intervention should not be delayed in order to obtain a scan. An unreducible spermatic cord torsion should be explored operatively to prevent infarction of the testis. At surgery, the testis is fixed to the scrotum, a procedure that usually prevents further difficulty.

Scrotal Masses

Evaluation of scrotal masses in male athletes is often necessary. Testicular cancer remains one of the most common malignancies in the 16- to 35-year-old male, which requires immediate urologic consultation. A testicular mass that is separate from the cord and epididymis is most likely due to a malignancy and demands prompt exploration. A mass separate from the testicles should be evaluated first by transillumination with a bright light. Masses that are unable to be transilluminated should be evaluated by ultrasound and possible surgical exploration.

Traumatic hydrocele involves a cystic mass that encompasses the testicle and epididymis. This mass is caused by decreased absorption of the normal tunica vaginalis secretions due to trauma, infection, or tumor. An acute hydrocele may contain an underlying malignancy and should be investigated by ultrasound or surgical exploration. Traumatic or infectious hydrocele may become large enough to cause significant pain and require surgical correction.

Varicoceles are present in 9% to 19% of all men (13). Varicoceles represent varicosity of the internal spermatic veins and often present in males without symptomatology. Seventy percent of varicoceles are found on the left side, 20% are bilateral, and 10% are on the right side. Surgical correction is indicated for pain control, diminished ipsilateral testicular size, or infer-

F I G U R E **11-9**

Missed testicular torsion. (A) Testicular dynamic flow study using intravenous technetium-99m pertechnetate. Sequential left-to-right gamma camera images show peripheral increased flow to the left hemiscrotum as compared with the right. (B) Delayed image shows a photopenic left testis (*arrow*) with peripheral hyperemia. This patient had symptoms for 2 days.

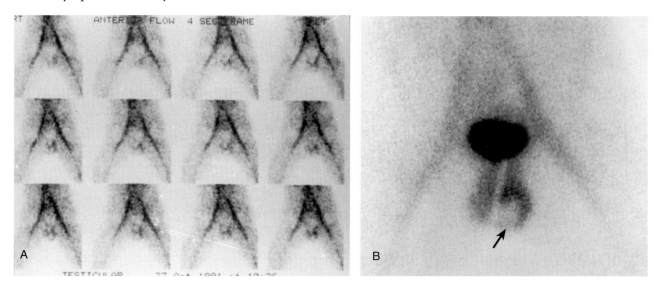

tility. Cystic masses within the epididymis or adjacent to the testicle are probably spermatoceles, caused by extravasation of sperm from the epididymis following trauma or infection. These usually require no further treatment unless they are extremely painful or large in size (11,13–15).

Penile Injuries

The erect penis is susceptible to acute trauma and fractures of the tunica albuginea. The area of fracture is swollen and ecchymotic, and the penis is bent to the affected side. This injury is a true urologic emergency necessitating evacuation of the hematoma and repair of the tunica tear. The athlete often attributes this fracture to work- or sport-related trauma and fails to mention his sexual activity that caused the injury. Direct blows to the flaccid penis or perineum may lead to vascular injuries and potential impotency. These are usually caused by straddle-type injuries or direct blows to the pubis such as spearing with football helmets. Injuries involving the penis that may disrupt the urethra should be evaluated with a retrograde urethrogram. Penile frostbite has been described in runners who wear inadequate clothing in cold weather. Consequently, adequate protection of the penis and perineum in extremely cold weather is mandatory.

Female Genitalia

Blunt trauma can damage the female genitalia, but this is an uncommon injury. The most common mechanism of injury involves straddle injuries that occur in gymnastics. The spectrum of injuries involves labial hematomas or tears, vaginal lacerations, clitoral tears, and urethral meatus injuries. Most of these injuries require proper imaging techniques as well as surgical consultation.

REFERENCES

1. Reid DC. Problems of the hip, pelvis, and sacroiliac joint. In: Sports injury: assessment and rehabilitation. New York: Churchill-Livingstone, 1992: 626–661.

2. Esposito PW. Pelvis, hip and thigh injuries. In: Mellion MB, Walsh WM, Shelton GL, eds. The physician's handbook. Philadelphia: Hanley & Belfus, 1990:410–411.

3. Sonzogni JJ, Gross ML. Biomechanics and soft-tissue insults. Emerg Med 1993;74–94.

4. Pearson RL. Osteitis pubis in a basketball player. Phys Sportsmed 1988;16:69–74.

5. O'Brien K. Bikers' bladder. N Engl J Med 1981; 304:1367.

6. Greenman PE. Principles of manual medicine. Baltimore: Williams & Wilkins, 1989:235.

7. Goldszer P, Parsee S, Segel T. Renal abnormalities during exercise. Your Patient and Fitness 1987;1:6–9.

8. McKeag D, Hough D. Primary care sports medicine. Iowa: Brown & Benchmark, 1993:383.

9. Sutton JM. Evaluation of hematuria in adults. JAMA 1990;263:2475–2480.

10. Hoover DL, Cromie WJ. Theory and management of exercise-related hematuria. Phys Sportsmed 1981;9:91.

11. Middleton WD, Siegel BA, Melson GA, et al. Acute scrotal disorder: prospective comparison of color Doppler vs testicular scintigraphy. Radiology 1990;177:177–181.

12. York JP. Sports in the male genital-urinary system. Phys Sportsmed 1990;18:92–100.

13. Noujain SC, Nagle CE. Acute scrotal injuries in athletes: evaluation by diagnostic imaging. Phys Sportsmed 1989;17:125–130.

14. Schneider RE. Genital urinary trauma. Emerg Med Clin North Am 1993;11:137–145.

15. Cass AS, Luxemberg N. Testicular injuries. Urology 1991;37:528–530.

CHAPTER 12

Thigh and Knee Injuries

LEIGH ANN CURL

HOLLIS G. POTTER

THOMAS WICKIEWICZ

lthough certainly not a replacement for astute history taking and physical examination skills, the clinician has an armamentarium of imaging possibilities at his or her disposal when treating patients with thigh or knee complaints. In choosing the most appropriate test in any given situation, a few key factors come into play. First, the physician must have a certain diagnosis or a list of diagnostic possibilities that he or she is entertaining based on the patient history and physical examination. "Shotgun" imaging is costly and, depending on the specific procedure done, is not always without risk to the patient. Second, each imaging tool has both advantages and limitations. Thus the selection of a specific imaging procedure requires both the ability to formulate a reasonable differential diagnosis based on the history and physical examination and an understanding of the imaging technique itself.

This chapter presents a "diagnosis-based" approach to various conditions of the thigh and knee. This will include pertinent comments on key points to be found in the clinical history and on physical examination, followed by a review of the imaging modalities as they apply to the particular condition being discussed.

Thigh

For the purposes of this chapter, discussion will include conditions of the thigh musculature (quadriceps and hamstrings) and associated soft tissues and the underlying femur. Conditions relating to the proximal femur and hip musculature are not addressed.

Muscle Strain and Rupture

Muscle *strain* is used to denote a condition in which partial or complete tears of the musculotendinous unit have occurred (1,2). A strain is felt to occur as a result of forceful muscle contraction opposing forces attempting to lengthen or stretch the muscle (3–5). Strains are usually graded by severity. In mild cases, complete tearing or separation does not occur, and therefore, the injury is either a *grade I* or *grade II strain*. Complete tearing or rupture is often referred to as a *grade III strain* (6). Clinically, patients with a grade I or grade II strain will present complaining of "muscle soreness." The pain experienced may be sudden or delayed until later during the activity or day. On examination, muscular tenderness to palpation can be elicited that may be maximal at the area of the musculotendinous junction. Ecchymosis may be present. Stretching will elicit discomfort of the involved musculature. The muscle will function, but strength will be limited due to associated pain (6,7).

In general, muscle strains usually are diagnosed on the basis of history and examination alone. Plain radiographs are not useful or required for diagnosis or treatment in an acute case. However, in a chronic situation, plain radiographs can be used to rule out the possibility of femoral stress fracture or myositis ossificans (discussed below). While myositis ossificans is probably more common after muscle contusions, it can be seen in any condition where there is muscle fiber disruption with secondary hemorrhage and hematoma. Advanced imaging modalities such as computed tomography (CT) or magnetic resonance imaging (MRI) are generally not indicated in cases of muscle strain.

Muscle rupture, grade III strain, occurs when the forces discussed above are of the magnitude to overcome the strength of the musculotendinous unit. Tearing occurs typically at the muscle-tendon junction or, in some cases, within the tendon itself. The myotendinous unit also may fail at the tendon insertion site. The patient may report that a "pop" or tearing sensation occurred coincident with the onset of acute pain. Most clinically significant quadriceps ruptures occur distally and will disrupt the extensor mechanism. This will be discussed later in the section on extensor mechanism injury.

Most hamstring ruptures occur proximally near the ischial origin and can be either medial (in the semimembranosus or semitendinosus) or lateral (in the biceps femoris). Usually, significant functional deficit occurs, limiting the patient's ability to actively flex or passively extend the knee. Clinically, a palpable defect within the musculotendinous unit is found. A painful mass (the retracted muscle belly) is also palpable. An attempt by the patient to contract the muscle is painful and demonstrates loss of continuity of the musculotendinous unit (loss of visible or palpable definition of the hamstring tendons).

While the clinical examination can be classic for a grade III or complete rupture, it can be difficult due to associated swelling and pain. In these instances, MRI examination may allow early identification of complete hamstring ruptures, particularly in tears involving the tendinous origins (7,8). The site of the tear and location of the involved ends (degree of retraction) can be demonstrated. MRI has a distinct advantage over CT, including improved soft tissue contrast, multiplanar imaging capabilities, and a lack of ionizing radiation. In acute injury, high signal on T2-weighted or high-contrast fat-suppressed images reflects edema and hemorrhage (9,10). In chronic injury patterns, MRI can localize the site of rupture, number of muscles involved, and degree of retraction (Fig. 12-1).

F I G U R E   **12-1**

(A) Coronal T2-weighted image through the hamstring muscles demonstrating abnormal signal and morphology on the left side, with evidence of nonacute injury in the semimembranosus and semitendinosus muscles, with retracted tendon edge (*arrow*). (B) Axial fat-suppressed, fast-spin-echo image demonstrating abnormal signal in the posterior compartment, as well as the markedly enlarged tendon of the semimembranosus (*arrow*), indicating retraction.

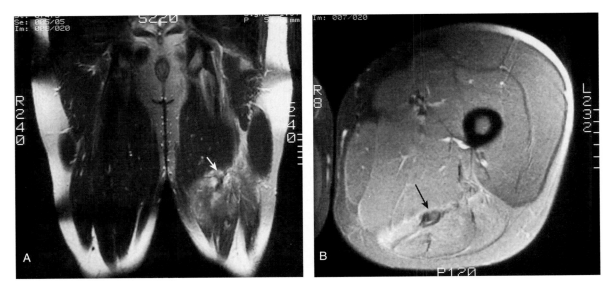

Chronic injuries are denoted by abnormal muscle architecture on high-resolution sequences, often with fatty infiltration. Comparison views of the unaffected side aid in assessing the injured side. Although unresolved, earlier recognition and surgical treatment of complete ruptures may afford a more beneficial outcome. We are currently reviewing our experience with such patients.

Muscle Contusion

Muscle contusion results from direct trauma to a muscle and is particularly common in contact sports. Most often the quadriceps is involved (*charley horse*) (5,7,11). The blunt trauma causes some disruption of muscle fibers, hemorrhage, and inflammation within the muscle, most of which occurs in the muscle fibers adjacent to the femur (6,12).

The patient is usually able to recall the specific time of injury and, depending on severity, may or may not have been able to continue playing. Clinically, the patient presents complaining of pain and tenderness of the involved muscle. On examination, swelling and tenderness to palpation are present. The presence of an intramuscular hematoma is sometimes palpable. Active extension will be painful, and knee range of motion in flexion will be limited to varying degrees depending on the severity of injury.

In this situation, plain radiographs are useful only to rule out an associated femoral fracture. If the patient presents late for diagnosis, radiographs will help evaluate for the presence of myositis ossificans (discussed below). MRI and CT scanning have no true role in the acute diagnosis and management of quadriceps or other muscle contusion and are not recommended routinely. However, in selected patients in whom symptoms are severe or response to rehabilitation is slow, MRI may be helpful to determine the extent of muscle tearing present. This information may lead to consideration of surgical decompression or repair and may guide the type and length of a patient's rehabilitation.

Myositis Ossificans

Myositis ossificans is a potential result of muscle injury with associated intramuscular hematoma. It represents ossification (heterotopic) at the site of the muscle injury (13). To date, there are no predicting factors to identify patients who will go on to develop myositis ossificans following muscle contusion.

Clinically, approximately 2 to 4 weeks following direct trauma and the formation of an intramuscular hematoma, a firm, hard mass will be palpable within the muscle (6). Tenderness and limited motion may persist but tend to stabilize and improve over time. Plain radiographs will show faint soft tissue mineralization and occasionally an underlying periosteal reaction. With time, the radiographs show a well-localized bone mass adjacent to the femoral cortex that consists of a sharply delineated cortical rim with a lacy or woven pattern centrally (Fig. 12-2). Separation from the adjacent cortex, characteristic of myositis, may or may not be clearly apparent.

Adjunctive radiographic studies, CT or MRI, are considered only in the situation in which the preceding radiographic findings are present and either 1) there is no known history of trauma or 2) the radiographic findings are not characteristic of myositis (i.e., femoral cortical or intramedullary involvement is suggested on plain films). In this situation, there may be concern for the possibility of an osteogenic sarcoma or other neoplasm. CT scanning can then be obtained. "Bone windows" in myositis will show separation of the soft tissue mass from the underlying femoral cortex and a zonal pattern to the mass with the mature cortical bone peripherally.

On MRI, the appearance of myositis varies with the sequential histologic change that occurs as the process progresses. Early (less than 4 weeks) to intermediate (several months) lesions may have an aggressive appearance on MRI images, simulating malignancy (14). For this reason, CT is preferred over MRI if myositis is suspected clinically, but plain radiographs are not diagnostic.

While technetium bone scintigraphy may show increased radiotracer deposition in the presence of a lesion (15), the technique has limited use in the current evaluation of myositis ossificans. However, if the lesion is functionally limiting and surgical excision is being considered, scintigraphy may assist in planning the timing of surgical excision. In lesions with a high level of radiotracer uptake, surgery is often delayed until a later date because persistently high or increasing levels of activity within a lesion are felt to be associated with an increased risk of recurrence following surgical excision. Thus sequential technetium studies, spaced 3 to

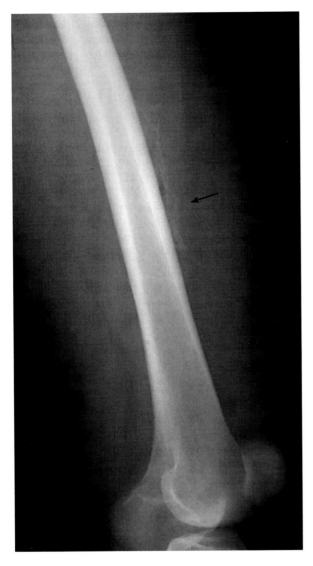

F I G U R E   **12-2**

Lateral radiograph of the femur demonstrating mineralization in the anterior soft tissues (*arrow*). Note the woven pattern of the mineralization and its separation from the anterior femoral cortex, both characteristic of myositis ossificans.

6 months apart, may be utilized preoperatively to plan the timing of surgical excision; operative resection is done when diminishing activity or a relatively inactive lesion is noted.

Ultrasonography early after injury may detect soft tissue changes indicative of myositis ossificans before plain radiographic changes can be seen (12). However, this potential for earlier diagnosis has not materialized into better or preventative treatment measures. Therefore, ultrasonography is rarely obtained.

Femoral Stress Fracture

Femoral stress fractures are relatively rare injuries. They occur in athletes who undertake sudden increases in training loads (particularly in runners) and can occur at any point along the femur (7). They represent fatigue failure of the bone under repetitive cyclic loading.

Patients usually present with complaints of persistent aching in the thigh or knee that is exacerbated by activity and often relieved by rest. Occasionally, nighttime aching is present, but this is not the predominant complaint. A history of recent increased training mileage or intensity may be elicited. Physical examination may demonstrate localizing tenderness to some aspect of the femur with pain on torsional testing or axial loading, but quite often this is fairly unremarkable.

Plain radiographs and technetium bone scan have been the traditional mainstay of diagnosis. Plain radiographs will be helpful only if the bone has entered the remodeling phase of the stress fracture in which reparative callus is present. This will appear as an area of endosteal and periosteal hyperostosis (Fig. 12-3A and B). A fracture line may be visualized within this zone. The plain radiographic findings may take anywhere from 2 to 6 weeks to develop following the onset of symptoms. Therefore, plain radiographs can be normal at the time of initial clinical evaluation (16).

For this reason, radionuclide scanning should be considered if the plain films are unremarkable in a patient whose history and examination are otherwise suspicious for stress fracture (17). A bone scan may demonstrate the presence of stress fracture as many as 3 weeks prior to the development of changes on plain films (18). The stress fracture will be seen as an area of increased activity on all three phases of the scan. On delayed images, the stress fracture appears as a solitary fusiform area of increased uptake (see Fig. 12-3C). With time and healing of the fracture, the blood flow and blood pool phases will show diminished activity, while the delayed phase remains positive. The delayed phase may show increased activity that persists past the time of clinical healing (17).

MRI also may be useful in the diagnosis of stress fracture (16,19) and may demonstrate occult fractures earlier than bone scintigraphy (20). On MRI, the cortical thickening associated with a "mature" stress fracture can be seen on

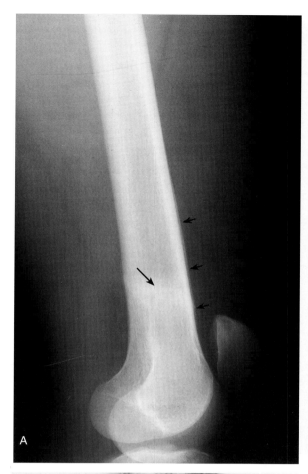

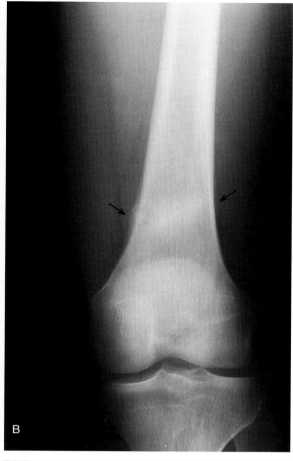

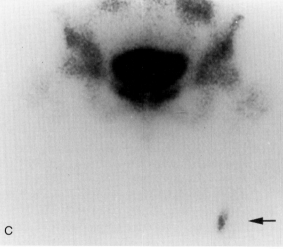

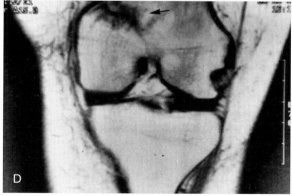

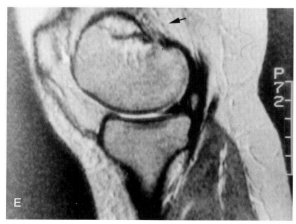

FIGURE **12-3**

AP (A) and lateral (B) views of the femur demonstrating sclerosis at the distal diaphyseal region of the femur (*arrows*) and indicating the presence of a stress fracture. Note the presence of periosteal reaction, particularly visible on the lateral view (*short dark arrows*), which extends both proximal and distal to the area of the stress fracture. (C) Technetium bone scan demonstrating increased uptake at the distal femur, consistent with stress fracture. Coronal T1-weighted (D) and sagittal T2-weighted (E) images demonstrating low-signal-intensity stress fracture of the supracondylar femur (different patient than in part A) surrounded by marrow edema (*arrows*).

T1-weighted images as a widened cortical signal. Early stress fractures appear as focal marrow edema, characterized by diminished signal intensity on T1-weighted images, with corresponding increased signal intensity on T2-weighted or fat-suppressed images (see Fig. 12-3D and E). While MRI may be more sensitive than either plain radiography or bone scintigraphy, current expense limits its practical use as a primary imaging modality in the management of most stress fractures.

Knee

Effusion

The presence of a knee effusion is a common finding in a multitude of conditions, both acute and chronic, that effect the knee joint. While the significance of the effusion is best related to associated findings on physical examination, a few brief comments on the radiographic findings as they pertain to the effusion itself can be made.

Knee effusions can be classified into one of a few major types: 1) serosanguineous (synovial fluid and plasma exudate or transudate), 2) hemarthrosis (blood), 3) lipohemarthrosis (fat droplets and blood), and 4) septic (pus). On plain radiography, each of the preceding will be apparent as an increased fluid density, most apparent in the suprapatellar pouch area (21) (Fig. 12-4). A lipohemarthrosis occasionally will demonstrate a fat-fluid level, especially apparent on a cross-table lateral view.

On MRI, very specific findings can be seen depending on the nature of the effusion. The serosanguineous effusion will have findings characteristic of normal joint fluid: intermediate signal intensity on T1 with marked increased signal on T2. This is the typical signal pattern of normal joint fluid, but an increased volume of fluid will be present. An acute hemarthrosis will show heterogeneous intermediate to diminished signal intensity, particularly on T2-weighted images. A lipohemarthrosis will show layering of the components on imaging; the hemarthrosis (protein and plasma) component assumes the dependent recesses of the joint and has a hypointense proteinaceous layer with an overlying hyperintense plasma layer, whereas the fatty droplets assume the most superficial position with a bright signal on T1-weighted images and

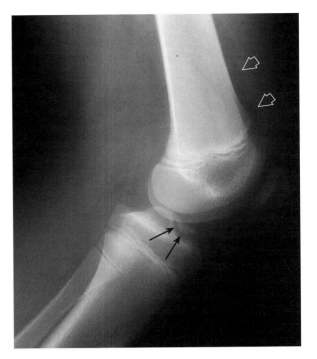

FIGURE **12-4**

Lateral radiograph of a skeletally immature individual who sustained a skiing injury to the knee. An effusion is noted in the suprapatellar pouch (*open arrows*), and an avulsion fragment of the tibial eminence is present (*dark arrows*).

intermediate signal on T2-weighted or gradient-echo images (Fig. 12-5). A septic effusion will have characteristics of a complex effusion, with thickening of the synovial lining and inflammatory debris producing an intermediate signal on both T1- and T2-weighted images.

While routine MRI imaging is obviously not recommended in every knee with an effusion, if an MRI has been obtained, the character of the effusion can be helpful to note in determining the underlying pathology. For example, a hemarthrosis may lead one to suspect an anterior cruciate ligament injury, whereas the presence of a lipohemarthrosis would lead one to search for the presence of an intra-articular fracture. Thickened synovium with foci of low signal on T2-weighted and gradient-echo sequences suggests pigmented villonodular synovitis (discussed below).

Meniscal Injury

Injuries to the menisci are some of the most common problems evaluated in clinical practice.

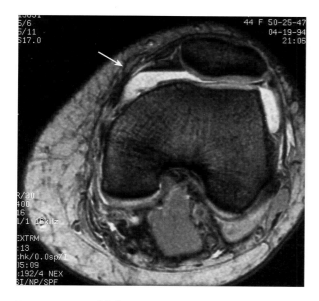

F I G U R E **12-5**

Axial gradient-echo sequence of the patellofemoral joint demonstrating a fluid level (*arrow*), representing a lipohemarthrosis, with the relative lower signal intensity of fat on the nondependent surface and blood products in the dependent portion.

While a torn meniscus can occur as an isolated problem, it is often seen in conjunction with other injury, anterior cruciate disruption being perhaps the most common (22).

The menisci are fibrocartilaginous structures interposed between the articular surfaces of the distal femur and the proximal tibia. They are essentially C-shaped or semilunar in appearance. Both the medial and lateral menisci are attached to the tibia centrally (near the tibial spines) and to the capsule peripherally. Their primary function is to protect the articular cartilage from excessive forces during daily and sporting activities. In essence, they act as intra-articular "shock absorbers." The menisci also play a role in nutrition of the articular cartilage and assist in stability of the knee joint.

Meniscal tears can be the result of either acute injury or degeneration with aging and can be either simple or complex. Simple tears most often occur in younger individuals following trauma and are directed either longitudinally or horizontally, thus paralleling the collagen fiber arrangement within the meniscus. Conversely, most complex tears are associated with aging of the meniscus and occur in older individuals with minimal or no history of trauma. While the preceding statements are only generalizations,

these two basic patterns of injury will be helpful to understand in terms of identifying the meniscal injury on various imaging studies.

Plain radiographs are useful in patients presenting with joint line pain and other findings suspicious for meniscal injury, since they will evaluate for any evidence of gross fracture, particularly if the symptoms developed following acute trauma. Recommended views include a standard AP in full extension and a lateral view in approximately 30 degrees of knee flexion. Standing or weight-bearing views are preferred. In a more chronic situation or in the older patient population, plain radiographs may demonstrate loss of joint space and other findings consistent with osteoarthritis (sclerosis, spur or osteophyte formation, and cyst formation). In this group of patients, an additional standing posteroanterior (PA) radiograph in 30 to 45 degrees of knee flexion can assist in evaluating for cartilaginous surface wear (23). This view is more sensitive for detecting loss of joint space compared with an AP view in full extension. The presence of gonarthrosis would make one suspicious of the possibility of a degenerative tear and, more important, would require further consideration as to how much of the patient's symptoms are attributable to a potential meniscal lesion. It has been shown that as many as 25% of the population in the second to eighth generations of life can have meniscal abnormalities on MRI images even though clinically asymptomatic (24).

While history, clinical examination, and plain radiographs can suffice to make the clinical diagnosis of a meniscal tear, in some situations further testing may be indicated. Historically, contrast arthrography was the mainstay for diagnostic imaging of meniscal injury, but now this has been replaced by MRI. The main advantage of MRI is the fact that it is noninvasive. Clinical experience and technical refinement in the quality of the MRI images have shown MRI to be highly accurate in the diagnosis of meniscal tears, with accuracy reported to be from 70% to 100% (25–31).

Contrast arthrography is still obtained occasionally, especially where MRI is of limited availability. For meniscal injury, double-contrast arthrography, in which radiopaque contrast and air are injected into the knee, is most useful (32). Accuracy in detecting meniscal tears is reported to be as high as 90% to 95% (31,33,34). A series of spot radiographs will show various segments of the meniscus in profile (34). Meniscal tears will be seen as contrast material extending into the triangular body or shadow of the meniscus, which is outlined by the contrast agent. Simple tears will demonstrate a single line or split within the meniscus, whereas complex tears will have a very irregular outline, often with multiple splits into the meniscal substance.

With MRI, the fibrocartilage of the meniscus yields a homogeneous low signal on both T1- and T2-weighted (or T2-equivalent) images, the margins of which should be sharp and well defined (Fig. 12-6). Meniscal tears will show disruption of the homogeneous low signal by areas of increased signal. While intrameniscal signal change representing myxoid or hyaline degeneration is easily recognized on MRI (termed *grade 1 globular* and *grade 2 linear signals*) (27), frank meniscal tears will show communication of the abnormal increased intensity signal with the articular surface of the meniscus (also termed a *grade 3 signal*) (Fig. 12-7).

The signal communication can be with either the femoral or the tibial surface of the meniscus, or both, depending on the anatomy of the tear present. It is not necessary to see the suspected tear on more than one image. Depending on slice thickness, the distance between image slices, and the size of the tear present, one image is all that may coincide with the location of the tear. Any high signal communicating with the meniscal surface, even if present on only one image, can be diagnostic of a tear. By careful evaluation of multiple images, it is usually possible to define the anatomy of a tear. Specifically, it is possible to determine if the tear is complex or simple, radial or longitudinal, horizontal, or if it involves the central or outer third of the meniscus.

Recognizing normal from abnormal meniscal morphology is also an important aid in recognizing meniscal pathology. On sagittal images, the posterior horn of the medial meniscus is larger (nearly two times) than its anterior counterpart (see Fig. 12-6B). Laterally, the horns are essentially the same size (see Fig. 12-6A). A small posterior horn of the medial meniscus,

F I G U R E   **12-6**

(A) Sagittal proton density–weighted image through the lateral meniscus demonstrating normal signal intensity within the fibrocartilage of the meniscus. Note is made of normal meniscal morphology, with equivalent size of both anterior and posterior horns (*long arrows*). The cortical signal of the tibial plateau is seen as a homogeneous dark line. Note the overlying intermediate signal of the articular cartilage. A similar pattern is seen for the cortex and articular surface of the distal femur. (B) Proton density–weighted sagittal image through the medial meniscus demonstrating that the posterior horn of the medial meniscus is larger than the anterior horn, reflecting normal meniscal morphology. An effusion is noted in the anterior aspect of the knee (*open arrow*).

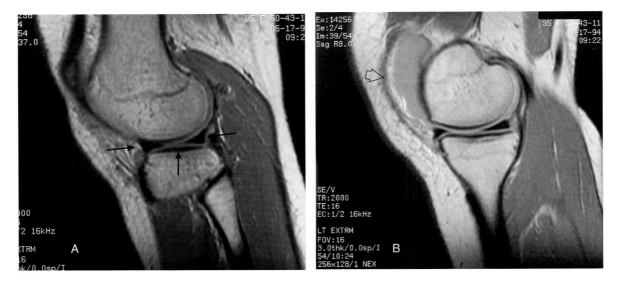

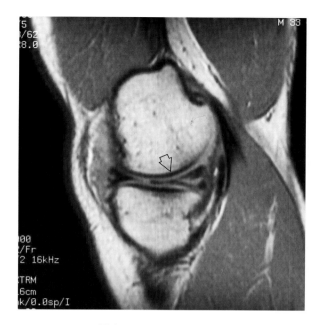

F I G U R E **12-7**

Sagittal proton density–weighted sequence through the medial meniscus demonstrating complex intrameniscal signal in the posterior horn reaching the articular surface, confirming the presence of tear (*open arrow*).

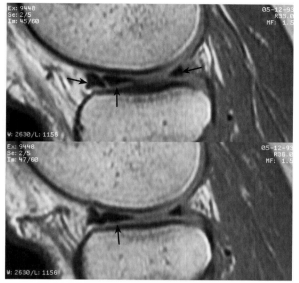

F I G U R E **12-8**

Proton density–weighted image through the lateral meniscus demonstrating small posterior horn with relative enlargement and abnormal signal in the anterior horn (*middle and right arrows*). This is a vertically oriented bucket-handle tear of the lateral meniscus, with a large portion of the posterior horn displaced adjacent to the anterior horn. The displaced fragment is denoted by the left most arrow.

particularly with loss of the sharp inner apex, should lead one to look for a displaced meniscal fragment. Similarly, disproportionate horn size can indicate the presence of a displaced lateral meniscus tear (Fig. 12-8).

With the preceding in mind, it is important to recognize normal anatomic structures that can be falsely interpreted as representing meniscal tears. Most commonly, the transverse ligament between the two anterior horns can be mistaken for tears on sagittal images (35) (Fig. 12-9). The transverse ligament can vary quite substantially in size between patients and will be visualized on sagittal images taken close to the notch. Similarly, the meniscofemoral ligaments of Humphrey and Wrisberg can be seen to pass from the lateral aspect of the medial femoral condyle to the posterior horn of the lateral meniscus and can appear as a tear in the posterior horn of the lateral meniscus (36) (Fig. 12-10). The popliteus tendon at the popliteal hiatus also can produce the appearance of a tear at the posterior horn of the lateral meniscus (Fig. 12-11). The inferolateral genicular artery can produce the appearance of a tear in the anterior horn of the lateral meniscus (35). All the pre-

F I G U R E **12-9**

Sagittal proton density–weighted image through the notch demonstrating the anterior horn of the medial meniscus (*bottom arrow*) and the overlying transverse ligament (*top arrow*).

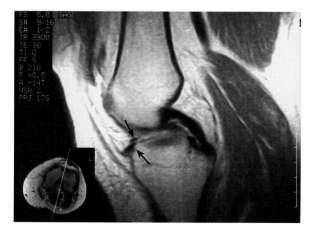

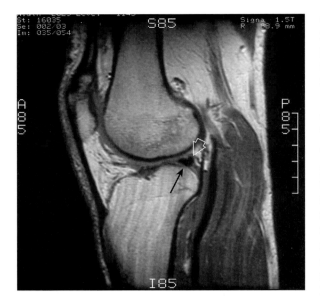

F I G U R E 12-10

Sagittal proton density–weighted image demonstrating the meniscofemoral ligament attachment to the posterior horn of the lateral meniscus. The meniscofemoral ligament is denoted by the large open arrow and appears almost as a contour irregularity or tear of the posterior horn of the meniscus (*solid dark arrow*).

ceding structures can be recognized by following their course on sequential images, by comparing findings on coronal and sagittal images, and most important, by being aware of their existence.

Cruciate Injury

The anterior and posterior cruciate ligaments are prime static stabilizers of the knee joint. The anterior cruciate ligament (ACL) extends anteromedially from the medial aspect of the lateral femoral condyle to its tibial attachment just in front of the anterior tibial spine. Its primary function is to prevent excessive anterior tibial translation during activity, primarily in the midrange of knee motion. The posterior cruciate ligament (PCL) extends posterolaterally from the lateral aspect of the medial femoral condyle to its posterior tibial attachment 1 cm below the joint line. Its primary function is to prevent excessive posterior tibial translation during activity, primarily with the knee in a position of 90 degrees of flexion.

Injury to the cruciate ligaments has received

F I G U R E 12-11

(A) Coronal fast-spin-echo T2-weighted image demonstrating the normal hiatus or recess between the popliteus tendon (*large open arrow*) and the lateral meniscus (*solid arrow*). The recess appears as a bright signal secondary to the presence of an effusion secondary to a tear in the anterior cruciate ligament. Note the attachment of the popliteus tendon to the lateral aspect of the femur. (B) T-2 weighted image demonstrating the appearance of the normal popliteus hiatus on a sagittal image (same patient as in part A). The popliteus tendon is marked by the large open arrow and the body of the lateral meniscus by the solid dark arrow.

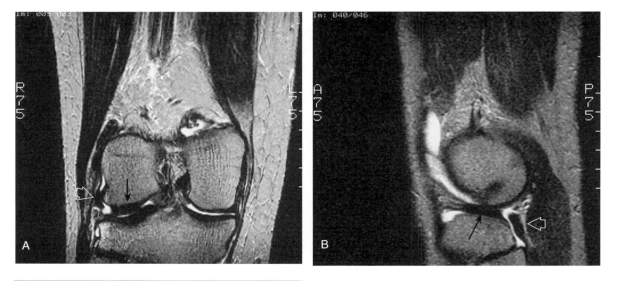

a great deal of attention over the past 20 years. Extensive research has been done looking at the diagnosis and treatment of these injuries. Immediate hemarthrosis following injury, subsequent clinical episodes of instability, and physical examination findings of increased anterior or posterior laxity can all help make the diagnosis. At times, however, further imaging studies are required and can be of great use in the clarification of what occasionally is an unclear clinical picture.

Plain radiographs (AP in extension, lateral at 0 to 30 degrees of flexion) should always be obtained following acute injury in which hemarthrosis is present. Aside from ruling out tibial plateau or other fractures, there are plain radiographic findings characteristic of some cruciate injuries. In younger patients (up to late adolescence), the ACL may avulse at its tibial insertion, and an avulsion fragment of the tibial eminence will be evident within the notch on the AP and/or lateral radiograph (see Fig. 12-4). While ACL avulsion injuries do occur in adults, their incidence is much less. Also less commonly, the PCL may avulse from its tibial insertion with a small bone fragment. Deepening of the lateral condylopatellar sulcus or terminal sulcus (greater than 1 mm as measured on a lateral radiograph of the knee) has been associated with ACL injury (37,38) (Fig. 12-12). A lateral capsular avulsion fragment (Segond's fracture) sometimes may be seen and is highly suggestive of ACL injury, with a reported association rate of as high as 100% (39) (Fig. 12-13).

As with meniscal injury, MRI has replaced contrast arthrography in the evaluation of cruciate injury. If arthrography is done, the normal cruciates will outline with contrast material, showing a straight, smooth edge (31,40,41). Since the cruciates are extrasynovial, however, this finding is not always classically present, and interpretation therefore may be limited. Some workers, however, have reported over 90% accuracy with this technique (40,41).

MRI is the current preferred technique to evaluate the anterior and posterior cruciates if their status is in question. It has been shown to be both sensitive and specific for the evaluation of cruciate injury (25,30,42). Studies have shown an accuracy of 95%, specificity of 98%, positive predictive value of 88%, and a negative predictive value of 96% of MRI in the evaluation of ACL injury (31). While evaluating the cruciates, MRI also will identify any associated injury to the menisci and collateral ligaments. The identification of these injuries can have significant im-

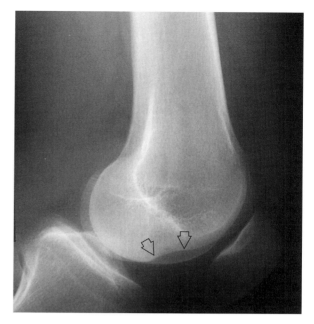

F I G U R E   12-12

Lateral radiograph of a patient with a torn anterior cruciate ligament demonstrating a large lateral condylopatellar sulcus (*open arrows*).

F I G U R E   12-13

AP view of the knee demonstrating a small avulsion fracture of the lateral portion of the proximal tibia (*arrow*), indicating a Segond injury.

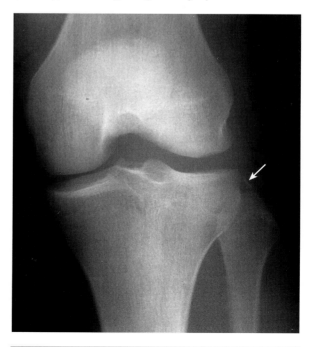

pact on the course of treatment subsequently chosen.

The intact anterior cruciate appears as a low signal band of fibers on both T1- and T2-weighted images (Fig. 12-14A). These low-signal bands are associated with linear areas of high signal secondary to interfascicular fat, particularly distally at the tibial attachment site. The fibers pass from the lateral femoral condyle to the tibia slightly medially and slightly obliquely from superior to inferior. The fibers should be smooth and of uniform signal, although the separate fiber bundles may be apparent, particularly anteriorly. Both sagittal and coronal images should be looked at to completely assess the ACL. An ACL that is not entirely within the plane of the sagittal image due to the obliquity of its course may be better visualized on the coronal sections (see Fig. 12-14B).

With partial ACL disruption, edema and hemorrhage will be seen within the ligament, but some continuity of fibers is evident. With complete ACL disruption, edema and hemorrhage will again be present, but there will be no continuity between femoral and tibial attachment sites. The ACL fibers may become "wavy" or assume a more horizontal position within the notch (Fig. 12-15A and B). In the chronic situation, ei-

ther the ACL will be replaced superiorly by fatty tissue and distinct ligament fibers will not be apparent or the fibers will have an abnormal horizontal course with an apparent proximal attachment over the posterior cruciate ligament (see Fig. 12-15C).

In addition to looking at the status of the ACL itself, there are other findings on MRI as there are on plain radiographs that correlate highly with ACL injury. Obviously, the lateral capsular avulsion, tibial eminence avulsion, and lateral notch sign discussed previously also can be seen on the MRI (Fig. 12-16A). Unique to MRI is its ability to demonstrate "bone bruising" of the femur and tibia. At the time of ACL injury, the forces associated with anterior subluxation and impaction of the tibia on the femur can lead to a bony contusion posteriorly on the lateral tibial plateau and at the middle aspect of the lateral femoral condyle. This will appear as a patchy or diffuse area of high marrow signal on T2-weighted images (43–45). While T1-weighted images may show a corresponding diminished signal void, they also may be unremarkable. This finding, termed *translational marrow edema,* is accentuated using fat-suppression techniques (see Figs. 12-15B and 12-16B). Acute angulation of the PCL (due to relative laxity from increased anterior

F I G U R E   **12-14**

(A) Sagittal proton density–weighted image demonstrating normal appearance of the anterior cruciate ligament in the intercondylar notch (*arrow*). (B) Normal appearance of the anterior cruciate ligament (*arrow*) is confirmed on this coronal fast-spin-echo image.

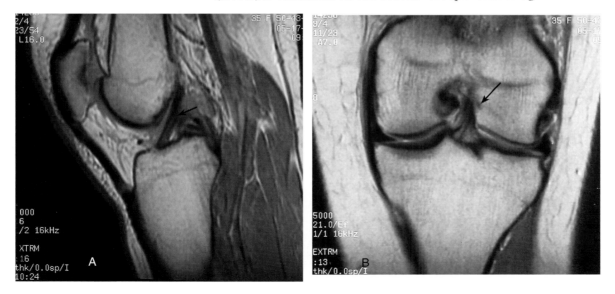

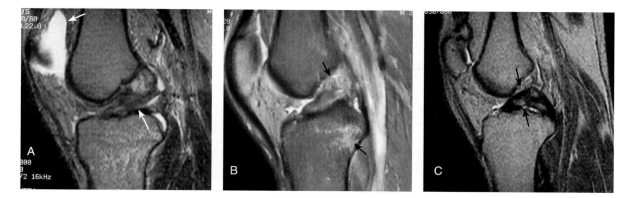

F I G U R E   **12-15**

(A) Sagittal T2-weighted image demonstrating proximal disruption of the anterior cruciate ligament (*long arrow*) as well as a joint effusion (*short arrow*). (B) Sagittal fat-suppressed image demonstrating proximal disruption of the anterior cruciate ligament (*top arrow*) as well as posterior contusion in the tibia (*bottom arrows*). (C) Sagittal T2-weighted image through the intercondylar notch demonstrating horizontal course of the anterior cruciate ligament, without evidence of acute injury pattern, and failure to identify an intact femoral insertion, indicating a chronic ACL disruption (*top arrow*).

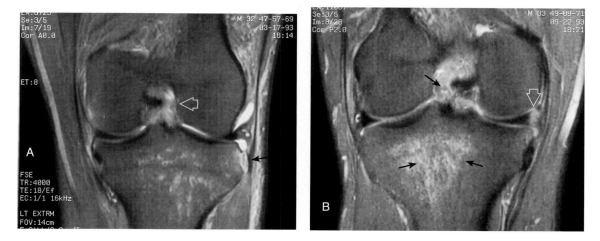

F I G U R E   **12-16**

(A) Coronal fat-suppressed, fast-spin-echo sequence confirming the presence of an anterior cruciate ligament tear (*open white arrow*) as well as an avulsion of the lateral margin of the proximal tibia (*black arrow*), indicating lateral capsular avulsion of the Segond type. (B) Coronal fat-suppressed, fast-spin-echo image demonstrating hemorrhage and edema within the intercondylar notch, with failure to identify normal ACL morphology, indicating an ACL tear (*open white arrow*). Increased signal in the proximal tibia reflects translational contusion (*black arrows*). Also of note is abnormal signal at the meniscal-capsular junction of the medial meniscus, adjacent to the medial capsular ligament (*top black arrow*), indicating concomitant meniscocapsular separation.

tibial translation) is a less reliable indirect sign of ACL injury.

The intact posterior cruciate ligament is a slightly larger structure than the ACL (approximately 2 to 3 mm wider at its midsection than the ACL). It appears as a very low signal structure on T1- and T2-weighted images and has a course that is slightly convex posteriorly (Fig. 12-17). Due to its size, it nearly always can be visualized in its entirety on a single sagittal image. As with the ACL, it is helpful to use both the sagittal and coronal images and follow its course.

The torn PCL will have findings similar to that of the ACL: hemorrhage with loss of fiber continuity (Fig. 12-18). With significant interstitial hemorrhage or subsequent scarring, a large "mass" may appear within the ligament.

Collateral Ligaments and Posterolateral Corner

As with the cruciate ligaments, the medial and lateral collateral ligaments are critical for knee stability. The medial collateral ligament (MCL) consists primarily of two components, *superficial* and *deep*. The superficial component extends from the medial epicondyle proximally to the anteromedial tibia distally, where it inserts 5

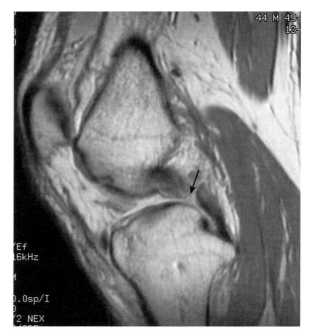

F I G U R E 12-18

Sagittal fast-spin-echo, proton density–weighted sequence through the knee demonstrating midsubstance disruption of the posterior cruciate ligament (*arrow*).

to 7 cm below the joint line just below the pes anserine. The deep medial collateral extends from the epicondyle proximally to the peripheral medial meniscus and proximal tibia distally. Thus it is composed of both meniscotibial and meniscofemoral components. The bursa of Voshell is located between the superficial and deep components of the MCL. The MCL is a prime stabilizer of the knee against valgus force, particularly with the knee at 30 degrees of flexion.

The lateral collateral ligament (LCL) and posterolateral corner or complex (PLC) are the prime stabilizers of the knee to varus and posterolateral force, respectively. Both complexes are primary stabilizers at 30 to 45 degrees of knee flexion. The LCL extends from the lateral epicondyle proximally to the fibular head distally. The PLC consists of (in addition to the LCL) the popliteal tendon, popliteofibular ligament, and posterior joint capsule. In addition, the distal insertion of the biceps femoris onto the fibular head and the iliotibial band onto the proximal tibia at Gerdy's tubercle also contribute to lateral knee stability.

Injury to the medial or lateral collateral ligaments can occur alone but often occurs in con-

F I G U R E 12-17

Sagittal proton density–weighted sequence through the knee demonstrating normal appearance of the posterior cruciate ligament within the intercondylar notch (*arrows*).

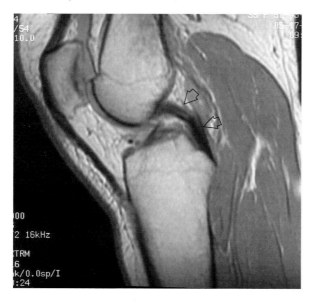

junction with other injury. The MCL is the most commonly injured knee ligament (46) and is occasionally injured in conjunction with the ACL and medial meniscus (O'Donoghue's triad) (47), whereas LCL injury often is found with injury to the PCL and posterolateral corner structures.

As with other suspected soft tissue injury about the knee, routine AP and lateral radiographs should be obtained to rule out the presence of fracture. This is particularly important in the younger patient with open physes, since a physeal fracture may mimic an MCL tear clinically. In this situation, stress radiographs will identify the source of the varus or valgus instability.

Disruption of the MCL may occur anywhere along the length of the ligament and involve either or both the superficial (tibial collateral) and deep (medial capsular) fibers. With complete or partial proximal injury, the torn ligament may undergo dystrophic calcification or ossification, which can be seen radiographically as the Pelligrini-Stieda lesion. On the lateral side, occasionally a small avulsion fragment of the proximal fibula will be seen with LCL and posterolateral corner injury.

If isolated injury to either the MCL or LCL is suspected clinically (localized tenderness over the ligament without excessive varus-valgus or anteroposterior laxity), additional imaging is not recommended routinely. However, if additional injury is suspected that would potentially alter patient management, such as combined ACL, MCL, and meniscal tears, further study may be warranted.

MRI is far superior to plain films in localizing the site of the ligamentous disruption and identifying associated injury. On the medial side, coronal imaging will show both the deep and superficial components of the MCL as linear low signal on both T1- and T2-weighted images. The tibial collateral or superficial component will extend from the epicondyle to its insertion below the joint line just deep to the pes tendons. A high signal (the interligamentous bursa of Voshell) may be seen separating the superficial from the deeper component, the latter of which arises from the condyle but inserts on the tibial margin (Fig. 12-19). Following complete injury, disruption of the normal superficial and deep fiber pattern will be seen, and T2-weighted images will identify associated hemorrhage and edema both within the ligament and overlying soft tissues (Fig. 12-20). With partial injury, the fibers will appear in continuity, but edema and

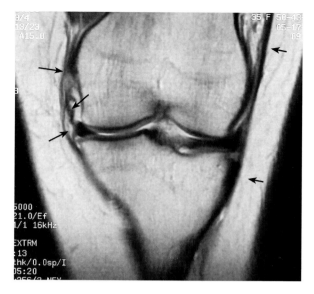

F I G U R E   **12-19**

Coronal fast-spin-echo sequence demonstrating the normal appearance of the anterior fibers of the medial collateral ligament. The superficial fibers are noted (*long dark arrows*), as well as the deep capsular ligament (*left middle arrow*). Also noted is the normal appearance of the iliotibial band, inserting on Gerdy's tubercle at the lateral aspect of the knee (*short dark arrows*).

F I G U R E   **12-20**

Coronal fat-suppressed, fast-spin-echo sequence demonstrating disruption of both the tibial insertion of the superficial medial collateral ligament (*large open arrow*) and the meniscotibial ligament (*small open arrow*). Note the normal appearance of the fibers of the superficial medial collateral ligament (*long black arrow*) and the meniscofemoral ligament (*short black arrow*) at their femoral insertions.

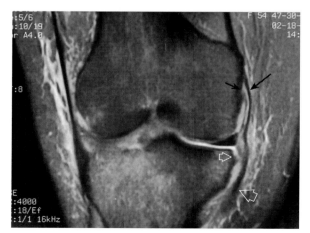

hemorrhage will be present. Injury can be limited to the medial capsular fibers and will show disruption here with an increased bursal signal, while the overlying tibial collateral component demonstrates normal signal characteristics.

The posterolateral complex consists mainly of the iliotibial band, the biceps femoris, the lateral (fibular) collateral ligament, the popliteus tendon, and the popliteofibular ligament. Each of these structures can be identified readily on MRI as distinct low-signal structures that can be followed on sequential images between their respective origins and insertions (48,49) (see Fig. 12-19). Edema and hemorrhage laterally and posterolaterally should prompt inspection of each of these structures individually, as should the finding of PCL injury, since they often occur in conjunction with each other.

The fibular collateral and popliteofibular ligaments are easiest seen on serial coronal images and should both insert on the proximal fibula. They may be avulsed with trauma. The popliteus tendon should be visualized along its course from the posterolateral tibia to its insertion near the lateral femoral epicondyle. Injury to this structure is recognized by an irregular contour (may become "wavy") or discontinuity in its course (50). Frequently, hemorrhage and edema may be found within the popliteus muscle belly, representing musculotendinous junction injury. In a similar fashion, both the tendon of the biceps femoris and the iliotibial band should be inspected for signs of injury.

Extensor Mechanism

The extensor mechanism of the knee includes the quadriceps muscle and its tendon, the patella and associated soft tissues, and the patellar tendon. Problems here can be generically divided into two major categories: 1) acute injuries including patellar fracture, patellar dislocation, and rupture of the quadriceps or patellar tendons, and 2) chronic conditions, including recurrent subluxation, various malalignment problems, patellofemoral chondromalacia, and other causes of patellofemoral pain. While entire texts have been devoted to the evaluation of these problems (51), we will address each of them here briefly, with emphasis on the acute injury.

Patellar Fracture

Patellar fracture occurs most commonly due to a violent blow to the anterior knee. Clinically,

focal tenderness is present with an associated effusion. Loss of extensor mechanism function is usually present.

The mainstay of diagnosis is plain radiographs, including a routine AP and lateral as well as a Merchant or "sunrise" infrapatellar view. The traditional axial or "sunrise" view is taken with the patient prone and the knee flexed to approximately 115 degrees. The cassette is positioned anterior to the knee, and the beam is angled 15 degrees cephalad from the vertical.

The Merchant view is obtained with the patient supine and the knee flexed 45 degrees in neutral tibial rotation. The x-ray beam is oriented from cephalad to caudad, at an angle of 30 degrees from the horizontal. The film cassette is placed at the midsection of the anterior tibia and held into place perpendicular to the x-ray beam. Typically, both knees are imaged simultaneously. Following significant trauma, pain often will necessitate that the infrapatellar view be taken in lesser degrees of flexion. In this situation, a Laurin view is appropriate. With the patient supine, the knee is placed in 20 degrees of flexion. The x-ray beam is oriented cephalad from the foot and aligned parallel to the anterior tibia. The patient holds the cassette perpendicular to the beam at the distal thigh (just proximal to the patella). Again, both knees can be imaged simultaneously.

In cases of fracture, the fracture lines and degree of fragment separation are usually readily apparent on the lateral and infrapatellar views to allow clinical decision making regarding treatment. If the articular step-off is greater than 2 mm, or if the proximal and distal fragments are separated by more than 4 or 5 mm, surgical reduction and fixation are typically recommended. Rarely, additional tomographic assessment will be required to determine if internal fixation is necessary and may be performed with either conventional tomography, CT scanning, or MRI. Plain film tomography is usually adequate and can be superior to CT because of the requirement of computer re-formation of axial data to obtain the sagittal and coronal images with CT. Because of the resulting step-off artifact generated with re-formatted images, which is compounded by any patient movement during the study, the actual degree of displacement may be difficult to determine. MRI avoids this problem and also allows assessment of the degree of associated retinacular injury but may be more expensive to obtain. A "limited" MRI study using fewer pulse sequences and less scan time can be obtained at a cost equivalent to that of a CT scan with image reconstruction.

Patellar Dislocation

Patellar dislocation may occur following a direct blow to the knee or, more commonly, due to a noncontact mechanism with simultaneous twisting and quadriceps contraction. The patient may present with the patella still dislocated, in which case the diagnosis will be obvious, or may give a history of dislocation followed by spontaneous reduction. Occasionally, patients describe reducing the patella themselves.

Clinically, a patient who has sustained an acute patellar dislocation will have a swollen knee with a moderate to severe effusion. The anterior retinaculum will be tender to palpation, and significant apprehension and pain will be obtained with passive patellar manipulation, particularly toward the direction of the dislocation (usually lateral). Knee flexion and extension typically are quite limited due to pain and apprehension, but the extensor mechanism should be intact to palpation and quadriceps contraction.

The role of imaging in patellar dislocation is twofold: 1) document the reduction, and 2) rule out any associated bone or osteocartilaginous injury. Plain films (AP, lateral, and infrapatellar views) should be obtained. The patella should be seen located within the femoral trochlea, and the surfaces should be inspected for evidence of fracture. An avulsion fracture or calcification along the medial edge of the patella is recognized as pathognomonic for patellar dislocation (52,53). Less commonly, a fragment is displaced from the lateral femoral condyle. Persistent malreduction and/or a large osteochondral fragment displaced within the joint should prompt early surgical intervention. Aside from plain radiographs, further diagnostic imaging is not routinely recommended following dislocation, although other imaging techniques have been studied (54–56). With MRI, an acute patellar dislocation will demonstrate retinacular injury. It is also possible to assess the articular surfaces for the presence of associated injury (Fig. 12-21).

Quadriceps and Patellar Tendon Rupture

Most extensor tendon ruptures occur in tendons that are under great tension, such as with maximal quadriceps contraction. A previous history of tendinitis and possibly steroid use is common (57,58). The patient will describe sudden severe

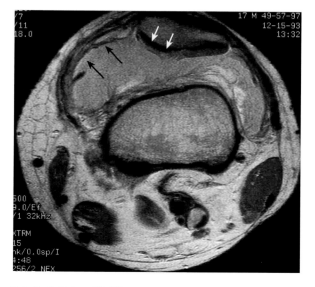

F I G U R E   12-21

Axial fast-spin-echo image through the knee demonstrating abnormal signal in the medial retinaculum with focal retinacular disruption (*black arrows*). Also of note is an acute chondral injury over the medial aspect of the patella (*white arrows*).

pain and weakness. The sensation of a sudden "pop" may have been experienced.

Physical examination usually shows generalized swelling and tenderness that may localize to either the quadriceps or the patellar tendon. With complete disruption, abnormal position of the patella may be noted on examination: patellar baja with quadriceps tendon rupture and patella alta with patellar tendon rupture. The degree of migration will be influenced by the degree of associated retinacular tearing. Attempted knee extension will be painful and, with complete rupture and significant retinacular injury, may be impossible.

Plain radiographs should be obtained. These should include AP, lateral, and infrapatellar views. Some advocate lateral views with the knee flexed from 45 to 90 degrees to place the extensor mechanism under some tension. However, pain often limits attempted imaging in this position. Any evidence of fracture, particularly sleeve fractures in younger patients, should be sought because these injuries can simulate the findings of a purely ligamentous injury clinically. In the absence of fracture, the position of the patella (baja or alta) should be noted, since it will correlate with the site of injury. The normal density of the quadriceps and patellar tendons, contrasted against the radiolucent subcutaneous fat, should be identified, since their absence is an indicator of potential injury.

With complete rupture and patellar migration, usually the plain radiographs and physical examination are sufficient for diagnosis and treatment. However, in the case of partial ruptures or in complete ruptures in which a significant component of the retinaculum remains intact, the diagnosis may be uncertain. Severe pain and localized tenderness may be noted by examination, yet some preservation of extensor function may be found and plain radiographs may be unremarkable. In this scenario, MRI can be obtained to evaluate the status of the tendons and the extent of the rupture, if present (59).

Both the quadriceps and patellar tendons are low-signal structures on T1- and T2-weighted images and are best inspected on sagittal and axial images. Loss of fiber continuity with associated edema and hemorrhage can be seen, and the percentage of the tendon involvement can be estimated (60). Wrinkling or laxity within the patellar tendon can be seen as a secondary indicator of extensor mechanism disruption (61) (Fig. 12-22). The degree of capsular and retinacular injury also can be visualized, particularly on axial images. Subsequent treatment decisions are then made.

Ultrasonography also has been used to evaluate extensor mechanism tendon rupture (62–64). We have no significant clinical experience with this technique.

Patellar Malalignment with Recurrent Subluxation

Patellar malalignment with recurrent subluxation is just one the many *chronic* conditions that can affect the patellofemoral joint. Exhaustive writings have reviewed these issues elsewhere (51,65–67), and here we will focus our efforts on this one condition. No effort will be made to detail the full evaluation of patellofemoral pain syndrome.

Patellar subluxation represents instability without frank dislocation. A history of previous frank dislocation may or may not be present. Patients will report "slipping" of the knee cap with activity, particularly with sudden motion or twisting. Clinically, extremity alignment, patellar mobility, and patellar tracking are evaluated. Most important is the finding of apprehension with mobility testing.

Nearly every possible imaging modality has

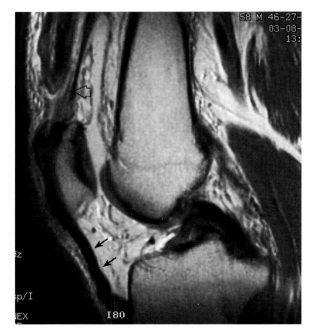

F I G U R E   **12-22**

Sagittal MRI demonstrating focal disruption of the quadriceps tendon at the superior aspect of the patella with retraction (*open arrow*). Surrounding soft tissue edema is seen, indicating relatively acute injury. The apparent redundancy in the patella tendon reflects the extensor mechanism disruption (*short black arrows*).

been evaluated regarding its usefulness in the evaluation of potential malalignment (31,68). Results are varied and sometimes conflicting. In general, our approach involves the use of plain radiographs as an initial step. These include AP, lateral, and infrapatellar Merchant or Laurin views. The AP and lateral views will assess patellar height. On the AP view, the inferior pole of the patella should be at the level of the roof of the intercondylar notch. On the lateral view (taken in 25 to 30 degrees of flexion), a number of indices can be calculated. The Insall and Salvati index is the ratio of the length of the patellar tendon to the length of the patella. A ratio of less than 0.8 is suggestive of patella baja, whereas a ratio of 1.2 or greater reflects patella alta (69) (Fig. 12-23). Patella alta is a contributing factor in patellar subluxation. An additional indicator of patella alta involves a lateral view taken in 90 degrees of knee flexion. If a line drawn across the anterior femoral cortex intersects the proximal pole of the patella, this is indicative of patella alta because this line intersects the patella in only 3% of the normal population.

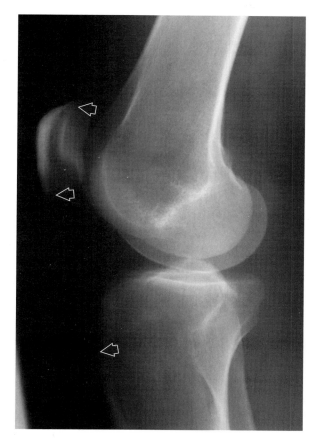

F I G U R E **12-23**

Lateral radiograph of the knee in a patient with anterior knee pain and a history of patellar subluxation. The Insall-Salvati ratio was determined to be 1.5, which is consistent with patella alta. The ratio is calculated by dividing the length of the patella tendon (distance between the bottom two arrows) by the length of the patella (distance between the top two arrows).

The infrapatellar radiograph will demonstrate the anatomy of the patellofemoral articulation. When interpreting these films, it is crucial to know the angle at which they were taken. Since nearly everyone will have seating of the patella within the trochlear groove at or above 90 degrees of flexion, views taken in this manner (such as the traditional "sunrise" or axial view) will not allow any inferences to be made regarding patellar congruence or tilt. The 45-degree Merchant view (70) and the 20- to 30-degree Laurin view (71,72) are more useful. While various angles and indices can be drawn and measured on these films and have been reported as predictive of patellofemoral pathology, in practice, they may not be that reproducible or reliable in patient management (73). They are useful, how-

ever, in that a hypoplastic trochlea, degenerative changes, and tendencies toward subluxation or tilt can be noted. It is important to image both knees simultaneously so that side-to-side comparisons can be made (Fig. 12-24). This can be particularly helpful if one knee is asymptomatic. We do not use CT or MRI routinely to evaluate for patellar congruency or tilt, although their use has been described and reviewed by others (55,58,65,68,74–81). Patellofemoral tracking has been evaluated more recently on cine MRI, allowing kinematic visualization of patellofemoral congruency and retinacular laxity (82,83).

Patellofemoral Chondromalacia

The term *chondromalacia* should be applied specifically to patients with known articular cartilage changes. It should not be used as a "wastebasket" term for all patients with clinical anterior knee pain (67,84,85). A specific diagnosis such as subluxation or excessive lateral pressure syndrome should be sought. There will be patients who present with anterior knee pain in whom examination and plain radiographs are unremarkable for evidence of malalignment or subluxation. At the time of arthroscopy, cartilage softening, fibrillation, and erosion have been found in such patients.

MRI can detect early cartilage changes and erosion consistent with a diagnosis of chondromalacia (86–88). The patellofemoral articulation is best evaluated on axial images. The normal cartilage will be of intermediate signal intensity on T1- and T2-weighted images (Fig. 12-25A). On high-contrast gradient-echo or fat-suppressed sequences, the cartilage will become hyperintense. The underlying subchondral bone is a low-intensity signal on both T1- and T2-weighted images.

The most reliable indicators of chondromalacia are focal contour irregularities and/or thinning of the hyaline cartilage associated with signal intensity changes within frank defects or contour irregularities on T2-weighted (87) and gradient-echo images (see Figs. 12-21 and 12-25B). Cartilage softening (grade 1 chondromalacia) is not reliably predicted on the basis of MRI findings but may be inferred by focal hyperintensity without an associated contour defect. While MRI may identify patellofemoral chondromalacia, the significance of these findings in each patient must be related to the individual patient's clinical symptoms, just as is the case with such findings when noted at arthro-

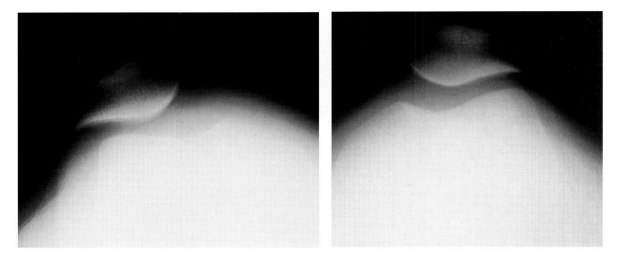

FIGURE **12-24**

Bilateral Merchant view of the knee demonstrating normal alignment on the right side with gross subluxation on the contralateral side.

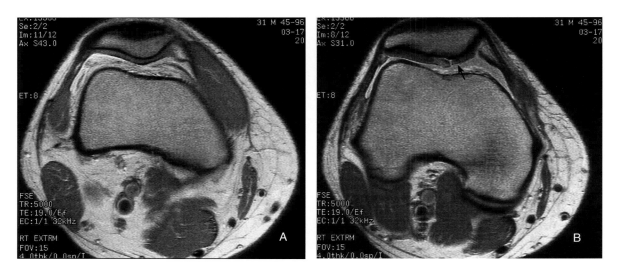

FIGURE **12-25**

(A) Normal uniform appearance of the patella cartilage is demonstrated on this axial high-resolution fast-spin-echo sequence. (B) Axial MRI demonstrating chondral flap tear, demonstrated by focal disruption (*arrow*) as well as adjacent signal hyperintensity within the lateral patella facet.

scopy (85). These same findings and statements apply to the femoral and tibial articular surfaces as well.

Bone Injury

Fracture

Fractures about the knee can be subdivided into stress fractures and complete injuries. The eval-

uation of stress fracture about the knee, although a relatively uncommon occurrence, should proceed in the fashion outlined earlier for femoral stress fractures.

With complete fractures about the knee, the critical determinants in management are whether or not the fracture is intra-articular and, if so, the degree of articular step-off present. Routine evaluation should start with plain film AP and lateral images. The lateral film can be taken in either full extension or slight flexion (20 to 30 degrees). Oblique views may help to identify the fracture lines in plateau fractures. In many cases, however, additional imaging will be required to ascertain the presence of significant articular step-off. This can be done with either trispiral tomography, CT scanning, or MRI (89,90).

Trispiral tomography is still useful in the evaluation of intra-articular fracture, although it has been replaced largely by current CT and MRI techniques. It allows imaging in both the sagittal and coronal planes and can provide the necessary detail for clinical decision making (91). Its major drawback is the time and significant radiation exposure involved.

CT can provide the necessary detail with less time and radiation exposure (90) and, currently, nearly similar expense. The one drawback of CT in this situation is that it requires image reconstruction to obtain sagittal views. The resulting step-off artifact can interfere with interpretation of the amount of articular incongruity present. Acquisition of images with smaller slice thicknesses can help reduce this difficulty but does increase the time and radiation exposure of the test. Still, it is probably the most commonly utilized test following conventional tomography in this situation.

There has been recent interest in the usefulness of MRI in evaluating intra-articular fractures. While the main drawback is cost, the MRI can obtain images directly in multiple planes without generating artifact like the CT and involves no radiation exposure. Once MRI was felt to be inferior for the imaging of bony fractures, but current techniques and experience suggest that it may be superior to CT for the evaluation of intra-articular fracture (92) (Fig. 12-26). Additionally, it allows for the evaluation of soft tissue injury that may be present.

Osteochondritis Dissecans

Osteochondritis dissecans (OCD) is a localized disease of the articular cartilage and its underlying bone. The etiology continues to be debated, with trauma and/or vascular ischemia being the leading theories. The clinical presentation of this condition is quite varied and in part depends on the size, location, and stability of the lesion. Intact lesions may present with only pain and effusion, whereas a loose or frankly displaced fragment will present with mechanical symptoms.

Plain radiographs should be obtained ini-

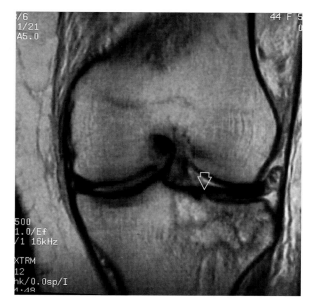

F I G U R E **12-26**

Coronal fast-spin-echo technique demonstrating the presence of a lateral tibial plateau fracture without depression of the articular surface (*arrow*). Aside from the presence of an effusion, plain films were unremarkable and did not show a fracture.

tially and should include a femoral notch or tunnel view. The notch view is an AP view taken with the knee in 40 to 45 degrees of flexion. The patient is positioned prone with the knee flexed and supported at the foot. The cassette is placed in front of the knee, and the beam is angled caudally at an angle of 40 degrees from the vertical. The notch view allows improved visualization of the posterior aspect of the femoral condyles, intercondylar notch, and intercondylar eminence of the tibia. The most common location of an OCD lesion is at the lateral aspect of the medial femoral condyle, and a standard AP view may not identify lesions in this location. Also, infrapatellar views should be obtained because lesions also can occur at this interface. On plain radiographs, an osteochondritic lesion will appear as an area of fragmentation or subchondral lucency that is well circumscribed by a sclerotic margin (Fig. 12-27A and B). Plain radiographs also may demonstrate frank dislodgment of the involved fragment, which then becomes a loose body in the knee.

The role of additional diagnostic studies is reserved for situations in which the degree of dislodgment or condition of the overlying articular cartilage is in question. Arthrography is invasive but will demonstrate any surface

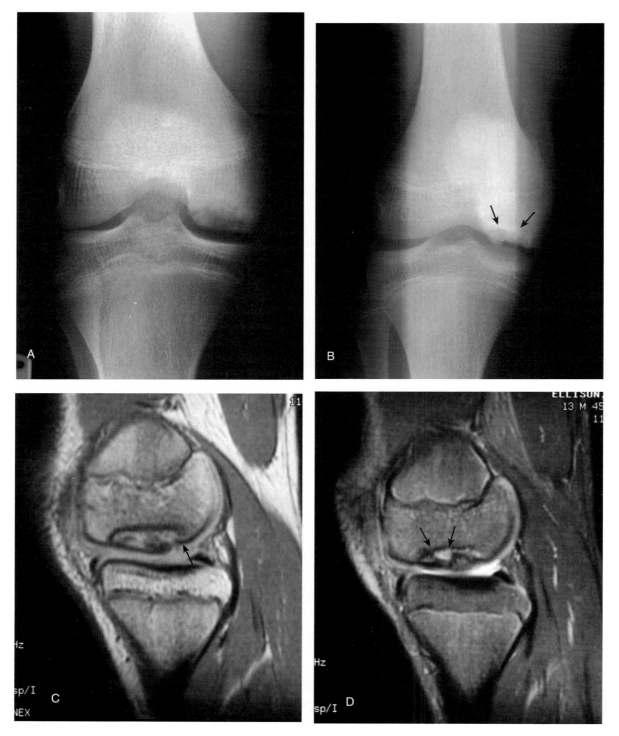

F I G U R E 12-27

AP (A) and notch (B) views of the left knee demonstrating an area of subchondral fragmentation in a patient nearing skeletal maturity. The lesion is primarily lucent with a surrounding sclerotic margin (*arrows*) and involves the weight-bearing aspect of the medial femoral condyle. This is the characteristic appearance of osteochondritis dissecans. (C) Sagittal proton density–weighted image of the same patient demonstrating contour irregularity of the surface of the medial femoral condyle with disruption of the subchondral plate at the posterior aspect of the lesion (*arrow*). (D) Sagittal fat-suppressed, fast-spin-echo sequence demonstrating cystic hyperintensity adjacent to the lesion (*arrows*). This indicates subchondral softening and, in conjunction with the disruption of the subchondral plate (part C), indicates a loose or partially detached osteochondritic fragment.

irregularity present at the site of the lesion. It also will show contrast material at the interface of the lesion and underlying bone if it is in fact partially separated with discontinuity of the overlying cartilage. These same findings can be identified on both arthrotomography and CT arthrography.

MRI is the preferable and noninvasive way of obtaining the same information (93–95). On T1-weighted images, the lesion may appear as a low to intermediate signal area within the subchondral bone, contrasted against the surrounding high signal of the normal fatty cancellous bone. The integrity of the overlying cartilage is best evaluated on T2-weighted, fat-suppressed, and gradient-echo images. The normal articular cartilage generates an intermediate signal intensity on T1-weighted images and a slightly increased intensity signal on T2-weighted and gradient-echo images. High signal within the cartilage or at the interface of the lesion and normal bone, indicating the presence of synovial fluid or granulation tissue at these areas, is consistent with loss of bone or cartilaginous integrity and suggests loosening (93,94) (see Fig. 12-27C and D). In our experience, prominent cystic changes at the interface between the native bone and the lesion often correlate with loosening at arthroscopic evaluation. In the extreme case, complete displacement of the fragment with a subsequent cavity in the articular surface may be apparent (94).

Loose Bodies

Loose bodies present clinically with intermittent mechanical symptoms. Their most common source is from pre-existing osteoarthritis, OCD, or osteochondral fracture. If they contain a significant amount of bone, they may be visualized on plain films. There position may be noted to change on sequential films, confirming the fact that they are free to move about the joint. One should be careful not to mistakenly identify the fabella, a sesamoid within the lateral head of the gastrocnemius, as a loose body.

If a loose body is suspected by history but not apparent by conventional radiography, further imaging may be indicated. In this situation it is likely that the fragment is completely cartilaginous. Historically, arthrotomography was useful in this situation. Currently, MRI offers a noninvasive choice. Additionally, MRI allows evaluation of other structures in the knee, particularly the menisci, which actually may be the cause of the patient's symptoms.

Detection of the loose body by MRI relies on the plane of the image coinciding with the location of the loose body at the time of scanning. In order to increase the sensitivity of MRI, imaging in all three planes (coronal, axial, and sagittal) should be done. Thus, while a "positive" MRI study is diagnostic, a poorly performed "negative" one may simply have skipped over the location of the fragment.

Pigmented Villonodular Synovitis

Pigmented villonodular synovitis (PVNS) is a localized, benign, proliferative disorder of the synovium. It can involve any joint, but the knee is the most common site (80% of cases). Patients can present with mechanical symptoms or with hemarthrosis that occurs spontaneously or following minimal trauma. Pain is the most common complaint. Plain radiographs should be obtained. Typically, they are negative, but occasionally they will demonstrate an area of well-circumscribed invasion or erosion at the joint surface, occasionally at both articular surfaces (96). Given the preceding patient presentation, when the lytic areas are observed on both sides of the joint, they are considered virtually pathognomonic for PVNS (97). The diagnosis can be confirmed by MRI (discussed next), or one can proceed with surgical intervention to resect the lesion.

If plain films are negative and PVNS is suspected, an MRI should be obtained. The MRI will show a low-intensity mass on T1-weighted images that becomes more hypointense on T2-weighted and gradient-echo images (98,99). This phenomenon, called *dephasing,* is due to the hemosiderin content of the lesion and is highly suggestive of PVNS (39) (Fig. 12-28). Following resection, the MRI is an easy way to evaluate for suspected recurrence.

Synovial Chondromatosis

Synovial chondromatosis represents a metaplastic condition of the synovial lining in which a focus of the synovial lining generates multiple osteocartilaginous loose bodies. Any synovial joint can be involved, but the knee and shoulder are the most common sites. Patients present with mechanical complaints due to the multiple loose bodies. Alternatively, if the productive

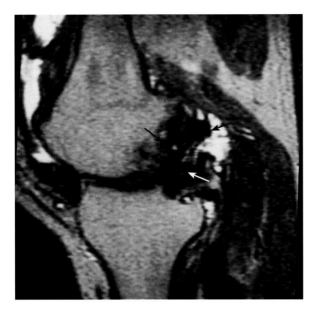

Sagittal T2-weighted image demonstrating markedly diminished signal intensity within the synovium, as well as extending through the intercondylar notch (*arrows*). This signal, indicating heavily pigmented synovium, represents a focal dephasing effect due to the presence of hemosiderin, which is characteristic of PVNS.

focus is located within a recess that does not communicate freely with the joint, symptoms relating to a subsequent mass effect may develop.

Plain radiographs are usually diagnostic. They will show multiple, sometimes hundreds, of variably sized mineralized lesions. Due to the cartilaginous nature of the process, the mineralization pattern will be that of stippled rings or lobules (97). The bony architecture of the knee joint itself usually remains undisturbed, but bony erosions rarely may be present. In the presence of nonmineralized bodies, CT arthrography or MRI will confirm the diagnosis by showing the multiple distinct cartilaginous bodies.

Cysts

Cysts frequently are found around the knee joint and usually are popliteal or meniscal in origin. Popliteal cysts develop in the semimembranous bursa and present as a posterior popliteal mass. Plain radiographs will be unremarkable or, with large cysts, may show a large fluid shadow posteriorly. Ultrasonography will easily confirm the

diagnosis if it remains in question after physical examination and plain radiography. MRI is more costly but also will readily demonstrate the cyst as a homogeneous low signal on T1-weighted images that becomes homogeneously hyperintense on T2-weighted images (31,100).

Meniscal cysts occur in conjunction with meniscus tears, most commonly laterally, and represent extravasation of joint fluid through the meniscal tear into the meniscocapsular junction. Like popliteal cysts, the diagnosis usually can be made based on history, physical examination, and plain radiography. Ultrasound can confirm the diagnosis. If an MRI is done, a meniscal cyst usually appears as a uniformly low-intensity signal on T1-weighted images and a hyperintense signal on T2-weighted images but may contain internal debris. The associated meniscus tear also should be evident (61,81).

REFERENCES

1. Burkett LN. Causative factors in hamstring strain. Med Sci Sport Exerc 1970;2:39–42.

2. McMaster PE. Tendon and muscle ruptures. J Bone Joint Surg 1933;15A:705–722.

3. Zarins B, Cuillo J. Acute muscle and tendon injuries in athletes. Clin Sports Med 1983;2:167–182.

4. Brewer BJ. Mechanism of injury to the musculotendinous unit. Instr Course Lect 1960;17:354–358.

5. Garrett WE. Basic science of musculotendinous injuries. In: Nicholas JA, Hershman EB, eds. The lower extremity and spine in sports medicine. St Louis: Mosby, 1986.

6. Young JL, Laskowski ER, Rock MG. Thigh injuries in athletes. Mayo Clin Proc 1993;68:1099–1106.

7. Brunet ME, Hontas RB. The thigh. In: De Lee JC, Drez D, eds. Orthopedic sports medicine: principles and practice. Philadelphia: WB Saunders, 1994.

8. Fleckenstein JL, Weatherall PT, Parkey RW, et al. Sports-related muscle injuries: evaluation with MR imaging. Radiology 1989;172:793–798.

9. DeSmet AA, Fisher DR, Heiner JB, Keene JS. Magnetic resonance imaging of muscle tears. Skeletal Radiol 1990;19:283–286.

10. Dooms GC, Fisher MR, Hricak H, Higgins CB. MR imaging of intramuscular hemorrhage. J Comput Assist Tomogr 1985;9:908–913.

11. Ryan AJ. Quadriceps strain, rupture, and charley horse. Med Sci Sports 1969;1:106–111.

12. Kirkpatrick JS, Koman LA, Rovere GD. The role of ultrasound in the early diagnosis of myositis ossificans: a case report. Am J Sports Med 1987; 15:179–181.

13. Baker BE. Current concepts in the diagnosis and treatment of musculotendinous injuries. Med Sci Sports Ever 1984;16:323–327.

14. Kransdorf MJ, Meis JM, Jelinek JS. Myositis ossificans: MR appearance with radiologic-pathologic correlation. AJR 1991;157:1243–1248.

15. Drane WE. Myositis ossificans and the three-phase bone scan. AJR 1984;142:179–180.

16. Lee JK, Yao L. Stress fractures: MR imaging. Radiology 1988;169:217–220.

17. Rupani HD, Holder LE, Espinola DA, Engin SI. Three-phase radionuclide bone imaging in sports medicine. Radiology 1985;156:187–196.

18. Wilcox JR, Moniot AL, Green JP. Bone scanning in the evaluation of exercise-related stress injuries. Radiology 1977;123:699–703.

19. Stafford SA, Rosenthal DI, Gebhardt MC, et al. MRI in stress fracture. AJR 1986;147:553–556.

20. Rizzo PF, Gould ES, Lyden JP, Asnis SE. Diagnosis of occult fractures about the hip. J Bone Joint Surg 1993;75A:395–401.

21. Hall FH. Radiographic diagnosis and accuracy in knee joint effusions. Radiology 1990;176:479–483.

22. Dehaven KE. Decision-making factors in the treatment of meniscus lesions. Clin Orthop 1990;252:49–54.

23. Rosenberg TD, Paulos LE, Parker RD, et al. The forty-five degree posteroanterior flexion weight-bearing radiograph of the knee. J Bone Joint Surg 1988;70A:1479–1483.

24. Kornick J, Trefelner E, McCarthy S, et al. Meniscal abnormalities in the asymptomatic population at MR imaging. Radiology 1990;177:463–465.

25. Jackson DW, Jennings LD, Maywood RM, Berger PE. Magnetic resonance imaging of the knee. Am J Sports Med 1988;16:29–47.

26. Polly DW, Callaghan JJ, Sikes RA, et al. The accuracy of selective magnetic resonance imaging compared with the findings of arthroscopy of the knee. J Bone Joint Surg 1988;70A: 192–198.

27. Crues JV, Mink J, Levy TL, et al. Meniscal tears of the knee: accuracy of MR imaging. Radiology 1987;164:445–448.

28. Kelly MA, Flock TJ, Kimmel JA, et al. MR imaging of the knee: clarification of its role. Arthroscopy 1991;7:78–85.

29. Reicher MA, Hartzman S, Bassett LW, et al. MR imaging of the knee: I. Traumatic disorders. Radiology 1987;162:547–551.

30. Mink JH, Levy T, Crues JV. Tears of the anterior cruciate ligament and menisci of the knee: MR imaging evaluation. Radiology 1988;167:769–774.

31. Berquist TH. Imaging of sports injuries. Gaithersburg, MD: Aspen, 1992.

32. Preston BJ. Arthrography. In: Galasko CSB, Isherwood I, eds. Imaging techniques in orthopedics. New York: Springer-Verlag, 1989.

33. Dumas JM, Edde DJ. Meniscal abnormalities: prospective correlation of double-contrast arthrography and arthroscopy. Radiology 1986; 160:453–456.

34. Freiberger RH, Pavlov H. Knee arthrography. Radiology 1988;166:489–492.

35. Herman LJ, Beltran J. Pitfalls in MR imaging of the knee. Radiology 1988;167:775–781.

36. Carpenter WA. Meniscofemoral ligament simulating tear of the lateral meniscus: MR features. J Comput Assist Tomogr 1990;14:1033–1034.

37. Warren RF, Kaplan N, Bach BR. The lateral notch sign of anterior cruciate ligament insufficiency. Am J Knee Surg 1988;1:119–124.

38. Cobby MJ, Schweitzer ME, Resnick D. The deep lateral femoral notch: an indirect sign of a torn anterior cruciate ligament. Radiology 1992;184: 855–858.

39. Goldman AB, Pavlov H, Rubenstein D. The Segond fracture of the proximal tibia: a small avulsion fracture that reflects ligamentous damage. AJR 1988;151:1163–1167.

40. Pavlov H. The cruciate ligaments. In: Freiberger RH, Kaye JJ, eds. Arthrography. New York: Appleton-Century-Crofts, 1979.

41. Pavlov H, Warren RF, Sherman MF, Cayea PD. The accuracy of double-contrast arthrographic evaluation of the anterior cruciate ligament. J Bone Joint Surg 1983;65A:175.

42. Lee JK, Yao L, Phelps CT, et al. Anterior cruciate ligament tears: MR imaging compared with arthroscopy and clinical tests. Radiology 1988; 166:861–864.

43. Speer KP, Spritzer CE, Bassett FH, et al. Osseous injury associated with acute tears of the anterior

cruciate ligament. Am J Sports Med 1992;20: 382–389.

44. Murphy BJ, Smith RL, Uribe JW, et al. Bone signal abnormalities in the posterolateral tibia and lateral femoral condyle in complete tears of the anterior cruciate ligament: a specific sign? Radiology 1992;182:221–224.

45. Nawata K, Teshima R, Suzuki T. Osseous lesions associated with anterior cruciate ligament injuries: assessment by magnetic resonance imaging at various periods after injuries. Arch Orthop Trauma Surg 1993;113:1–4.

46. Fetto JF, Marshal JL. Medial collateral ligament injuries of the knee: a rationale for treatment. Clin Orthop 1978;132:206–217.

47. O'Donoghue DH. Surgical treatment of fresh injuries to the major ligaments of the knee. J Bone Joint Surg 1950;32A:721.

48. Mink JH, Deutsch AL. The knee. In: Mink JH, Deutsch AL, eds. MRI of the musculoskeletal system: a teaching file. New York: Raven Press, 1990:251–387.

49. Mink JH. The ligaments of the knee. In: Mink JH, ed. Magnetic resonance imaging of the knee. New York: Raven Press, 1987.

50. Burstein DB, Fischer DA. Isolated rupture of the popliteus tendon in a professional athlete. Arthroscopy 1990;6:238–241.

51. Ficat RP, Hungerford DS. Disorders of the patellofemoral joint. Baltimore: Williams & Wilkins, 1977.

52. Bassett FH II. Acute dislocation of the patella, osteochondral fractures, and injuries of the extensor mechanism of the knee. Instr Course Lect 1976;25:40–49.

53. Freiberger RH, Kozier LM. Fracture of the medial margin of the patella: a finding diagnostic of lateral dislocation. Radiology 1967;88: 902–904.

54. Virolainen H, Visuri T, Kuusela T. Acute dislocation of the patella: MR findings. Radiology 1993;189:243–246.

55. Koskinen SK, Kujula UM. Patellofemoral relationships and the distal insertion of the vastus medialis muscle: a magnetic resonance imaging study in nonsymptomatic patients and in patients with patellar dislocation. Arthroscopy 1992;8:465–468.

56. Lance E, Deutsch AL, Mink JH. Prior lateral patellar dislocation: MR imaging findings. Radiology 1993;189:905–907.

57. Kelly DW, Carter VS, Jobe FW, Kerlan RK. Patellar and quadriceps tendon ruptures—jumper's knee. Am J Sports Med 1984;12:375–380.

58. Tarsney FF. Catastrophic jumper's knee: a case report. Am J Sports Med 1981;9:60–61.

59. Kuivila TE, Brems JJ. Diagnosis of acute rupture of the quadriceps tendon by magnetic resonance imaging: a case report. Clin Orthop 1991;262:236–241.

60. Zeiss J, Saddemi SR, Ebraheim NA. MR imaging of the quadriceps tendon: normal layered configuration and its importance in cases of tendon rupture. AJR 1992;159:1031–1034.

61. Berlin RC, Levinsohn EM, Chrisman H. The wrinkled patellar tendon: an indication of abnormality in the extensor mechanism of the knee. Skeletal Radiol 1991;20:181–185.

62. Fornage BD, Rifkin MD, Touche DH, Segal PM. Sonography of the patellar tendon: preliminary observations. AJR 1984;143:179–182.

63. Kalebo P, Sward L, Karlsson J, Peterson L. Ultrasonography in the detection of partial patellar ligament ruptures (jumpers knee). Skeletal Radiol. 1991;20:285–289.

64. Karlsson J, Kalebo P, Goksor L, et al. Partial rupture of the patellar ligament. Am J Sports Med 1992;20:390–395.

65. Fulkerson JP, Shea KP. Disorders of patellofemoral alignment. J Bone Joint Surg 1990;72A: 1424–1429.

66. Leach RE. Malalignment syndrome of the patella. Inst Course Lect 1976;25:46–54.

67. Merchant AC. Classification of patellofemoral disorders. Arthroscopy 1988;4:235–240.

68. Ghelman B, Hodge JC. Imaging of the patellofemoral joint. Orthop Clin 1992;23:523–543.

69. Insall J, Goldberg V, Salvati E. Recurrent dislocation and the high-riding patella. Clin Orthop 1972;88:67–69.

70. Merchant AC, Mercer RL, Jacobsen RH. Roentgenographic analysis of patellofemoral congruence. J Bone Joint Surg 1974;56A:1391–1396.

71. Laurin CA, Levesque HP, Dussault R, et al. The abnormal lateral patellofemoral angle: a diagnostic roentgenographic sign of recurrent subluxation. J Bone Joint Surg 1978;60A:55–60.

72. Laurin CA, Dussault R, Levesque HP. The tangential x-ray investigation of the patellofemoral angle. Clin Orthop 1979;144:16–26.

73. Minkoff J, Fein L. The role of radiography in the evaluation and treatment of common arthritic disorders. Clin Sports Med 1989;8:203–260.

74. Inoue M, Shino K, Hirose H, et al. Subluxation of the patella: computed tomographic analysis of patellofemoral congruence. J Bone Joint Surg 1988;70A:1331–1337.

75. Schutzer SF, Ramsby GR, Fulkerson JP. Computed tomographic classification of patellofemoral pain patients. Orthop Clin North Am 1986;17:235–248.

76. Shellock FG, Mink JH, Fox JM. Patellofemoral joint: kinematic MR imaging to assess tracking abnormalities. Radiology 1988;168:551–553.

77. Kajula UM, Osterman K, Kormano M. Patellar motion analyzed by magnetic resonance imaging. Acta Orthop Scand 1989;60:13–16.

78. Ghelman B, Hodge JC. Imaging of the patellofemoral joint. Orthop Clin North Am 1992;23: 523–543.

79. Shellock FG. Patellofemoral joint abnormalities in athletes: evaluation by kinematic magnetic resonance imaging. Top Magn Reson Imaging 1991;3:71–95.

80. Inoue M, Shino K, Hirose H, Ono K. Subluxation of the patella: computed tomography of patellofemoral congruence. J Bone Joint Surg 1983;70A:1331–1377.

81. Shellock FG, Mink JH, Deutsch AL, Fox JM. Patellar tracking abnormalities: clinical experience with kinematic MR imaging in 130 patients. Radiology 1989;172:799–804.

82. Brossman J, Muhle C, Schroder C, et al. Patellar tracking patterns during active and passive knee extension: evaluation with motion-triggered cine MR imaging. Radiology 1993;187:205–212.

83. Shellock FG, Deutsch AL, Mink JH. Patellofemoral joint: advanced kinematic MRI techniques. Appl Radiol 1994;23–31.

84. Hughston JC. Patellar subluxation: a recent history. Clin Sports Med 1989;8:153–162.

85. Royle SG, Noble J, Davies D, Kay PR. The significance of chondromalacic changes on the patella. Arthroscopy 1991;7:158–160.

86. Ochi M, Sumen Y, Kanda T, et al. The diagnostic value and limitation of magnetic resonance imaging on chondral lesions in the knee joint. Arthroscopy 1994;10:176–183.

87. Brown TR, Quinn SF. Evaluation of chondromalacia of the patellofemoral compartment with axial magnetic resonance imaging. Skeletal Radiol 1993;22:325–328.

88. Hayes CW, Sawyer RW, Conway WF. Patellar cartilage lesions: in vitro detection and staging with MR imaging and pathologic correlation. Radiology 1990;176:479–483.

89. Apple JS, Martinez S, Allen NB, et al. Occult fractures of the knee: tomographic evaluation. Radiology 1983;148:383–387.

90. Rafii M, Firooznic H, Golimbu C, Bonamo J. Computed tomography of tibial plateau fractures. AJR 1984;142:1181–1186.

91. Elstrom J, Pankovich AM, Sasson H, Rodriguez J. The use of tomography in assessment of fractures of the tibial plateau. J Bone Joint Surg 1976;58A:551–555.

92. Kode L, Leiberman JM, Motta AO, et al. Evaluation of tibial plateau fractures: efficacy of MR imaging compared with CT. AJR 1994;163:141–147.

93. DeSmet AA, Fisher DR, Graf BK, Lange RH. Osteochondritis dissecans of the knee: value of MR imaging in determining lesion stability and the presence of articular cartilage defects. AJR 1990;155:549–553.

94. Mesgarzadeh M, Sapega AA, Bonakdarpour A, et al. Osteochondritis dissecans: analysis of mechanical stability with radiographic scintigraphy and MR imaging. Radiology 1987;165:775–780.

95. Nelson DW, DiPaola J, Colville M, Schmidgall J. Osteochondritis dissecans of the talus and knee: prospective comparison of MR and arthroscopic classification. J Comput Assist Tomogr 1990;14: 804–808.

96. Dorwart RH, Genant HK, Johnston WH, Morris JM. Pigmented villonodular synovitis of synovial joints: clinical, pathologic and radiologic features. AJR 1984;143:877–885.

97. Murray RO, Jacobson HG. Benign neoplasms. In: The radiology of skeletal disorders. New York: Churchill-Livingstone, 1977.

98. Kottal RA, Vogler JB III, Matamoros A, et al. Pigmented villonodular synovitis: a report of MR imaging in two cases. Radiology 1987;163:551–553.

99. Poletti SC, Gates HS, Martinez SM, Richardson WJ. The use of magnetic resonance imaging in the diagnosis of pigmented villonodular synovitis. Orthopedics 1990;13:185–190.

100. Burk DL, Dalinka MK, Kanal E, et al. Meniscal and ganglion cysts of the knee: MR evaluation. AJR 1988;150:331–336.

CHAPTER *13*

Lower Leg Injuries

ROBERT MONACO

BRIAN HALPERN

E. LEE RICE

MICHAEL A. CATALANO

The lower leg, between the knee and the ankle, is a frequent site of injury in athletics. These injuries comprise up to 30% of the conditions seen at some sports medicine clinics (1,2). Thorough history and physical examination skills are often all that are required to make the correct diagnosis. However, physicians have a variety of imaging modalities at their disposal to help with diagnosis, prognosis, and treatment.

Plain films, including anteroposterior (AP) and lateral views, are simple, readily available, relatively inexpensive, and often suffice to help make the correct diagnosis. Bone lesions not apparent on plain film x-rays often may be assessed by triple-phase radionuclide bone scanning. Magnetic resonance imaging (MRI) is unsurpassed in its evaluation of soft tissue lesions and is increasingly useful for bony lesions such as stress fractures. Computed tomography (CT) can help better determine the extent of bony involvement. Ultrasound also plays a role in specific conditions, especially with the use of Doppler to diagnose vascular problems.

Chronic and Overuse Injuries

Injuries to the lower leg are often secondary to overuse phenomena. The most common of these are medial tibial stress syndrome (MTSS) and stress fractures. Chronic exertional compartment syndrome also must be considered in the differential diagnosis of these conditions, which are discussed below.

Medial Tibial Stress Syndrome

Medial tibial stress syndrome (MTSS) is a more specific diagnosis for the older term *shin splint syndrome* (3). It consists of pain over the posterior medial tibia in the middle and distal thirds of the leg. It may result from muscle weakness, anatomic malalignment, or errors in training technique (e.g., sudden increase in activity, excessive mileage, poor footwear, inappropriate surface). Many feel that it results from inflammation of the soleus muscle at its insertion into the posteromedial border of the tibia (4). The flexor digitorum longus muscle also may play a significant role (5). The syndrome, by definition, excludes stress fractures, compartment syndromes, and ischemic disease.

Medial tibial stress syndrome accounts for about 13% of injuries in runners (6). Patients usually have diffuse pain with exertion over the posteromedial tibia about 4 to 12 cm proximal to the medial malleolus (3,7). Active resisted plantar flexion or toe raises may exacerbate the pain (4).

Routine x-rays of the leg (AP and lateral) are often normal. However, they occasionally may show hypertrophy of the posteromedial cortex of the tibia or a faint periosteal reaction. Triple-phase bone scans show a characteristic pattern in medial tibial stress syndrome that clearly distinguishes it from a stress fracture (8–15). Typically, there is a moderate diffuse increased uptake of radionuclide along the posterior aspect of the tibia on *delayed* images. Phases one (radionuclide angiograms) and two (blood-pool images) are always normal. Figure 13-1 depicts the classic bone scan findings of MTSS. The

bone scan differences between MTSS and stress fractures are noted in Table 13-1. MTSS responds extremely well to a conservative treatment plan.

Stress Fractures

Stress fractures of the lower leg are extremely common in athletes. In a population of runners, the incidence ranges from 4% to 16% (16,17). A stress fracture is a partial or complete fracture of a bone resulting from its inability to withstand nonviolent stress that is applied in a rhythmic, repeated subthreshold manner (18). The repetitive stress exceeds the bone's normal remodeling response of hypertrophy and results in microcortical fracture(s). Stress fractures are associated most commonly with a sudden change (increase) in activity. They are also clearly multifactorial in etiology. Other associated factors include hard surfaces, poor footwear, lower limb malalignment, amenorrhea, poor calcium intake, and eating disorders (1,19).

Tibial Stress Fractures

In athletes, the tibia (49%) is the most common bone to have a stress fracture (16). Tibial stress fractures may represent 10% of the injuries that present to a sports medicine practice (18). When stress fractures occur in the tibia, they are commonly in the posteromedial area in the proximal or distal third. They are classically on the compressive side of the bone in the posteromedial region and rarely in the central region. This location helps distinguish these injuries from more ominous stress fractures, which occur on the anterior central portion of the tibia and medial

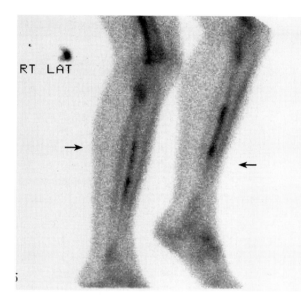

F I G U R E   **13-1**

Bone scan findings in medial tibial stress syndrome. Delayed bone scan imaging shows diffuse moderate increased uptake (*arrows*) along the posteromedial distal third of the tibia, consistent with medial tibial stress syndrome.

T A B L E   **13-1**

Bone Scan Appearance of Medial Tibial Stress Syndrome Versus Stress Fracture

	MTSS (Fig. 13-1)	**Stress Fracture (Fig. 13-4)**
Phase	Only positive on delayed images	Any phase can be positive
Shape	Linear/vertical	Round/fusiform
Location	Posterior medial tibia	Anywhere in lower leg
Intensity	1+ to 3+ with varying uptake along length	Can be 1+ or 3+
Length	Nearly one third of the bone	Less than 20% of the bone

SOURCE: Adapted from Matire JR. The role of nuclear medicine scans in evaluating pain in athletic injuries. Clin Sports Med 1987;6:713–737; and Rupani H, Holder L, Espinola D, Engin S. Three phase radionuclide bone imaging in sports medicine. Radiology 1985;156:187–196.

malleolus. These two stress fractures carry a much worse prognosis and are discussed in detail below.

In the early stages, stress fractures can be confused easily with MTSS. However, if the offending exercise persists, the athlete begins to note pain during routine activities of daily living. The pain is often localized to a particular focal point over the tibia.

Imaging evaluation of suspected stress fractures should begin with plain AP and lateral x-rays of the lower leg. Oblique views also may prove to be useful. Findings on x-rays are variable, since usually 2 to 3 weeks of symptoms are required for bone changes to be observed (20,21). Initial findings may include subtle blurring of the trabecular margins and small, fluffy densities corresponding to new bone formation (21). As the stress fracture begins to mature, typical findings, when present, include slight periosteal reaction, sometimes associated with scalloping or subperiosteal resorption. Occasionally, a small fracture line can be seen. Figure 13-2 reveals early x-ray findings in a distal tibial stress fracture. As the process continues and the stress fracture matures, x-rays usually reveal periosteal new bone formation, with endosteal thickening and cortical hypertrophy. Features of a well-healed stress fracture are shown in Figure 13-3.

If initial x-rays are negative, the clinician can either manage clinically or repeat serial x-rays beginning at 2 weeks to see if bony changes are now revealed. It often takes 10 to 21 days for a lesion that is positive on a bone scan to show up on standard x-rays (21,22). However, up to 50% of bone scan–positive stress fractures may continue to demonstrate normal plain x-rays (21).

A more definitive diagnosis can be made promptly with the use of triple-phase technetium bone scanning (8–14,23). Bone scans are clearly far more sensitive and reliable than plain x-rays. The bone scan may be positive as early as 6 hours after symptoms but usually takes 2 to 8 days (16,21,24,25). False-negative nuclide studies with stress fractures are exceedingly rare and may be most likely due to technical factors (26).

Bone scans show characteristic focal fusiform uptake, which is readily distinguishable from the linear diffuse uptake of MTSS (23) (see Table 13-1). Bone scan findings in a posteromedial tibial stress fracture are shown in Figure 13-4. Bone scans also can help determine the

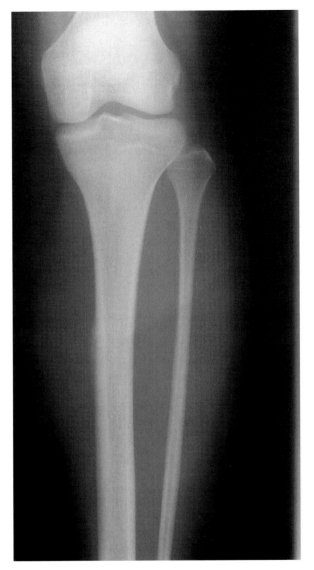

FIGURE   13-2

Radiographic findings in early stress fractures. Anteroposterior x-rays reveal increased periosteal reaction with cortical thickening on the posteromedial tibia consistent with an early stress fracture.

age of stress fractures. At the 2- to 4-week period, all phases of a bone scan (dynamic, blood pool, and delayed) will be positive. As healing progresses, dynamic angiogram (phase 1) and eventually blood-pool phases become negative. Delayed activity persists for about 3 months and then slowly decreases from 3 to 8 months. It can still be positive at 12 months or more. Table 13-2 summarizes the dating of stress fractures by bone scan (13,23).

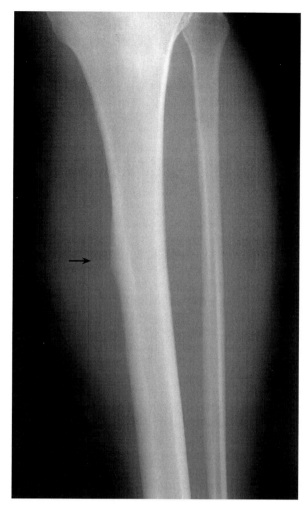

F I G U R E   13-3

Radiographic findings in mature stress fractures. Anteroposterior x-rays reveal periosteal new bone formation (*arrow*) with endosteal thickening and cortical hypertrophy. This is consistent with a mature stress fracture.

It is not uncommon to find multiple areas of increased uptake on bone scans in these patients. Studies show that approximately 40% of the positive findings are not symptomatic (11,14). These may represent subclinical areas of increased bone strain or "stress remodeling" consistent with the continuum of bony stress changes (12,27,28). They may go on to frank stress fracture if the repetitive loading is not interrupted. Full lower extremity triple-phase bone scans are thus ordered so as to help assess these other areas of bone strain that can go on to a full stress fracture. Clinicians also must remember that not all focal bone abnormalities on

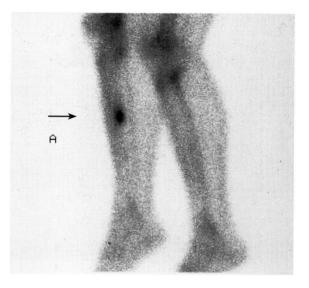

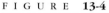

F I G U R E   13-4

Bone scan findings in tibial stress fractures. Delayed images of the lower leg show focal fusiform uptake (*arrow*) in the posteromedial tibia consistent with a stress fracture.

radiographs and bone scans are stress fractures. They also may represent other bony pathologies, such as osteomyelitis, osteogenic sarcoma, osteoid osteoma, Paget's disease, exostoses, or tumors that result in periosteal reaction or peripheral bone destruction (22,29,30). Clinical history often helps distinguish these conditions.

MRI is becoming increasingly utilized for the evaluation of bone stress injuries. It can be extremely useful and is appealing because it is noninvasive and lacks radiation exposure. Compared with bone scans, MRI remains expensive and may not, at this time, provide additional information that changes clinical management. MRI may, however, demonstrate occult fracture earlier than bone scintigraphy and help provide a biologic assessment of the state of the fracture (31,32). It also may help increase specificity, since it can improve the ability to determine conditions such as osteomyelitis and bone tumor (33).

Typically, early stress fractures on MRI reveal focal marrow edema, characterized by diminished signal intensity on T1-weighted images with corresponding increased signal intensity on T2-weighted or fat-suppressed images (Fig. 13-5) (30,32,34,35). Figure 13-6 reveals MRI findings in a tibial stress fracture. Arendt and colleagues further defined four clinical categories based on the bone scan and MRI

T A B L E **13-2**

Dating of Stress Fractures by Bone Scan

Phase	0–4 Weeks	4–8 Weeks	8 Weeks to 12 Months
Dynamic	+ to ++	—	—
Blood pool	+ to ++	+	Gradually decreases
Delayed	+++	+++	+++ to 12 weeks ++ from 3–8 months + up to 12 months

Note: + = minimally increased activity, barely perceptible above the normal soft tissue or bone; ++ = moderately increased activity obviously greater than the adjacent soft tissue or bone and easily visualized; +++ = intense activity, equaling that of growth plate regions in younger patients.

SOURCE: Adapted and modified from Matire JR. The role of nuclear medicine scans in evaluating pain in athletic injuries. Clin Sports Med 1987;6:713–737; and Rupani H, Holder L, Espinola D, Engin S. Three phase radionuclide bone imaging in sports medicine. Radiology 1985;156:187–196.

image (34,36). These correlated with the pathologic spectrum from bone strain and stress to frank fracture. Grades I and II included early marrow edema, which progressed to grade III (osseous stress phenomena with periosteal changes) and on to grade IV (frank cortical breaks). Table 13-3 summarizes these findings. Attempts are being made to correlate MRI findings with prognosis and treatment plans.

MRI, at certain centers, appears to be quickly becoming the imaging modality of choice for specific stress fractures. These stress fractures usually include those more difficult to diagnose, such as femoral neck and pelvic stress fractures, and those in flat bones such as the metatarsals. However, at this time, MRI of potential stress fractures of the long bones of the tibia and fibula appears more technically challenging, is costly, and cannot be recommended routinely over plain films or bone scans. Future changes in techniques, such as, for example, limited imaging protocols with STIR images, may address the issues of cost. Further research using MRI may lead to earlier and more precise diagnosis, allowing for accelerated rehabilitation programs and quicker return to competition. The future of MRI is very promising for stress fracture assessment.

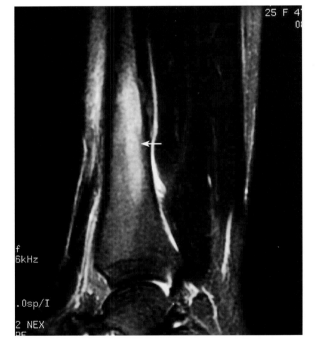

F I G U R E **13-5**

MRI of stress fracture. T2-weighted sagittal images show a longitudinal hyperintense signal in the bone marrow of the distal tibia and disruption of a thickened posterior cortex. This is diagnostic of a stress fracture.

Anterior Tibial Stress Fractures

Pain on the anterior central region of the tibia is suggestive of an anterior tibial stress fracture. The etiology is believed to be due to the repetitive forceful contraction of the flexor leg muscles, and this injury occurs primarily in athletes who perform jumping activities (1,37,38). These lesions are located on the tension side of the

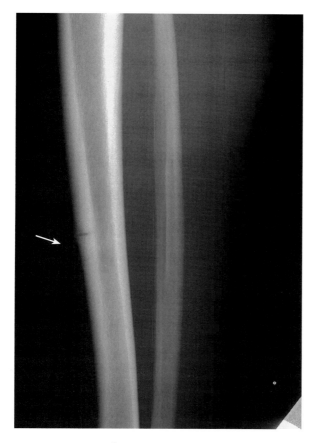

FIGURE **13-6**

Anterior tibia stress fracture. Lateral radiographs of the leg reveal the dreaded black line on the anterior tibial cortex (*arrow*). These stress fractures are noted for their long healing time and high rate of nonunion.

bone and have poor vascular supply. They take extensive time to heal (months), especially if not diagnosed early. When diagnosed late, histopathologic findings have been consistent with nonunion (38). Surgery is often required for these debilitating stress fractures.

As in most stress fractures, initial x-rays are often negative. Mature anterior tibial stress fractures, however, often will reveal anterior cortical thickening and the "dreaded black line" of a horizontal fracture (see Fig. 13-6). Clinicians must have a high level of suspicion for this stress fracture and proceed quickly with the appropriate imaging modalities to confirm the diagnosis. Bone scans may be used, but when used late, they may show only a minimally or mildly positive study despite obvious radiographic abnormalities (29). Negative scans may be secondary to bone infarct in the area of initial stress (25,39). MRI therefore may play a larger role for these fractures. These fractures need to be followed closely and reimaged, especially if pain persists or worsens. They carry one of the worst prognosis of all stress fractures of the lower leg.

Another anterior tibial stress fracture occurs proximally on the tibia and many times has a larger posteromedial component. This stress fracture carries a much better prognosis than the aforementioned lower anterior tibial stress fracture. This stress fracture is often mistaken for a pes bursitis. It should be highly suspected in the well-trained athlete, especially a distance runner, who gives the classic history of a stress fracture,

T A B L E **13-3**

Radiologic Grading of Stress Fractures

	X-Ray	**Bone Scan**	**MRI**
Normal	Normal	Normal	Normal
Grade I	Normal	Poorly defined area of increased activity	Positive STIR; negative T1, T2
Grade II	Normal	More intense but still poorly defined	Positive T2; negative T1
Grade III	Discrete line; discrete periosteal reaction	Sharply marginated area of increased activity (focal or fusiform)	Positive T1, T2; no definite cortical break; periosteal changes
Grade IV	Fracture or periosteal reaction	More intense transcortical uptake	Positive T1, T2 with fracture line

SOURCE: Adapted from Arendt EA, Clohisy DR. Stress injuries of bone. In: Hershman EB, Nicholas JA, eds. The lower extremity and spine in sports medicine. Vol 1. St Louis: Mosby, 1995:65–79.

as discussed previously. Pain and swelling over the pes bursa may be noted on examination. The workup should begin with routine AP and lateral radiographs. These are almost always negative. Precise diagnoses can be made by use of MRI or bone scans. MRI will clearly distinguish a pes bursitis from an underlying stress fracture. Bony edema will be prominent on T2-weighted images, as noted in Figure 13-7. Bone scintigraphy also will be positive in a stress fracture but lacks the superior soft tissue evaluation of MRI.

Medial Malleolus Stress Fractures

Medial malleolar stress fractures are another atypical stress fracture of the leg that deserve special attention. The clinical picture is similar to that of other lower leg stress fractures, except pain is located directly over the medial malleolus. These fractures usually extend obliquely beginning at the tibial plafond. They may be unstable and may require extensive casting or surgery for satisfactory healing (40). Patients who present with the clinical picture of a medial malleolus stress fracture with negative plain x-rays should be imaged with a triple-phase bone scan or MRI to help confirm the diagnosis. Although these stress fractures are uncommon, the physician needs to carry a high level of suspicion and implement the appropriate therapy immediately.

Fibular Stress Fractures

The fibula represents between 6% and 24% of all stress fractures (16,18). Fibular stress fractures typically occur in the distal third, 5 cm above the lateral malleolus (41). Clinical and radiographic presentations are similar to posteromedial tibial stress fractures. Figure 13-8 shows a healing fibular stress fracture. Prognosis is excellent.

Proximal third fibular stress fractures are much rarer and are believed to be secondary to repetitive jumping stress. They are more common in basketball players, hurdlers, gymnasts, and ballet dancers (29,42). Runners are less commonly affected. Radiographic and bone scan presentations are similar to those of other stress fractures. These stress fractures require a more extensive time to heal than distal fibular stress fractures.

Chronic Exertional Compartment Syndrome

A *compartment syndrome* is defined as a condition where an elevated tissue pressure in a closed fascial space results in reduced capillary blood perfusion and compromised neurologic function (1,30,43). These syndromes can be acute (usually associated with trauma) or chronic. Acute compartment syndromes are less common in sports and not discussed here. Chronic exertional compartment syndrome always must be considered in the differential diagnosis of chronic lower leg pain that occurs with activity. There are at least four well-described fascial compartments in the leg (1,30,43). These include the anterior, lateral, superficial posterior, and deep posterior compartments. In addition, the tibialis posterior is often considered to be a compartment of its own. Each compartment contains a specific sensory nerve and particular muscles. Table 13-4 lists the compartments and their respective nerve. The anterior and deep posterior compartments are the two most commonly affected and account for approximately 80% of all cases (43). Treatment often requires surgical fascial release.

Patients complain of pain with prolonged activity when using the muscles over the affected compartment. Numbness and weakness in the distribution of the nerve of the affected

FIGURE   **13-7**

Stress fracture versus pes bursitis. The underlying bony edema seen in a stress fracture on the anteromedial tibia at the hamstring insertion. These stress fractures are often mistaken for a pes anserine bursitis.

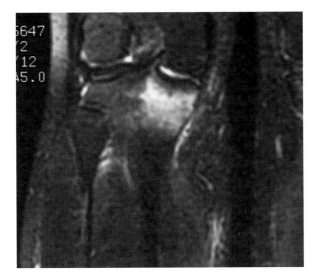

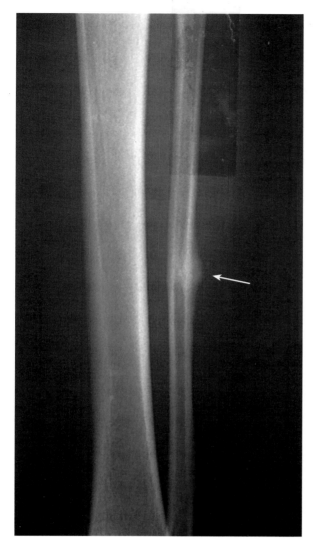

FIGURE **13-8**

Fibular stress fracture. Anteroposterior radiographs reveal periosteal reaction and new bone formation (*arrow*) at the middle to distal third of the fibula consistent with a stress fracture.

compartment also may be noted. Diagnosis is best made with direct measurement of intracompartmental pressure, although no standard protocol exists.

Plain x-rays should be obtained to rule out associated problems such as fracture or heterotopic ossification. CT and bone scan serve no practical role, except to possibly exclude other problems. They should not be obtained routinely unless the history and physical examination suggest a diagnostic dilemma requiring specific studies. Ultrasound evaluation has been used, but the relationship to intracompartmental pressures is not clearly established (44). It is extremely technician dependent, not readily reproducible, and not obtained routinely for this diagnosis at many centers. Preliminary studies with MRI have been disappointing, but further modifications of protocols may hold future promise (45). Neither MRI, ultrasound, CT, nor technetium bone scanning can be recommended routinely at this time. Recent research with thallium scanning done in Australia seems to hold future promise for diagnoses by noninvasive imaging (46). However, this work currently remains experimental.

Acute Injuries

Muscle Strains

Muscle strains are especially common in the lower leg. Strains refer to a partial or complete tear of the musculotendinous unit. A strain usually occurs in response to powerful contractions combined with forced lengthening of the muscle (47). For example, a sudden violent gastrocnemius contraction of an already lengthened muscle overwhelms the muscle-tendon unit. This results in a sudden, painful injury near the myotendinous junction (47,48).

Gastrocnemius Strains

The medial gastrocnemius is one of the most common muscles to be strained in the body. Inherent properties of this muscle may make it particularly susceptible (49,50). The condition is most common in recreational athletes who make a sudden movement and feel a "pop" in the back of the leg. It is occasionally referred to as *tennis leg*. Rarely, if ever, is the plantaris involved, as previously believed (30,51).

Clinical examination is consistent with the degree of strain described above and almost always suffices to make the diagnosis. Radiologic assessment for acute injuries is usually not required. Plain films are of limited value in soft tissue evaluation because of the intrinsic low contrast they provide. They should, however, be performed prior to other imaging tests to exclude bony abnormality or soft tissue calcification. Gastrocnemius strains almost always respond favorably to conservative management and infrequently require further work-up.

TABLE 13-4

Main Lower Leg Compartments

Compartment	Muscles	Nerve	Deficit
Anterior	Extensors (TA, EDL, EHL)	Deep peroneal	Weak ankle and toe extension; decreased sensation over first web space
Lateral	Peroneals	Superior peroneal	Weak ankle eversion; decreased sensation, lateral leg
Superficial posterior	Gastrocnemius-soleus	Sural	Decreased ankle plantar flexion; decreased sensation, lateral foot
Deep posterior	Flexors (FHL, FDL)	Tibial	Decreased toe flexion; decreased sensation, sole of foot
Posterior tibialis		Tibial	Decreased ankle inversion

However, examination sometimes can be difficult due to associated swelling and pain. Thrombophlebitis or deep venous thrombosis also can be mistaken for a gastrocnemius tear. If the diagnosis remains in question, MRI and/or Doppler can be extremely helpful. MRI also can show the exact site of the tear, as well as the degree of muscle retraction.

In chronic injuries, plain radiographs need to be performed first to rule out bony lesions as well as myositis ossificans. MRI also may be of further help in chronic injury, where the diagnosis can be more difficult. MRI reveals abnormal muscle architecture on high-resolution sequences, often with atrophy and fatty infiltration. Comparison views of the unaffected side can be of significant value. MRI once again also helps to rule out other possible pathology.

Other Strains

Other muscles of the lower leg may be injured and require imaging. When the clinical history, physical examination, and standard radiographs do not suffice, MRI can once again provide better definition of these soft tissue lesions. Please see the discussion in Chapter 14 for further details.

Contusions

Acute Contusions

Muscle contusions are extremely common in athletics, particularly contact sports. While the quadriceps is most often involved, the gastrocnemius-soleus complex also can be contused. Blunt trauma results in hemorrhage, inflammation, and disruption of muscle fibers (48). The effects parallel the events in muscle strain, with the only exception being the location. Strains predominantly affect the myotendinous junction, while contusions can affect any part of the muscle.

Radiographs should be ordered in severe contusions to rule out associated tibia and fibula fractures. They may become helpful at 2 to 4 weeks in the evaluation of a developing myositis ossificans (52). Patients who present late from contusions also require radiographs to rule out myositis ossificans (discussed below). As noted before, MRI and ultrasound may play a limited role in defining the hematoma extent but are rarely required. Their acute use, along with that of CT, is not routinely recommended.

Myositis Ossificans

Myositis ossificans is a potential result of any muscle trauma, especially when intramuscular hematoma is present. Clinically, a firm, hard mass will be palpable between 2 and 4 weeks after injury. The radiographic changes over time have been well documented (53). Initial x-rays at the time of trauma are negative. By the third to fourth week, flocculated densities are seen within the soft tissue mass, with the underlying bone demonstrating a periosteal reaction. By 3 to 6 months, the bony mass usually stabilizes or even decreases in size. The lesion can be confused with an osteosarcoma but can be differentiated by various means, including history, course of radiographic stabilization, age of the patient, and alkaline phosphate levels (52). Figure 13-9 shows the classic x-ray findings in a mature myositis ossificans.

Fractures

Mechanism

Traumatic tibial and fibular shaft fractures are one of the most common long bone fractures (54). These fractures occur as a result of either a direct blow or high-velocity rotation with the foot in a fixed position. Both the tibia and fibula alone or together may be involved.

Direct blows to the tibial shaft causing fracture are common because the exposed subcutaneous location offers minimal protection. These fractures are seen much more often in high-energy trauma such as motor vehicle accidents but do occur in sports such as soccer or football. Sports injuries are considerably different in that these fractures are almost always closed, with little damage to the surrounding soft tissues.

Many lower leg fractures seen in sports medicine are secondary to indirect forces. If the fixed ankle/foot is subjected to a high-velocity rotation, force is directed up the tibia and fibula and can lead to a fracture. This type of mechanism usually results in a longitudinal fracture line, either spiral or oblique, most frequently involving the distal to middle thirds of the tibia/fibula. Please see Chapter 14 for detailed discussion of these injuries.

Imaging

Imaging of possible tibia and fibula fractures should begin with routine anteroposterior and lateral radiographs. The entire tibia/fibula should be visualized. One should be especially careful not to overlook associated injuries of the ankle or knee and obtain the appropriate views when necessary. A mortise view is mandatory if any ankle pathology is even remotely suspected. Initial x-rays may be obtained with the limb splinted, as long as fracture lines are not obscured. Postreduction views should be taken after any manipulation of the extremity and should include both the knee and ankle joints on the same radiographic plate so that alignment can be appropriately determined (55). Serial x-rays often are required to help assess

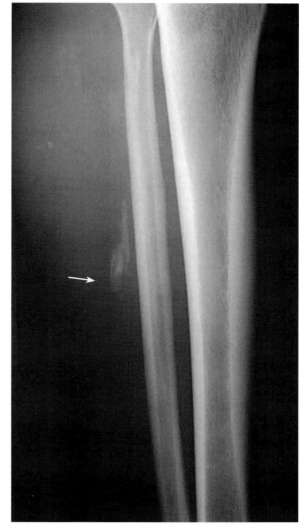

FIGURE 13-9

Myositis ossificans. Lateral x-rays of the lower leg reveal soft tissue calcification (*arrow*) in the gastrocnemius-soleus muscles consistent with a mature myositis ossificans.

fracture healing, alignment, and return to participation.

Routine radiographs should help provide the necessary anatomic information to assess the fracture. Fractures should be described in the classic manner, including 1) open or closed, 2) anatomic location (proximal, middle, distal), 3) fracture configuration (transverse, oblique, spiral, segmental, comminuted with or without butterfly or multiple fragments), 4) angulation (distal fragment in relationship to the proximal),

5) displacement (expressed as the percentage of the diameter of the proximal fragment, e.g., 25%, 50%, 75%), 6) shortening, and/or 7) rotation (55).

Additional studies such as CT can be useful to evaluate angulation, the position of fragments after spiral fracture, and for subtle injuries (56). MRI can be of use for analysis of soft tissue injury and further anatomic definition but is rarely required.

Fibula Fractures

Most fibula shaft fractures result from the same injury associated with the tibia fracture. The type of fibula fracture associated with the tibia fracture helps indicate the degree of trauma to the soft tissues. Severe comminution of the fibula or diastases between the interosseous membrane between the fibula and tibia indicates an unstable fracture (55). Isolated fibula fractures, with the exception of the Maisonneuve injury, are uncommon. They usually result from direct force over the fibula. They may have relatively minor pain and can be mistaken for a contusion. Figure 13-10 shows a comminuted fracture at the middle third of the fibula. The fracture occurred secondary to direct trauma from another opponent (kick) during a soccer game. These fractures do particularly well with conservative treatment plans.

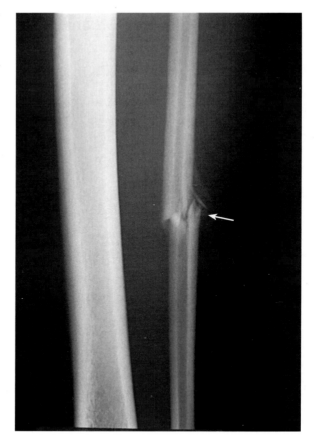

FIGURE **13-10**

Isolated fibula fracture. Anteroposterior x-rays of the lower leg reveal an isolated fracture of the middle third of the fibula (*arrow*).

Tibia Fractures

The isolated tibial shaft fracture usually occurs secondary to direct impact and is immediately apparent. Pain and swelling localized to the site of the fracture are severe. The fracture is usually in an excellent alignment and position. Combined fractures of the tibia and fibula are usually secondary to indirect forces and are discussed further in Chapter 14. These fractures also can occur secondary to direct impact. Figure 13-11 shows a healing fracture of the middle third of the tibia and fibula.

The treatment of a particular fracture of the tibial shaft must be determined by the morphology (location, comminution, and pattern) of the fracture, the presence of associated injuries, and the general patient/athlete profile (55). Most series support the use of conservative, closed weight-bearing treatment for the majority of these low-energy fractures with minimal soft tissue damage. Clinical examination and serial x-rays are required to help assess fracture healing and determine the athlete's return to competition.

Conclusion

In conclusion, this chapter has discussed the common sports medicine problems that affect the lower leg. A good clinical history, physical examination, and standard x-rays should provide the diagnosis in the majority of cases. When required, the imaging modalities discussed above (bone scan, MRI, CT, and ultrasound) should help confirm the diagnosis and

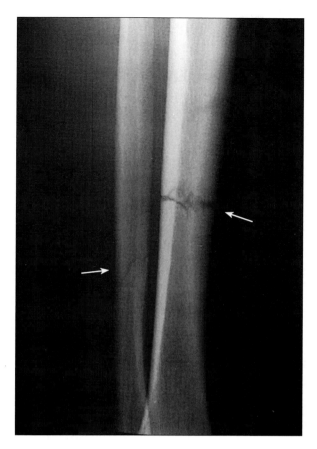

FIGURE **13-11**

Tibia and fibula fracture secondary to direct impact. Healing fracture is noted through the cast in the middle third of the tibia and fibula. The fracture healed well with conservative measures.

allow for the appropriate treatment plans and quick return to the sports activity.

REFERENCES

1. Andrish JT. The leg. In: DeLee JC, Drez D, eds. Orthopedic sports medicine: principles and practices. Vol 2. Philadelphia: WB Saunders, 1994: 1603.

2. Deveraux MD, Lachmann SM. Athletes attending a sports injury clinic—a review: Br J Sports Med 1983;17:137–142.

3. Mubarak SJ, et al. The medial tibial stress syndrome: a cause of shin splints. Am J Sports Med 1982;10:201–205.

4. Michael RH, Holder LE. The soleus syndrome: a cause of medial tibial stress (shin splints). Am J Sports Med 1985;13:87–94.

5. Garth W, Miller S. Evaluation of claw toe deformity weakness of the foot intrinsics and posteromedial shin pain. Am J Sports Med 1989;17:821.

6. James SL, Bates BT, Osternig LR. Injuries to runners. Am J Sports Med 1978;6:40–50.

7. Detmer DE. Chronic shin splints: classification and management of medial tibial stress syndrome. Sports Med 1986;3:436.

8. Milgrom C, Giladi M, Stein M, et al. Medial tibial pain. Clin Orthop 1986;213:167–171.

9. Norfray J, Schlachter L, Kernahan W Jr, et al. Early confirmation of stress fractures in joggers. JAMA 1980;243:1647–1649.

10. Nusbaum A, Treves S, Micheli L. Bone stress lesions in ballet dancers: scintigraphic assessment. AJR 1988;150:851–855.

11. Rosen PR, Micheli LJ, Treves S. Early scintigraphic diagnosis of bone stress and fractures in athletic adolescents. Pediatrics 1982;70:11–15.

12. Roub LW, Gumerman LW, Hanley EN, et al. Bone stress: a radionuclide imaging perspective. Radiology 1979;132:431–438.

13. Rupani H, Holder L, Espinola D, Engin S. Three phase radionuclide bone imaging in sports medicine. Radiology 1985;156:187–196.

14. Zwas S, Elkanovitch R, Frank G. Interpretation and classification of bone scintigraphic findings in stress fractures. J Nucl Med 1987;28:452–457.

15. Holder LE, Michael RH. The specific scintigraphic pattern of "shin splints" in the lower leg. J Nucl Med 25:865–869.

16. Matheson GO, Clement DB, McKenzie DC, et al. Stress fractures in athletes: a study of 320 cases. Am J Sports Med 1987;15:46–48.

17. Orava S, Hulkko A. Stress fracture in athletes. Int J Sports Med 1987;8:221–226.

18. McBryde AM. Stress fractures in athletes. Am J Sports Med 1976;5:212.

19. Barrow GW, Saha S. Menstrual irregularity and stress fractures in collegiate female distance runners. Am J Sports Med 1988;16:209–216.

20. Devas M. Stress fractures. London: Churchill-Livingstone, 1975:56–91.

21. Greaney RB, et al. Distribution and natural history of stress fractures in US Marine recruits. Radiology 1983;146:339.

22. Berquist TH. Tibia, fibula, and calf. In: Imaging of sports injuries. Gaitherberg, MD: Aspen, 1992:155–165.

23. Martire JR. The role of nuclear medicine scans in evaluating pain in athletic injuries. Clin Sports Med 1987;6:713–737.

24. Siddiqui AR. Bone scans for early detection of stress fracture. N Engl J Med 1978;298:1033.

25. Wilcox JR Jr, Moniot AL, Green JP. Bone scanning in the evaluation of exercise-related stress injuries. Radiology 1977;123:699–703.

26. Milgron C, Chisin R, Giladi M, et al. Negative bone scans and impending tibial stress fractures. Am J Sports Med 1984;12:488–491.

27. Matheson GO, et al. Scintigraphic uptake of technetium at nonpainful sites in athletes with stress fractures: the concept of bone strain. Sports Med 1987;4:65–75.

28. Chisin R, et al. Clinical significance of nonfocal scintigraphic findings in suspected tibial stress fractures. Clin Orthop 1987;220:200.

29. Martire JR, Levinsohn ME. The lower leg. In: Imaging of athletic injuries. New York: McGraw-Hill, 1992:45–78.

30. Bachner EJ, Friedman MJ. Injuries to the leg. In: Hershman EB, Nicholas JA, eds. The lower extremity and spine in sports medicine. Vol 1. St Louis: Mosby, 1995:523–580.

31. Stafford S, Rosenthal D, Gebhardt M, et al. MRI in stress fracture. AJR 1986;147:553–556.

32. Lee JK, Yao L. Stress fractures: MR imaging. Radiology 1988;169:217–220.

33. Castillo M, Tehranzadeh J, Morillo G. Atypical healed stress fracture of the fibula masquerading as chronic osteomyelitis. Am J Sports Med 1988;16:185–188.

34. Arendt EA, et al. The MR spectrum of stress injury to bone and its clinical relevance. Am J Sports Med (in press).

35. Vogler JB, Murphy WA. Bone marrow imaging. Radiology 1988;168:679.

36. Arendt EA, Clohisy DR. Stress injuries of bone. In: Hershman EB, Nicholas JA, eds. The lower extremity and spine in sports medicine. Vol 1. St Louis: Mosby, 1995:65–79.

37. Rettig A, Shelbourne D, McCarroll J, et al. The natural history and treatment of delayed union stress fractures of the anterior cortex of the tibia. Am J Sports Med 1988;16:250–255.

38. Green N, Rogers R, Lipscomb B. Nonunions of stress fractures of the tibia. Am J Sports Med 1985;13:171–176.

39. Blank S. Transverse tibial stress fractures: a special problem. Am J Sports Med 1981;9:322–325.

40. Shellbourne K, Fisher D, Rettig A, McCarroll J. Stress fractures of the medial malleolus. Am J Sports Med 1988;16:60–63.

41. Blair WF, Manley SR. Stress fractures of the proximal fibula. Am J Sports Med 1980;8:212–213.

42. Symeonides PP. High stress fractures of the fibula. J Bone Joint Surg 1980;62(B):192–193.

43. Pedowitz R, Hargens A, Mubarak S, Gershuni D. Modified criteria for the objective diagnosis of chronic syndrome of the leg. Am J Sports Med 1990;18:35–40.

44. Gershuni D, Gosink B, Hargens A, et al. Ultrasound evaluation of the anterior musculo-fascial compartment of the leg following exercise. Clin Orthop 1982;167:185–190.

45. Amendola A, Rorabeck C, Vellett D, et al. The use of magnetic resonance imaging in exertional compartment syndromes. Am J Sports Med 1990;18:29–34.

46. Hayes A, Bower G, Pitstock K. Chronic (exertional) compartment syndrome of the legs diagnosed with thallous chloride scintigraphy. J Nucl Med 1995;36:1618–1624.

47. Garrett WE. Basic science of musculotendinous injuries. In: Nicholas JA, Hershman EB, eds. The lower extremity and spine in sports medicine. St Louis: Mosby, 1986.

48. Garrett WE, Lohnes J. Cellular and matrix response to mechanical injury at the myotendinous junction. In: Leadbetter WB, Buckwalter JA, Gordon SL, eds. Sports-induced inflammation. Park Ridge, IL: American Academy of Orthopedic Surgeons, 1990:215–224.

49. Sutro C, Sutro W. The medial head of the gastrocnemius: a review of the basis for the partial rupture and for intermittent claudication. Bull Hosp Joint Dis Orthop Inst 1985;45:150–157.

50. Frominson A. Tennis leg. JAMA 1969;209:415–416.

51. Speer KP, Lohnes J, Garrett WE. Radiographic imaging of muscle strain injury. Am J Sports Med 1993;21:89–96.

52. Brunett ME, Hontas RB. The Thigh. In: DeLee JC, Drez D, eds. Orthopedic sports medicine: principles and practices. Vol 2. Philadelphia: WB Saunders, 1994:1106–1108.

53. Noran A, Dorfman HD. Juxtacortical circum-

scribed myositis ossificans: evolution and radiographic features. Radiology 1970;96:301–306.

54. Leach RE. Fractures of the tibia and fibula. In: Rockwood CA, Green DP, eds. Fractures in adults. Philadelphia: JP Lippincott, 1984:1593–1663.

55. Russell TA, Taylor JC, La Velle DG. In: Rockwood CA, Green DP, eds. Fractures in adults. Philadelphia: JB Lippincott, 1992:1915–1981.

56. Gershuni DH, Skyhar MJ, Thompson B, et al. A comparison of conventional and computed tomography in the evaluation of spiral fractures of the tibia. J Bone Joint Surg 1985;67A: 1388–1395.

CHAPTER *14*

Ankle and Foot Injuries

JONATHAN T. DELAND
LANCE A. MARKBREITER

*S*ports-related injuries of the foot and ankle are extremely commonplace in the office of the orthopedist, sports medicine practitioner, and primary care physician. As a general rule, the history and physi-cal examination are paramount in importance. However, imaging modalities give confirmation of the diagnosis or exclude other diagnoses. With all the advances in imaging technology, the plain radiograph remains the most useful tool for the vast majority of foot and ankle injuries. Plain films are the stepping stones for radiologic diagnosis, and the majority of patients do not require more extensive studies. It is therefore necessary to obtain high-quality routine films. The physician should be knowledgeable of the special plain radiographic views that can be ordered to help define the various injuries encountered in this complex anatomic region. There are certain musculoskeletal disorders for which further studies such as computed tomography (CT) and magnetic resonance imaging (MRI) are very helpful, and these will be discussed below.

Ankle Sprains

The sprained ankle is the most common sports-related injury that the orthopedist or primary care physician will encounter. Most are mild to moderate inversion sprains that usually make a full recovery with conservative treatment in-

cluding rest, ice, compression, and elevation (RICE). The more severe injuries often require physical therapy to regain strength and range of motion. A good physical therapy program will strengthen the musculature of the lower extremity and increase proprioception, making for a fuller and quicker recovery. A few of these "routine" sprains actually represent more significant injuries that should be treated differently. An accurate diagnosis relies on the patient's history, physical examination, and radiologic findings.

One must be aware of the anatomy and function of the ankle ligaments. Inversion in plantarflexion is limited by the anterior talofibular ligament (ATFL) and, in dorsiflexion, by the calcaneofibular ligament (CFL) (1). The mechanism of injury in a routine ankle sprain is most commonly inversion and plantarflexion. Therefore, it is most often primarily an ATFL injury. However, occasionally the foot is inverted and dorsiflexed (primarily CFL injury). With enough inversion, both ligaments fail, and fractures of the distal fibula or medial malleolus can occur. Sprains are graded as mild (grade I), moderate (grade II, where some functional stretching out of the ligaments is present), and severe (grade III, where there is complete ligamentous rupture).

The deltoid ligament on the medial side of the ankle is the main guard against excessive eversion. It can be injured independently or associated with injury to the syndesmotic or lateral ligaments. Often undiagnosed is the syndesmotic or "high" ankle sprain. This is an injury to the anterior tibiofibular ligament in addition to the ligaments mentioned above. Tenderness is therefore also located at the anterolateral corner of the ankle joint. It is an eversion or combination inversion-eversion injury. It often causes pain and discomfort far in excess of the more common routine "low" ankle sprains. A syndesmosis injury will constitute injury to the anterior tibiofibular ligament but also can include the posterior tibiofibular and interosseus membrane, since these structures make up the syndesmosis. General knowledge of ankle anatomy will allow the physician, by palpation and testing of these ligaments, to decipher which ligaments have been sprained (i.e., high versus low ankle sprains). Stress radiographs will be discussed below and can confirm the presence of completely torn ligaments or chronic laxity. However, stress x-rays may not be necessary if the examiner is experienced in the foot and ankle examination.

The patient who presents with an acute grade I or II ankle sprain is best treated with rest, ice, compression, and elevation (RICE), followed by exercise and rehabilitation. Radiographs are required to rule out bony pathology if sufficient tenderness is present over the bones. Routine anteroposterior (AP), lateral, and mortise views of the ankle should suffice to rule out most fractures. The mortise view is obtained by internally rotating the lower leg 20 degrees to bring the medial and lateral malleoli parallel to the plane of the cassette, thereby placing the ankle mortise joint space in full view. One should appreciate on the film an equal joint space on all three sides of the talus. Any significant widening (greater than 2 mm) in the medial joint space is consistent with complete rupture of the syndesmotic ligaments (Fig. 14-1). No further radiographic investigations are warranted in the acute setting unless tenderness is present elsewhere in the foot, ankle, or leg. Detection of a lateral talar process fracture can be difficult on routine ankle films. If impressive bony tenderness is present in the talus or a fracture is suspected for other reasons, a CT scan should be performed (Fig. 14-2). Similarly, fractures in the foot near the ankle can simulate ankle sprains. Foot x-rays should be obtained if there is any unusual bony tenderness in the foot. Often misdiagnosed as an ankle sprain is a fracture of the base of the fifth metatarsal or a fracture of the anterior process of the calcaneus.

Treatment of grade III injuries remains controversial. Studies show that if a late repair is necessary, the results are as effective as an immediate ligamentous reconstruction (2). Most surgeons will reserve surgical treatment for those patients who continue to have chronic instability after a lengthy trial of conservative treatment. Therefore, stress films are rarely needed in acute ankle sprains.

If the athlete continues to complain of ankle pain or gives a history of multiple episodes of the ankle "giving way," it becomes imperative to confirm that instability exists. At this point, radiographic stress views can be used if deemed necessary after the physical examination. The

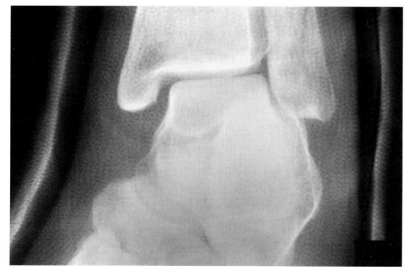

FIGURE **14-1**

X-ray in a cast showing mild widening of the medial joint space. A true mortise view can only be taken out of a cast and is the best view to judge widening of the medial joint space.

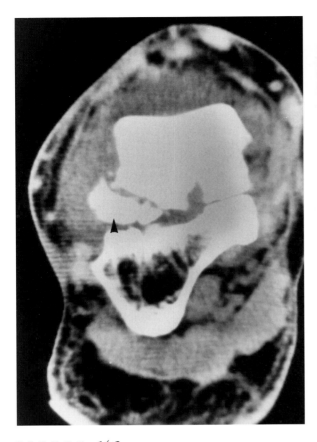

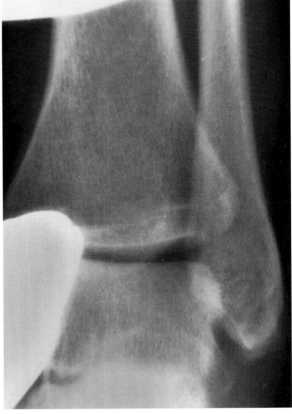

F I G U R E **14-2**

CT scan showing old fractured lateral process of lateral process of the talus that was not apparent on routine ankle films.

F I G U R E **14-3**

Lateral tilt AP stress view. This amount of opening was within 5 degrees of the opposite ankle and therefore does not represent instability.

two types of stress views generally employed are the inversion and the anterior drawer tests. It is imperative to examine the contralateral ankle for comparison. These stress views can be obtained by using a specially produced device or, more commonly, by the examiner using lead gloves and directly applying the stress. An inversion stress film is a mortise view taken with maximal inversion stress applied to the ankle and subtalar joints, stabilizing the tibia and attempting to tilt the talus medially (Fig. 14-3). An anterior drawer stress radiograph is a lateral film with an anterior force applied to the heel and a posterior force applied to the distal tibia. A true lateral film (not with the ankle rotated into internal or external rotation) must be obtained so that the measurement is accurate. Landmarks for measuring anterior displacement of the talus on the tibia can be difficult to locate. The most posterior point of the articular surfaces of the talus

and tibia are usually readily identifiable landmarks. Because of difficulty in assessing landmarks and the need for true lateral films, accurate stress films for anterior displacement of the talus can be harder to obtain than the talar tilt films. An anterior drawer stress film with greater than 4 mm of difference between the normal ankle and the opposite ankle is consistent with an ATFL injury. A talar tilt film with more than 5 degrees difference indicates increased laxity.

Rarely, the instability can be located primarily at the subtalar joint. If ankle instability cannot be demonstrated and subtalar instability is suspected, special subtalar stress views (Broden) can be obtained. These are performed by placing the foot in 45 degrees of internal rotation and shooting the beam with a 20-degree caudal tilt as the subtalar joint is being stressed. Any difference in the opening of the posterior facet is considered to be abnormal and consistent with subtalar instability. This instability without concomitant ankle instability is very rare in our experience.

If plain radiographs fail to make a diagnosis and the patient's pain continues to persist, a CT scan should be obtained to rule out occult bony pathology. These pathologies would include osteochondral defects of the talus, fractures of the lateral or posterior talar process, or a fracture of the anterior process of the calcaneus (Fig. 14-4). Fractures of the lateral talar process and anterior process of the calcaneus, however, most often can be detected on the mortise ankle x-ray and oblique plain films of the foot, respectively. An MRI also can be used to rule out these bony diagnoses and has the additional advantages of depicting cartilage lesions. An MRI is best used when cartilage or other soft tissues need to be visualized. The quality of the MRI and its interpretation are more variable than CT scans.

F I G U R E **14-4**

Oblique view of foot showing a radiolucent line (*arrow*) across the anterior process of the calcaneus documenting an anterior process fracture.

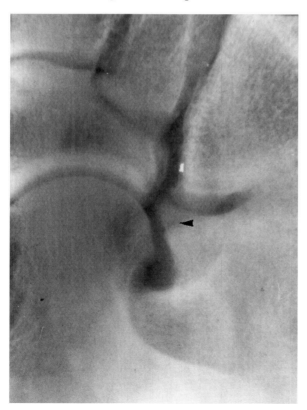

Ankle Fractures

Most ankle fractures are a combination of soft tissue and bony injuries. The physical examination in combination with radiographs will determine the extent of bony and ligamentous disruption.

Routine ankle views (AP, lateral, and mortise views) should be ordered whenever there is any suspicion of a possible fracture (i.e., exquisite bony tenderness). The mortise view should show both the medial and lateral joint spaces well. Any widening of the joint space or fracture displacement by more than 2 mm is significant displacement and should be reduced. The mortise view also may reveal widening of the medial clear space without an associated ankle fracture, a finding that can occur only with disruption of the syndesmosis and a fibular fracture at the calf or knee. In this disruption, no fracture may be seen on ankle films yet the fibula, talus, and foot are displaced laterally. If not stabilized surgically, there is a high risk for progressive arthritis of the ankle.

If the patient notes tenderness over the fibula in the calf or near the knee, a Maisonneuve high fibula fracture along with syndesmosis injury should be suspected. This tenderness should be checked for, and AP and lateral views of the entire tibia and fibula should be ordered when tenderness is present. Routine ankle films usually do not show the middle or proximal fibula, and therefore, the Maisonneuve fracture and the associated instability can be missed if the calf is not examined. The presence of this fracture points to probable disruption of the syndesmosis even when widening is not present on initial films. Suspected injuries of the syndesmosis can be further evaluated by external rotation stress views. These are obtained by external rotation of the foot while holding the leg stabilized with the knee flexed to 90 degrees. This will reproduce pain at the syndesmosis and widening between the medial malleolus and talus. General or spinal anesthesia may be required. Syndesmotic injuries with displacement are important injuries that are often overlooked. At the least, patients suspected of a syndesmotic injury without a fracture should be brought back and x-rayed again in 2 weeks with weight-bearing views.

Salter fractures occur through the physis in children. In a Salter I injury no viable fracture line is present, since the fracture is entirely at the physis or growth plate. The epiphysis is often not displaced, and therefore, the diagnosis is made clinically by tenderness over the physis. X-rays should be checked for bony extension of the fracture, which would indicate a different injury (Salter II or III) and the need for reduction as well as casting.

In general, open reduction and internal fixation are indicated for ankle fractures with greater than 2 mm of displacement. Good plain films are therefore critical for the proper treatment of these injuries. A comminuted distal tibia fracture that involves the tibial plafond is a much more complex problem and is called a *pilon fracture* (Fig. 14-5). These injuries usually require a CT scan for preoperative planning.

Anterior Ankle Pain

Anterior ankle pain is very common in the athlete. The most common etiology is mechanical impingement, which is reported in 45% of football players and 59% of dancers (3). Anterior impingement is caused by osteophyte formation on the distal anterior lip of the tibia and a corresponding portion of the dorsal talar neck. The injury occurs by one of two mechanisms, chronic

FIGURE **14-5**

Fracture of the tibial plafond easily apparent on plain x-ray, but the CT scan is often necessary for preoperative planning.

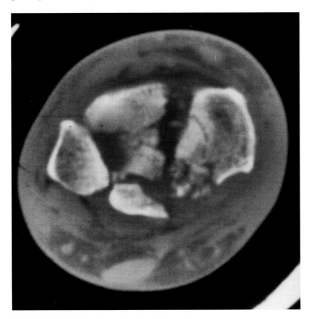

hyperdorsiflexion, as seen in ballet dancers performing a grand plie, or plantarflexion causing a tear in the anterior capsule.

Diagnosis should be made by the history, physical examination, and x-ray studies. A lateral film of the ankle generally will show the spur formation (Fig. 14-6). In the normal ankle, the angle or line along the anterior lip of the tibia and dorsal aspect of the talus should be greater than 60 degrees. However, with anterior impingement, this angle is usually smaller. If the diagnosis is in question, a weight-bearing forced dorsiflexion lateral (relevé) film should show the impingement between the "kissing" osteophytes. A medial talar neck osteophyte may not be seen on x-rays except possibly on the mortise view. It can generally be palpated on the medial neck of the talus.

Another cause of anterior ankle pain is an osteochondral lesion of the talar dome. The mechanism of this injury remains controversial. Most commonly, the athlete presents with chronic ankle pain that has failed to improve with conservative treatment. A high index of suspicion is necessary because the diagnosis is difficult to obtain by history and physical examination. Plain ankle radiographs generally will demonstrate the lesion. The physician may have to look very carefully to locate the defect in the talar dome, and sometimes the lesion cannot be seen on the plain films. Those lesions located in the posteromedial dome are generally nondisplaced and cup-shaped as compared with anterolateral lesions, which tend to be displaced, shallow, and wafer-shaped (Fig. 14-7). To fully evaluate the condition of the cartilage and the bony fragment or to diagnose the lesion, an MRI is the definitive study. Many osteochondral lesions are asymptomatic. These lesions can be classified by their appearance on the MRI or CT scan. A grade 1 lesion has an intact roof, grade 2 has a disrupted cartilage roof, grade 3 has the fragment separated but not displaced out of its bed, and grade 4 is a lesion with a displaced fragment. Operative intervention is recommended for symptomatic grade 3 and grade 4 lesions.

Posterior Ankle Pain

The athlete who presents with pain in the posterior aspect of the ankle may have a posterior impingement syndrome (os trigonum syndrome). The most posterior portion of the talus consists of medial and lateral tubercles, between

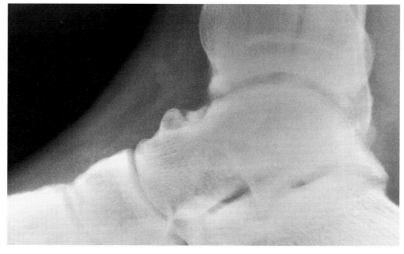

FIGURE **14-6**

Spurs at anterior talar neck and lateral calcaneus that caused pain in this patient. Tomograms or a CT scan are only necessary if there is a question as to location of spurs in the coronal (medial/lateral) plane.

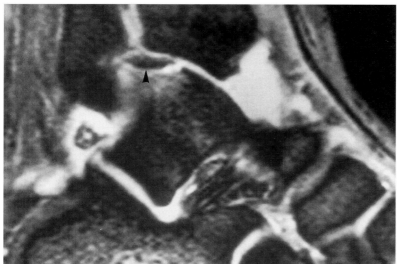

FIGURE **14-7**

Osteochondral lesion (*arrow*) in the posterior talar dome with the MRI demonstrating the lesion as a separated fragment.

which the flexor halluces longus tendon courses. The os trigonum is an ununited lateral tubercle of the posterior talus. In the vast majority of cases it is not painful. This radiographic finding is present in 7% to 10% of the population, and it is bilateral in half the cases (1).

The posterior impingement syndrome most often affects ballet dancers, whose art relies on the ability to perform on point (maximal or abnormal amounts of ankle plantarflexion). The os trigonum is best seen on the lateral radiograph (Fig. 14-8). A fully plantarflexed lateral view can demonstrate the impingement. It is important to note that the presence of an os trigonum does not automatically diagnose the cause of the patient's posterior ankle pain. The differential diagnosis includes a stress fracture of the os trigonum, flexor hallucis longus tendinitis (com-

mon in dancers), peroneal tendinitis, tarsal coalition, Achilles tendinitis, posterior ankle spurs, and an osteoid osteoma (4). These diagnoses should be considered before the os trigonum is chosen as the cause of the pain.

Osteoid Osteoma

An osteoid osteoma is a benign lesion that causes a painful inflammatory reaction within the bone unrelated to athletic activity. The presenting symptom is pain without traumatic origin, and these lesions can occur in bones all over the body. The radiograph of a typical lesion shows a dense osteoblastic reaction surrounding an osteolytic nidus (Fig. 14-9). These lesions are small (less than 1 cm) and may not be seen on a plain

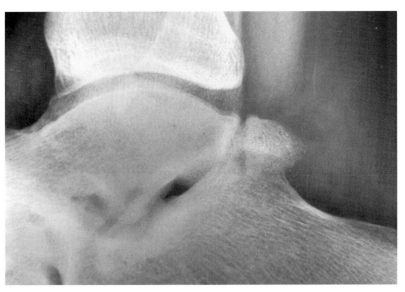

FIGURE **14-8**

An unusually large os trigonum, which in this instance caused pain with plantarflexion.

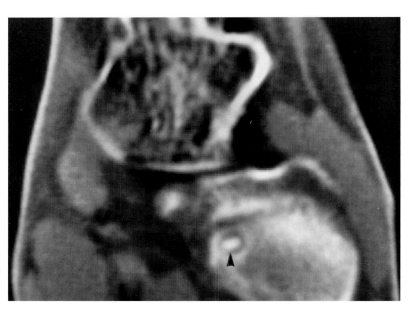

FIGURE **14-9**

Osteoid osteoma, indicated by the white osteoblastic area (*arrow*) on the CT scan. The lesion was not visible on plain films.

film. A technetium bone scan will have markedly increased uptake and, if negative, excludes the diagnosis. In patients in whom there is an index of suspicion, a CT scan (rather than an MRI) will demonstrate the lesion. An MRI may not visualize this lesion. Dramatic relief of pain after taking aspirin or other anti-inflammatory medications greatly increases the index of suspicion. If necessary for pain control, treatment is surgical removal of the central nidus, following which the osteoblastic reaction resolves.

Achilles Tendon

The Achilles tendon is the largest tendon in the body and is part of the strongest musculotendinous complex in the lower leg. Achilles pain is very common in the running athlete, with an incidence ranging from 6.5% to 18.5% (5). It can be from bursitis (inflammation of the bursa), tendinitis (inflammation around the tendon), and tendonosis (degeneration of the tendon) (6). Patients who localize their pain to the tendon's insertion on the calcaneus can have a posterosuperior prominence of the calcaneal tuberosity (Haglund's deformity) and/or Achilles spur. The Haglund's deformity is a prominence that produces an irritation that leads to bursitis and possibly tendonosis. Plain radiographs also may demonstrate calcification within the Achilles tendon near its insertion, or there may be a spur at this insertion. The athlete with chronic insertional Achilles pain at the heel may benefit from excision of the Haglund's deformity and/or removal of the spur/calcific deposits from within the tendon if the pain has not resolved with 3 to 6 months of conservative management (Fig. 14-10). Haglund's deformity can be measured, but this is not necessary in making a treatment decision. Prominent calcifications and spurs

should be removed only after failure of conservative therapy (rest, heel lift, protective pads, physical therapy).

In most instances, Achilles ruptures tend to occur in the middle age "weekend warrior" as a result of sudden dorsiflexion of the ankle or, less commonly, plantarflexion against resistance. Radiographs are not necessary in making the diagnosis but can suggest a rupture if fat lines next to the Achilles tendon are obscured. The positive physical findings include difficulty in going up onto the toes with the other foot already off the ground, a positive Thompson's sign (squeezing of the prone calf fails to produce plantarflexion of the dangling foot and ankle equal to the opposite side), and tenderness (7). Less than careful clinical examination has missed ruptures, and partial ruptures can occur. Questionable cases should be re-examined within 1 week. There is rarely a question after careful physical examination, and an MRI therefore is usually not necessary. If performed, it should be done at a facility that is used to performing orthopedic (musculoskeletal) studies, or mistakes can be made (Fig. 14-11).

The MRI has become more valuable in chronic tears and in patients managed conservatively with serial casts (8). The MRI can document the apposition of the tendon ends. It also can distinguish between peritendinitis, tendonosis, incomplete rupture, and complete rupture.

F I G U R E   **14-10**

Achilles spur with two calcifications superior and anterior to the spur.

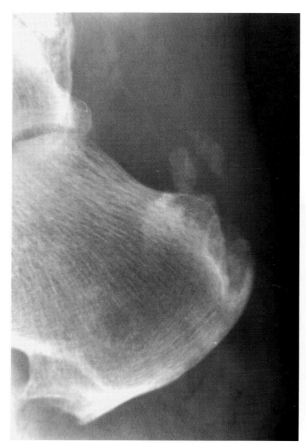

F I G U R E   **14-11**

MRI scan of an Achilles rupture (*arrow*), which was incorrectly read as normal.

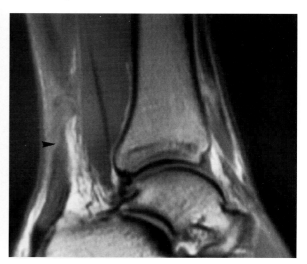

Posterior Tibial Tendon

The athlete with posterior tibial "tendinitis" will present with pain, tenderness, and swelling around the medial malleolus. Occasionally, the pain is localized to the tendon insertion at the navicular. The patient will have good active inversion of the foot, and the pain most often resolves with rest. In some of these cases an accessory navicular may be present. If an accessory navicular is not seen on routine foot films, a medial oblique view (i.e., opposite to the normal oblique) will demonstrate if it is present (Fig. 14-12). If an acute injury or symptoms continue, it may suggest posterior tibial dysfunction, and MRI can be used to assess the tendon for degeneration or partial rupture. An accessory navicular is usually asymptomatic but can cause pain, especially after trauma. Symptoms are usually caused by acute pull on the ossicle or from progressive flattening of the longitudinal arch.

Excision of the accessory navicular is necessary only when anti-inflammatory drugs, orthotics, and 6 weeks of cast immobilization fail to relieve the pain.

Rupture of the posterior tibial tendon is most frequently a chronic process associated with a slowly progressive flatfoot deformity (Fig. 14-13). These are usually patients over 40 years of age. An inciting episode of trauma may be superimposed on or begin the chronic process. A deformity is often already present and is best seen by viewing the standing foot, heel valgus, and forefoot abduction. Patients have difficulty in accomplishing single-foot heel rise with the other foot already off the floor. Also, the heel may not invert well even if same-heel rise is accomplished. The diagnosis is made on physical examination. Early in the course of the disorder there will be pain at the site of posterior tibial tendon distal to the medial malleolus, tenderness at that site, weakness on inversion testing, and difficulty in heel rise. A standing lateral ra-

FIGURE **14-12**

Medial oblique view (opposite to normal oblique of foot) showing an accessory navicular. On occasion only this view will show the accessory navicular.

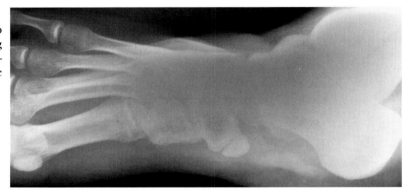

FIGURE **14-13**

Lateral standing view to assess the medial longitudinal arch. Note the plantar angulation of the talar head and neck relative to the longitudinal axis of the first metatarsal.

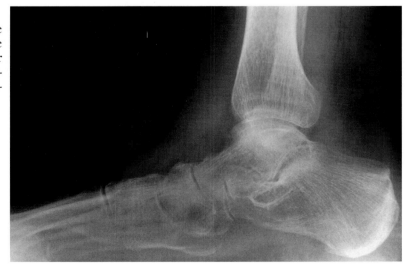

diograph often will demonstrate a decreased medial arch in comparison with the opposite foot. This sag in the arch can be subtle and at the level of the talonavicular, naviculocuneiform, and metatarsal tarsal joints or any combination thereof. An MRI usually can differentiate between tenosynovitis and tendonosis (degeneration) or partial rupture. It is not necessary in the majority of cases because muscle weakness and collapse of the arch make the failure of the tendon obvious. The MRI can be useful in treatment decisions involving the differentiation of tenosynovitis, tendonosis, and partial tear with the tendon (Fig. 14-14).

Rupture of the peroneus longus has been associated with pathology at the level of the os peroneum and often can be documented on plain films by proximal displacement or fracture of the os perineum. If present, the os peroneum is seen on the lateral or oblique radiograph of the foot (Fig. 14-15). The os peroneum is present normally in about 10% of feet (4). Its presence does not indicate peroneus longus pathology, but fracture or displacement of the os peroneum does. Tears of the peroneal brevis can be difficult to document even on an MRI and most often present as chronic pain at the distal fibula. Care must be taken to make the MRI cuts perpendicular to the longitudinal axis of the tendon.

Tarsal Coalition

This entity, known in the literature under other headings such as *peroneal spastic flatfoot* and *rigid flatfoot,* is a congenital fusion or failure of segmentation between tarsal bones (9). The development of symptoms is most often associated with calcification of the cartilaginous fibrous union in early adolescence. The onset of symptoms may occur with a minor athletic injury or no particular injury. The most common coalitions are calcaneonavicular and talocalcaneal, both of which lead to decreased subtalar joint motion and are associated with various degrees of pronation. The restriction of motion places abnormal stress on the tarsal bones, resulting in discomfort from stiffness as well as discomfort at the site of the coalition (10).

Any patient with decreased subtalar motion and associated pain should have appropriate radiographs of the foot. Most calcaneonavicular coalitions are visible on the routine oblique view of the foot. In others, the bridge has not ossified, and the diagnosis of a calcaneonavicular coalition is suggested by an elongation of the anterior calcaneal process of the navicular, "anteater" deformity (Fig. 14-16). If any question remains, a CT scan can be ordered but is most often not necessary.

The talocalcaneal coalition is more difficult to visualize on plain radiographs. A suggestive sign on the radiograph is beaking of the superior talar head seen on the lateral radiograph. The most common location of the lesion is at the middle facet of the subtalar joint. A posterior tangential (Harris) view can be helpful in visualization but may fail to show it clearly. Narrowing or obliteration of the middle facet joint space is present.

The test that best visualizes a talocalcaneal coalition is a CT scan (Fig. 14-17). In studies comparing radiography, arthrography, scintigraphy, and computed tomography, CT was clearly superior to the other modalities in coalition recognition (11). If surgery is being contemplated, CT provides a precise outline of the coalition. Coro-

F I G U R E **14-14**

MRI of the posterior tibial tendon (*arrow*) showing degeneration (*gray area*) within the tendon (tendonosis) rather than just fluid around the tendon (tendinitis).

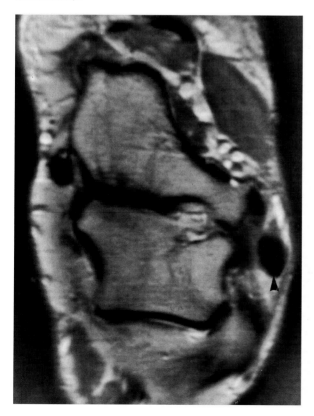

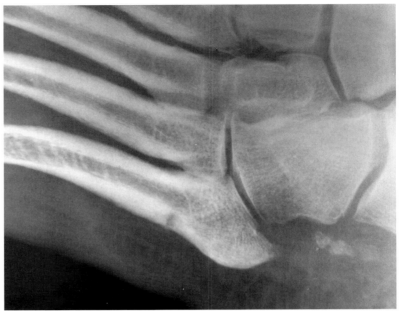

FIGURE **14-15**

Old fracture of os perineum that was not causing symptoms at the time of presentation of the lateral stress fracture at the metaphysis of the fifth metatarsal.

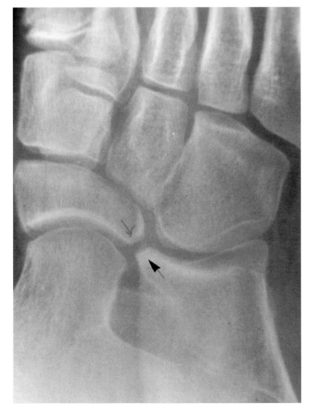

FIGURE **14-16**

Calcaneonavicular coalition with the arrows marking the coalition.

nal sections will best demonstrate the talocalcaneal bar. MRI is costly and adds little, if any, information to that obtained by the CT scan.

Calcaneus

Calcaneal fractures can be divided into two major categories, extra-articular and intra-articular. The extra-articular group is made up of fractures of the anterior process, tuberosity, medial process, body, and sustentaculum tali. These generally occur in the athlete by an indirect mechanism such as a twisting force or, in the case of tuberosity fractures, by a muscle avulsive force. Falls from a height or high-velocity accidents are responsible for the majority but not all intra-articular fractures (12).

The diagnosis of a calcaneal fracture is suspected by exquisite tenderness over the calcaneus and is made by radiographic studies. The initial x-ray examination of the patient who complains of rear foot pain following trauma should include supine AP and lateral views of the foot and an axial calcaneal (Harris) view (Fig. 14-18). The AP view will demonstrate the talonavicular joint and the calcaneocuboid joint, which may have associated injuries. The lateral view will outline the calcaneal tuber angle and the posterior facet. The axial view delineates the tuberosity, body, and sustentaculum. An AP view of the ankle is also helpful to show the

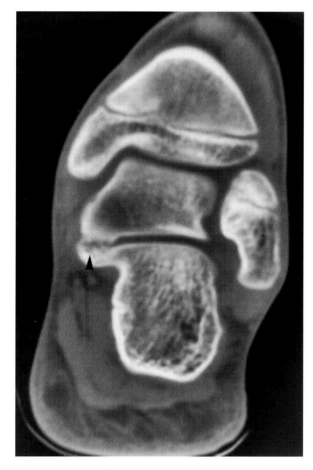

FIGURE   **14-17**

Talocalcaneal coalition demonstrating sclerosis and narrowing of the middle facet (*arrow*) of the talocalcaneal (subtalar joint) on CT scan.

widening of the calcaneus with respect to the lateral malleolus and to rule out ankle pathology. Any patient with a calcaneal fracture due to a fall from a height should have radiographs of the lumbosacral spine, pelvis, and contralateral foot unless alert mental status and a normal physical examination do not suggest any injury to the area. Studies have shown that 10% of calcaneal fractures are associated with compression fractures of the lumbar spine and 26% with other injuries of the lower extremity. Associated injuries can occur in up to 60% of patients (13).

Special oblique views (Broden's views) have been helpful in the past, but today, any patient with suspected articular involvement should have a CT scan (14) (Fig. 14-19). Coronal cuts of the posterior articular surface will demonstrate the number of fragments, the amount of displacement, and the extent of any impingement. This information is critical for deciding if the fracture should be treated operatively and for the preoperative planning itself. The general goals of operative treatment are to reestablish the posterior facet joint surface, narrow the heal, regain calcaneal length, and support this reduction with internal fixation.

LisFranc Injuries

Trauma to the tarsometatarsal joint can result in sprains, fractures, dislocations, or any combination thereof. The mechanism of injury to the athlete can be either direct impact or an indirect

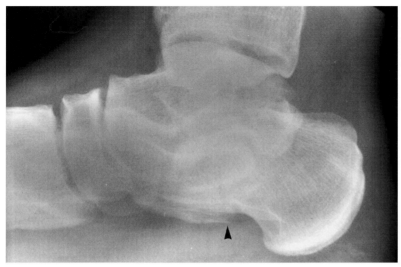

FIGURE   **14-18**

Lateral view showing the calcaneal fracture (*arrow*) at the inferior border of the calcaneus.

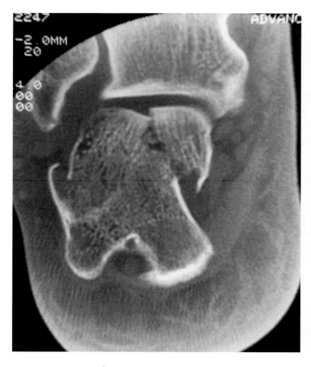

F I G U R E **14-19**

CT scan of same patient as in Fig. 14-18 showing the fracture in better detail with displacement and angulation of the posterior facet of the subtalar joint.

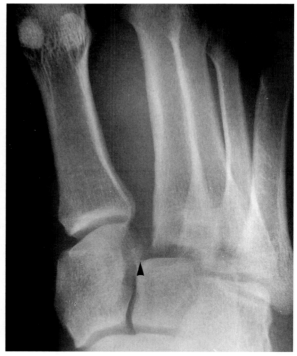

F I G U R E **14-20**

LisFranc fracture-dislocation showing lateral displacement of a second metatarsal on the middle cuneiform (*arrow*). These lesions can be subtle and easily missed unless carefully looked for.

force. Usually the athlete will have immediate pain and swelling, but he or she may be able to bear some weight on the foot.

As for most trauma, the diagnosis is suggested by tenderness on physical examination and confirmed by x-rays. The radiographs can have a variety of findings but no one particular feature. When viewing the AP x-ray of a normal foot, the medial borders of the second metatarsal and middle cuneiform should in the normal foot form a line without a step-off. Besides a step-off, the physician also should look for widening between the first and second metatarsal bases (Fig. 14-20). Two millimeters of widening in comparison to the opposite foot is significant displacement. One may find a fracture of one or more of the metatarsal bases or an avulsion fracture of the LisFranc ligament. This ligament is the strong plantar ligament extending from the medial base of the second metatarsal to the medial cuneiform. An avulsion fragment may be seen between the first and second metatarsals or the middle and medial cuneiforms (Fleck sign). Displacement also may be appreciated between the other metatarsals, the medial and middle cunei-

forms, and the base of the fourth metatarsal and the cuboid. Any dorsal displacement of a metatarsal is considered significant (Fig. 14-21). If no displacement is seen but tenderness is exquisite, repeat x-rays with weight-bearing views should be performed in 1 to 2 weeks, since displacement can occur after weight bearing. An alternative when the tenderness is highly suggestive is stress radiography under anesthesia. The forefoot should be held in abduction for an AP view and in plantar flexion against a neutral hind and midfoot for the lateral view. An MRI can document disruption of the ligament but needs to be performed by a radiologist experienced in performing this examination.

The proper treatment of a LisFranc injury is operative reduction and fixation if significant displacement (2 mm or more) is present. When surgery is contemplated, a CT scan may be necessary to further outline the details of the fracture-dislocation or injuries involving the intercuneiform and naviculocuneiform articulations but is not routinely necessary. A properly performed MRI with the use of a shoulder coil can

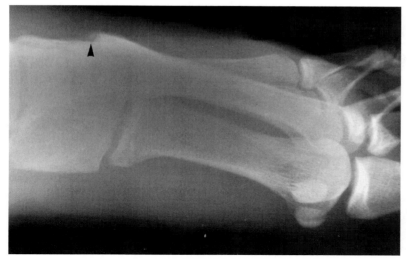

FIGURE   **14-21**

Dorsal displacement (*arrow*) of the second metatarsal in a Lis-Franc fracture-dislocation.

identify rupture of the LisFranc ligament if repeat x-rays are equivocal.

Stress Fractures

Stress fractures (March fracture) were described originally in Prussia in 1855 because of swollen feet in young military recruits. This was before the advent of radiology. With the tremendous recent interest in physical fitness, particularly running, stress fractures of the foot have become more commonplace (5).

During the early stages, the athlete will suffer from localized swelling and pain. While the swelling may lessen over time, there will remain a discrete area of bony tenderness. Unless the athlete has been having pain for several weeks, x-ray evaluation is not diagnostic. The films often will be normal. The most useful diagnostic modality at this stage is a technetium bone scan, which will demonstrate increased uptake as early as 48 hours after the onset of symptoms (15). Bone scanning is expensive and time-consuming. It therefore should only be used when the diagnosis is in question and will change the course of treatment. Tenderness on a metatarsal shaft in an individual who has been unusually active on his or her feet and who has initially normal x-rays should be considered a stress fracture until proven otherwise. Since the history and bony tenderness is so characteristic, a bone scan is most often not necessary.

The athlete who presents with symptoms of greater than 2 weeks may have positive radiographic findings. These include the presence of reactive bone formation, bone resorption at the fracture line, and endosteal thickening (Fig. 14-22). The fracture can be difficult to see even at 3 or 4 weeks. At long-term follow-up, plain films can show large quantities of callus formation. This confirms the original diagnosis. If the tenderness has dissipated, the athlete may very gradually return to full activity but should avoid the schedule or factor that originally caused the physical overload of that bone.

Stress fractures commonly occur in the second metatarsal, fibula, calcaneus, and distal tibia. They also can occur in the other metatarsals, as well as in the navicular, cuboid, cuneiforms, talus, and sesamoids. Most stress fractures can be treated by elimination of the stressful activity and protected ambulation with a supportive shoe or ankle brace. A few troublesome fractures include the navicular stress fracture and the Jones fracture, which is at the diaphyseal-metaphyseal junction of the proximal fifth metatarsal. These particular stress fractures should be treated non-weight-bearing and in a cast. If the physical examination and x-ray are equivocal, a bone scan can be useful to document the stress fracture. Especially if not properly treated, stress fractures can have delayed or nonunions resulting in prolonged disability for the athlete. At minimum, they require 6 weeks of non-weight-bearing in a short leg cast. Patients should be warned that these fractures could require internal fixation. When sclerosis and resorption are noted at the diaphyseal-metaphyseal junction of the fifth metatarsal, the treating physician must be highly suspicious of a chronic stress fracture that eventually can require surgical treatment. A navicular

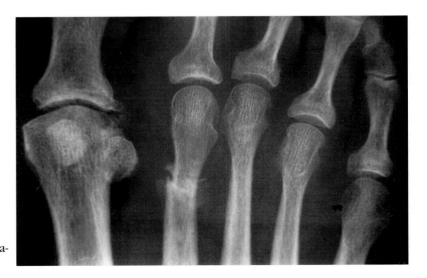

FIGURE 14-22

Stress fracture of the second metatarsal with callus formation.

stress fracture may not be visible on plain films and may be a cause of anterior ankle pain (Fig. 14-23). AP tomograms or a CT oriented along the dorsal aspect of the foot is often necessary for making this diagnosis. A bone scan can be used early in the course of the disease to document the need for the non-weight-bearing cast treatment.

If a stress fracture of the sesamoids is suspected, sesamoid views should be ordered. These are obtained by hyperextending the toes and directing the beam tangentially to the plantar surface of the metatarsal heads. Osteonecrosis of the sesamoid may be present. Both the AP and tangential views should be inspected for lucencies in or fragmentation of the bone.

Hallux Rigidus

Hallux rigidus is a painful degenerative process of the first metatarsophalangeal joint associated with a significant limitation of dorsiflexion. The limited motion is attributable to arthritis in the joint and the dorsal proliferation of bone around the articular surface of the first metatarsal head (Fig. 14-24). This entity can greatly debilitate an athlete who requires dorsiflexion of the first metatarsophalangeal joint, such as a runner or dancer.

The diagnosis is made on physical examination by restricted painful dorsiflexion of the first metatarsophalangeal joint. X-rays should be a routine foot series (AP, lateral, and oblique). Dorsal osteophyte formation is best seen on the lateral x-ray, with joint space narrowing looked

for on all three views. Additional findings include flattening of the metatarsal head, cyst formation, and additional osteophyte formation on the medial and lateral aspects of the metatarsal and proximal phalanx. A CT scan or MRI is not necessary in these patients.

Conservative treatment is directed toward limiting motion at the joint, thereby decreasing the pain. This can be accomplished with a stiff sole or a rocker-bottom shoe that has a large toe box to accommodate the dorsal exostosis. In athletes with mild arthritic change, cheilectomy (resection of the spurs) and an osteotomy of the proximal phalanx can be used to lessen the discomfort.

Freiberg's Disease

Freiberg's disease occurs in lesser metatarsal heads (most commonly the second) and is considered to be a form of avascular necrosis. It is often seen in the adolescent athlete, more commonly in females. The patient usually complains of pain and decreased motion relieved by rest. Physical examination demonstrates swelling, mild erythema, and decreased motion. The differential diagnosis includes instability of the joint, infection, and stress fracture of the metatarsal shaft.

Plain radiographs are usually all that is needed to confirm the diagnosis, since most patients present after weeks of symptoms. Irregularity and flattening of the metatarsal head are characteristic (Fig. 14-25). Sclerosis of the head,

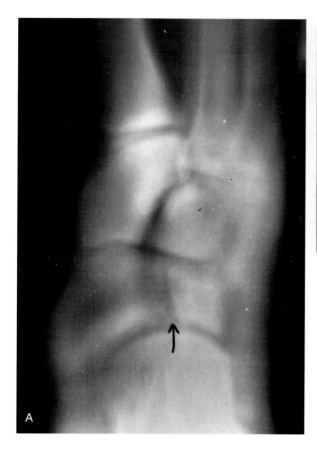

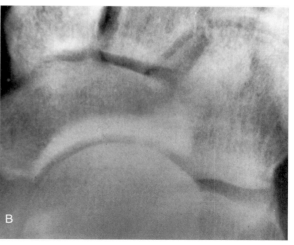

FIGURE   **14-23**

AP tomograms (A) along the axis of the midfoot showing a navicular stress fracture (*arrow*) that could not be seen on the plain radiograph (B).

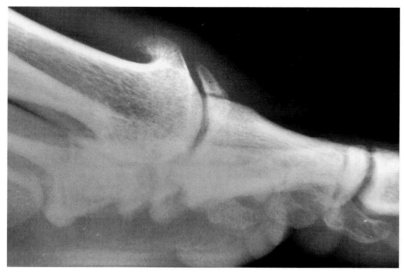

FIGURE   **14-24**

Hallux rigidus with dorsal spurring of metatarsal head and proximal phalanx.

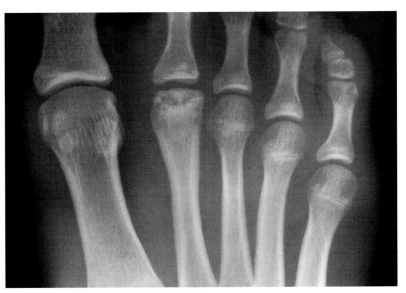

F I G U R E **14-25**

Flattening and irregularity of the second metatarsal head in Freiberg's disease.

dorsal spurring, loose body formation, and secondary thickening of the metatarsal shaft also can be found (16). Unless there are no radiographic findings, an MRI is not necessary.

This disorder has been classified into four stages based on the x-ray findings (17). These are 1) normal, 2) flattened head, 3) deformed head or loose body, and 4) severe degenerative joint disease. Generally, the early stages can be treated conservatively with activity modification and stiff shoes that limit joint motion. Patients with more advanced stages or athletes who cannot restrict activity are generally treated surgically with debridement of osteophytes and loose bodies. In the patient for whom there exists a high suspicion of Freiberg's disease and who had normal x-ray findings (stage 1), a bone scan will confirm that the process is in the metatarsal head, and if more detailed visualization of the cartilage or joint fragment is necessary to decide on surgery, an MRI by a radiologist experienced in MRI of the foot and ankle is helpful.

Sesamoid Injuries

The sesamoids of the hallux act as weight-bearing surfaces for the first metatarsal, points of insertion for multiple intrinsic muscles, and protectors of the flexor hallucis longus. Sesamoid problems often develop in runners from repetitive stress. The range of pathologies includes bursitis over the tibial sesamoid, sesamoiditis,

osteochondritis, chondromalacia, degenerative arthritis, and fracture. Pain localized to the sesamoid should be evaluated with standard radiographs of the foot as well as a sesamoid view. The special sesamoid view can be obtained, as mentioned in the section on stress fractures.

It can be important to differentiate between a bipartite sesamoid and a fracture. The fractured sesamoid usually divides the bone into equal parts with irregular edges, whereas the bipartite sesamoid has round, smooth edges and if put together is larger than a normal sesamoid. A stress fracture of the sesamoid often begins as a mild diffuse pain that becomes more localized and acute with successive trauma. Radiographs usually are not helpful in the first month. During this early phase, a bone scan can be performed, but a good physical examination with tenderness directly over the sesamoid can make the scan unnecessary.

Most sesamoid injuries are treated with lengthy conservative treatment (6 months). While this seems to be lengthy conservative treatment, sesamoids have become asymptomatic after long periods of conservative therapy with orthotics or padding in the shoes and limited activity. In the high-level athlete after 6 months of conservative treatment without significant improvement, either partial or total surgical excision can be offered with the realization that pain relief may not be full. MRIs and CTs can be helpful when excluding infection or detecting osteonecrosis in questionable cases (Fig.

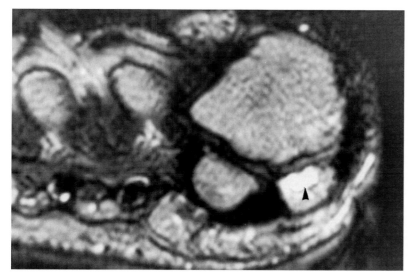

F I G U R E **14-26**

MRI showing signal change in the medial sesamoid with a subchondral cyst in a sesamoid that appeared normal on routine radiographs. Surgical exploration for pain of over 1 year's duration revealed severe arthritis of the sesamoid, necessitating removal.

14-26). These should be ordered in the rare cases where lengthy conservative treatment has failed and the plain x-rays are not sufficiently helpful in making the diagnosis.

REFERENCES

1. Grant JCB. A method of anatomy. Baltimore: William & Wilkins, 1958.

2. Cass JR, Morrey BF, Yoshihisa K, Chao EY. Ankle instability: comparison of primary repair and delayed reconstruction after long-term follow-up study. CORR 1985;198:110–116.

3. Stoller SM. A comparative study of the frequency of anterior impingement exostosis of the ankle in dancer and non-dancer. Foot Ankle 1984; 4:201.

4. Hamilton WG. Foot and ankle injuries. In: Mann RA, ed. Surgery of the foot and ankle. 6th ed. St Louis: Mosby, 1993:1266.

5. Clement DB, Tauton E, Smart GW. A survey of overuse running injuries. Phys Sportsmed 1981;9: 47–58.

6. Plattner P, Mann RA. Disorders of tendons. In: Mann RA, ed. Surgery of the foot and ankle. 6th ed. St Louis: Mosby, 1993:810.

7. Thompson TC. A test for rupture of the tendoachilles. Acta Orthop Scand 1962;32:461–465.

8. Weinstabl R, Stisical M, Neubeld A, et al. Classifying calcaneal tendon injury according to MRI findings. J Bone Joint Surg 1991;73A:683.

9. Davidson R. Deformity of the child's foot. In: Sammarco GJ, ed. Foot and ankle manual. Philadelphia: Lea and Febiger, 1992.

10. Harris RI, Beath T. Etiology of peroneal spastic flatfoot. J Bone Joint Surg 1948;30B:624.

11. Herzenberg JE, Goldner JL, Martinez S, Silverman PM. Computed tomography of talocalcaneal tarsal coalition: a clinical and anatomical study. Foot Ankle 1986;6:273.

12. Cave EF. Fracture of the os calcaneus: the problem in general. Clin Orthop 1963;30:64–66.

13. Gage JR, Premer R. Os calcis fractures: an analysis of 37. Minn Med 1971;54:169–176.

14. Stephenson JR. Treatment of displaced intra-articular fractures of the calcaneus using medial and lateral approaches, internal fixation and early motion. J Bone Joint Surg 1987;69A:115–130.

15. Forrester DM. Sports injuries in imaging of the foot and ankle. Gaithersburg, MD: Aspen Publications, 1988.

16. Spreul J, Klaaren H, Mannarino F. Surgical treatment of Freiberg infarction in athletes. Am J Sports Med 1993;21:381.

17. Gauthier G. Freiberg's infarction: a subchondral bone fatigue fracture. A new surgical treatment. Clin Orthop 1979;142:93–95.

Index